Redesigning the Medicare Contract

Redesigning the

MEDICARE CONTRACT

Politics, Markets, and Agency

Edward F. Lawlor

The University of Chicago Press
Chicago and London

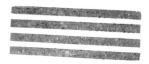

Edward F. Lawlor is dean of and professor in the School of Social Service
Administration, professor in the Irving B. Harris Graduate School of Public
Policy Studies, faculty associate at the Center for Health Administration
Studies, and senior scholar at the MacLean Center for Clinical Medical Ethics
at the University of Chicago. He is the founding editor of the *Public Policy and
Aging Report*.

The University of Chicago Press, Chicago 60637
The University of Chicago Press, Ltd., London
© 2003 by The University of Chicago
All rights reserved. Published 2003
Printed in the United States of America
12 11 10 09 08 07 06 05 04 03   1 2 3 4 5

ISBN: 0-226-47034-2 (cloth)

Library of Congress Cataloging-in-Publication Data

Lawlor, Edward F.
    Redesigning the Medicare contract : politics, markets, and agency /
Edward F. Lawlor.
        p.   cm.
    Includes bibliographical references and index.
    ISBN 0-226-47034-2
    1. Medicare. I. Title.

RA412.3.L39 2003
368.4′26′00973—dc21

                                                                2003008541

♾ The paper used in this publication meets the minimum requirements of the
American National Standard for Information Sciences—Permanence of Paper
for Printed Library Materials, ANSI Z39.48-1992.

CONTENTS

ACKNOWLEDGMENTS

This book had a long gestation and owes its completion to the support and wisdom of my family, friends, and colleagues. Much of the early development of the ideas in this book occurred while Betsy Lawlor and I were editing the *Public Policy and Aging Report,* originally a very humble publication created on the kitchen table with the then-new technology of a personal computer and laser printer. As my partner in all the important things in life, she has provided hard work, insight, and support that have propelled this project from start to finish. Our children—Matt, Abby, and Casey—also deserve great credit for supporting an all-too-hectic lifestyle that included completing this manuscript while I had a day job as a dean and professor.

This book bears the imprint of many outstanding colleagues and students. My original mentor in policy analysis, Larry Lynn, has been a source of both intellectual and personal support throughout my career. David Dranove and Will White originally introduced me to agency theory and its potential application to health policy in a series of Center for Health Administration Studies (CHAS) workshops and papers in the mid-1980s. Jack Meyer provided me with an opportunity to study and understand purchasing models during his work with the Midwest Business Group on Health. Katie Merrell has been the resident Medicare guru at CHAS and taught me a great deal about reimbursement and policy design for more than twelve years. Colleen Grogan provided excellent comments and helped with the political science of the book as chapters went through revisions. I also had the benefit of an extraordinary group of Chicago faculty colleagues who provided important feedback over the entire gestation of the book. My thanks to Ron Andersen, Kate Cagney, Carol Carter, Christine Cassel, Marshall Chin, Nicholas Christakis, Tom D'Aunno, Michael Koetting, John Lantos, John La Puma, Helen Levy, Will Manning, David Meltzer, Steven Miles, Ralph Muller, Bill Pollak, Kristiana Raube, Lainie Ross, Mark Siegler, and Henry Webber. Many of my doctoral students have also been my teachers. I hope Christina Bethell, Joel Cohen, William Dale, Julie Darnell, Scott Geron, Carlos Gomez, David Grabowski, Stuart Hagen, Kenneth Langa, Kyung Sook Park, and Jolyne Gannon Rowley will all see the legacy of our conversations together in this work. Finally, the book benefited from an extraordinarily thoughtful set of comments by Joseph White and an anonymous reviewer. Tanya Nimocks and Eileen Fitzsimons brought exceptional care, good spirit, and energy to the task of finally preparing this manuscript for publication.

CHAPTER ONE

Why Medicare Needs Good Agency

The Problem

Exciting new therapies are being developed and tested for patients who have suffered strokes, brain injuries, or spinal cord injuries.[1] These experimental therapies are low tech and labor intensive, requiring weeks of hands-on work between physical therapists and patients to retrain the brain, the nervous system, and muscles. Medicare does not pay for these therapies, and its coverage of other rehabilitative services has been reduced in recent years in response to rapidly escalating costs.

Is it a smart decision to deny Medicare beneficiaries coverage for these therapies? Truth is, we do not know, because the Medicare program does not embody the tools—the political, economic, and administrative arrangements—to make these decisions in a way that simultaneously and effectively represents the interests of society and the individual beneficiaries of the program. In the parlance of this book, the Medicare program lacks good *agency*.

Solving agency problems in Medicare is not a panacea—there are still difficult cost and equity issues that will face the program, particularly as the baby boom generation ages—but the tools and frameworks of an agency approach provide a fresh approach to thinking about issues of representation, incentives, information, and organization in the program.

The Idea

This book proceeds from a very simple idea. Medicare policy design can be thought of as an exercise of writing a contract for purchasing health care for older and disabled persons. In this simple view, Medicare policy is designed to carry out the desires of beneficiaries (the individuals who are covered by Medicare) as well as other taxpayers, who pay for a significant portion of the expenses covered by Medicare. Thus, the contract has elements of social policy, because the interests of society need to be carried out, and elements that address private features between a Medicare beneficiary and his or her providers of care.

In order for this complex Medicare contract to be effective, appropriate mechanisms of agency must be created. Good agency requires that the preferences and demands of Medicare beneficiaries and society (i.e., the "principals" in this contract) are carried out in the details of service delivery, that patients and taxpayers get the highest quality care for their purchase. In some cases, this agency function is carried out by organizations. For example, administrative agencies carry out tasks designated by the Congress, such as assuring the quality of Medicare services. If these agencies do not operate under a clear mandate, with sufficient resources, or with appropriate delegation and administrative discretion, then the goals of the Medicare program will not be realized. In other cases, the agency function will be carried out by professionals, such as physicians or social workers, who represent the interests of Medicare beneficiaries in decisions as diverse as plan choices or establishing advance directives for end-of-life care. In still other cases, proper agency helps resolve dual or multiple interests in service delivery, such as conflicts between an individual beneficiary's interest and the public interest.[2] Managed care organizations have the potential to perform this kind of dual agency, where they simultaneously serve as providers of care for individuals and stewards of a fixed budget established by the Congress.

Agency in Medicare is defined in a political context. At the highest levels, the Congress serves the public interest in Medicare through a set of institutions (e.g., committee structure, analytic supports) that are weak, accountability over the program that is diffuse, and relationships to the administration of the program that are often ill-defined. As chapter 2 will demonstrate, congressional decision making about Medicare is the result of the program's special political history, in which the vendors and their interests in its services have come to dominate the agenda. At the administrative level, the organizations charged with managing and overseeing Medicare services have been criticized for not carrying out congressional mandates for the program or realizing a high level of accountability and oversight of services. In its defense, the Centers for Medicare and Medicaid Services (CMS), the administrative agency charged with financing and managing the program, lacks resources, has not been delegated the requisite administrative authority by the Congress, and does not exhibit the organizational structure to be an effective principal for the Medicare program.

At the level of managed care contracts, the Medicare program has not been able to implement a regime of payment, coverage, information, and accountability that has either satisfied policy and political expectations for managed care or demonstrated significant growth and expansion in the marketplace. This is most recently made apparent in the experience of the Medicare+Choice program, in which enrollment and coverage have actually declined. Finally, agency breaks down at the level of individual beneficiaries (and their families), where the complexity of the program, the cognitive and functional limitations of many beneficiaries, and the inherent difficulties of making medical decisions undermine the ability of vulnerable older and disabled people to control their care—to act as effective principals in the Medicare contract.

Five Realities

A large body of literature about the Medicare program already exists, discussing its politics, its performance as a program, the characteristics of its beneficiary population, and its agenda for reform.[3] In addition to the ongoing formal oversight the program receives from the Congress, interest groups, think tanks, and researchers, there are a number of major task forces and commissions that have tackled a broader agenda of reform principles and design. It turns out that many of the ideas for reform of the program have fresh currency in the contemporary debate, though our politics tends to have a very short attention span. Indeed, many "old" ideas for Medicare reform (such as social health maintenance organizations) will be revisited in the contractual framework presented in this book.

While it would be unproductive to provide still another overview or literature review of the Medicare program, it is important to briefly assert five broad realities that describe the Medicare program, its providers, and its beneficiaries and that frame the approach taken in this book: (1) beneficiaries are vulnerable; (2) everything varies by geography; (3) administration of the program is halting; (4) providers are nimble and quick; and (5) Medicare is big and complicated.

These realities provide the context for the entire reform discussion of the book, as well as motivate particular approaches to reform. For example, the idea that many *beneficiaries are vulnerable* motivates the emphasis on creating new forms of agency for beneficiaries to support plan choice and decision making for Medicare services. The idea that *everything varies by geography* provides an important context for the analysis of Medicare managed care and helps motivate the regional approach to reform that is developed at the end of this book. Like the political history of Medicare described in chapter 2, these realities provide an important foundation for the policy design, contractual, and institutional discussions of this book.

Reality 1: Beneficiaries Are Vulnerable

The modern Medicare population presents a particularly subtle problem of interpretation in demography, epidemiology, and socioeconomic status. On the one hand, through the magic of improved standards of living and models of "successful aging," the Medicare population has never been healthier, enjoyed the fruits of economic success more, or exhibited higher levels of social and physical functioning. Indeed, Medicare itself is credited with at least some of the improved life expectancy and elevated level of functioning of the older population.[4]

Alongside this mental image of societal aging, however, there needs to be another image of vulnerable beneficiaries who have not enjoyed these benefits of prosperity and improved life experiences of health, education, and social support. A significant group of beneficiaries have experienced hardships, such as serious illness or the loss of a spouse, that leave them without the resources to successfully manage their health care. Many examples could be presented,[5] but a few are especially salient for understanding alternative models of Medicare reform.

Briefly, consider the following indicators of vulnerability in the Medicare population:

- Thirty percent of beneficiaries live alone. Of these beneficiaries, 60 percent had incomes of less than $15,000 in 1996. Almost three-quarters of those living alone are women, and 17 percent of this group are over the age of 85.[6]
- In a Kaiser/Commonwealth survey of Medicare beneficiaries, more than half of the respondents living below the poverty line reported

their health status as fair or poor. Roughly one-quarter of this poverty group reported having heart disease, one-quarter reported diabetes, and one-quarter reported having difficulty with one or more activities of daily living (ADLs).[7]

- More than half of the Medicare population has difficulty using comparative health information to make health plan choices. In a study of health-plan decision making (based on thirty-five decision tasks), the average participant made errors in 25 percent of the tasks.[8]

The interaction of beneficiaries with the health system is a dynamic one, meaning that changes in cognitive or financial wherewithal may occur as a beneficiary goes through the aging process, illness, or other life events. The environment of health care coverage and provision is also constantly changing, forcing beneficiaries to chase a moving target of coverage options, providers, and plans. The much-publicized managed care plan withdrawals are the most dramatic example of the shifting environment of coverage for beneficiaries, but more common are changes in plan names and organizations; movements of providers in and out of plans; and shifting, complex changes in coverage and copayments such as those that have occurred with prescription drug coverage in recent years. From a beneficiary perspective, the turbulence and change of the health care market is bewildering.

In Medicare managed care, the policy concern has been that beneficiaries with poor health status, those with functional limitations, or the very old may experience problems with access. In traditional Medicare, vulnerability to access problems appears to be related to race, indicators of need for care, income, and coverage by supplemental forms of insurance.[9] Rural beneficiaries present still other problems of vulnerability, where low income and inadequate insurance coverage are compounded by transportation difficulties, distance from care, and a relative lack of providers.[10] While Medicare provides nominal coverage for the aged and the disabled, it does not guarantee that certain groups will not face systematic disadvantage in their realized access to health services. For example, an analysis of clinical care (in particular, clinical services that are demonstrably related to poor outcomes in chronic, acute, and surgical conditions) found significant underuse for beneficiaries who are African American, residents of poverty areas, and residents of health professional shortage areas.[11]

The implications of these vulnerabilities are numerous, including the obvious and much-discussed need for Medicare to improve its targeting and subsidies for the most economically disadvantaged beneficiaries. Despite

Medicare's universal coverage for older and disabled beneficiaries, important problems of access and underuse of services still exist. It is also important to recognize that the vulnerability of many beneficiaries has root causes way beyond the purview of Medicare, or even of social insurance more broadly.

The most important implication of this reality for the contractual approach in this book, however, is that *significant agency will be required for vulnerable Medicare beneficiaries.* As a group, Medicare beneficiaries cannot be left simply to the exigencies of the market. They will require supports in information, decision making, and management of health care services in order to effectively participate in the contemporary health care marketplace, and to utilize available health services effectively.[12] A low-income beneficiary—who would often also be disadvantaged by having less than a high school education, chronic conditions, or no familial or other supports—cannot reasonably be expected to make optimal decisions about plan choices, provider selection, and treatment choices without assistance. Many Medicare reform schemes, such as those that rely heavily on choice or on instruments like medical savings accounts, do not fully appreciate the level and kind of assistance that many beneficiaries require.

An appreciation of the diversity of the Medicare population, as well as its pockets of underlying risk and vulnerability, should inform both the debate about what is possible to achieve through reform and the proper design of institutional arrangements to support optimal plan decision making by beneficiaries and effective utilization of health resources. While work on the development of informational tools for beneficiaries (to compensate for literacy and decision-making deficits) has begun in the wake of Medicare+Choice, significant gaps remain between the profile of risks and vulnerability for beneficiaries and the design of cost-sharing arrangements, coverage, information, and other program elements.[13]

Reality 2: Everything Varies by Geography

A large literature in health services research has documented the existence of small-area variations in practice patterns and services.[14] This literature, stimulated by a set of papers by John Wennberg and colleagues, raised fundamental questions about the empirical bases for clinical practice, the role of physician training and practice patterns in determining the particular clinical treatment decisions, and the overall efficiency and effectiveness of medical services. One body of geographic variations research emphasizes the role of supply-side resources, such as the number of hospital beds, in producing practice variations.[15] A second literature emphasizes the role of underlying differences in population epidemiology and demand for medical services.[16]

Other research has investigated the role of payment policy in producing or re-inforcing geographical variations in Medicare practice.[17] The most recent and extensive analyses of regional variations in Medicare spending conclude that these differences are primarily explained by higher intensities of specialist and inpatient care (in high-spending places). In high-spending regions, Medicare patients receive 60 percent more services, without apparent benefit in access, quality of care, satisfaction with care, or outcomes.[18] A related literature, the studies of medical appropriateness pioneered by Robert Brook and colleagues at RAND, also raised questions about the known clinical indications for medical services and the actual treatment decisions made by physicians.[19] For the public, these variations in practice for Medicare services were most graphically and dramatically illustrated in the *Dartmouth Atlas*,[20] which showed regional and local variations in Medicare resources (e.g., hospital beds and physicians), utilization (e.g., rates for mammography and radical prostatectomy), and outcomes.

This small-area variations literature helped spawn a generation of outcomes and medical effectiveness research.[21] Business groups on health used variations data as a tool for developing quality and information approaches to purchasing. The government supported a regime of research and dissemination based on responding to variations, particularly through the Agency for Health Care Policy and Research. However, this regime soon faced political opposition and waning policy enthusiasm as the difficulties of mounting a national program of outcomes-based research and practice became apparent.

Although the small-area variations and outcomes research agenda has in some respects been eclipsed, the existence of variations is still a reality with important implications for Medicare reform. Many versions of Medicare variation could be presented, but indicators at the state level illustrate the basic story.[22] Medicare inpatient hospital use ranged from a low of 244 discharges per 1,000 beneficiaries in Utah to a high of 452 discharges per 1,000 beneficiaries in Mississippi. Rates for specific procedures vary significantly from state to state: 5 percent of Medicare beneficiaries underwent echocardiography in Oregon in 1995, versus 15 percent in Michigan.[23] Home health and skilled nursing facility use shows similar geographic variation.[24] For home health services, the number of home health visits per 1,000 beneficiaries varies four-fold from the lowest using state (Oregon) to the highest (Louisiana). The number of home health users (per 1,000 Medicare fee-for-service beneficiaries) varies threefold across states.[25] These differences in utilization cannot simply be explained away by differences in the underlying epidemiology of the Medicare population—differences in health status or other risks—nor do they appear to explain differences in outcomes in morbidity or mortality.

Similarly, the financing and organization of Medicare services varies tremendously by geography. Underlying coverage and measures of access (e.g., retiree health coverage, prevalence of Medigap policies, Medicaid secondary coverage) show considerable variation by state and region. For example, only 12.7 percent of beneficiaries had individually purchased Medigap policies in the Pacific Northwest, versus 41.9 percent in the East North Central Region. The distribution of Medicare managed care plans and participation also shows dramatic regional, state, and local variation, a topic of considerable importance in chapter 4.

What Medicare pays for the care of each beneficiary also varies tremendously by place, a function of both differences in prices paid and the volume of services delivered. Overall, the difference in Medicare spending per capita in 1998 ranged from $3,380 per beneficiary in Vermont to $11,801 in the District of Columbia. Historically, Medicare has substantially varied its payment for hospitals, physicians, and HMOs from place to place, but not necessarily on the basis of "true" costs, quality, performance, or outcome criteria. Recently, as a result of payment changes initiated by the Balanced Budget Act (BBA) of 1997, payment variations for managed care plans have begun to shrink nationally.

As important for our story as these indicators of variation in the organization and finance of the program, are indicators of variation in quality of clinical care actually received by Medicare beneficiaries. A recent study by Stephen Jencks and colleagues showed significant variation in the quality of clinical practice from place to place (although an equally significant message from this study might be the relatively low overall national rates for certain clinically indicated services). For example, the rate at which antibiotics are administered to Medicare beneficiaries within eight hours of the time of admission with the diagnosis of pneumonia varied from 38 percent in Puerto Rico to 93 percent in Montana. The median difference across states for these quality performance indicators was 33 percentage points.[26] This means that the likelihood that a Medicare beneficiary will receive a relatively straightforward and accepted clinical intervention depends a great deal on where he or she lives. The authors of this study argue that these results provide the basis for "HCFA [the Health Care Financing Administration; since 2001 CMS] to move beyond its historical emphasis on individual cases and providers and to take responsibility as a purchaser for the care delivered to the population of Medicare beneficiaries." More broadly, the weight of the evidence about geographic variations argues for much more systematic attention to quality issues and management of the Medicare delivery system by geography, a departure from Medicare's tradition of largely national administration.

Even end-of-life care, the topic of chapter 6, exhibits this same kind of regional variation. A study by Jonathan Skinner and John Wennberg on Medicare spending in the last six months of life illustrated the profound differences in treatment approaches and ultimate costs that result from geographic differences in practice patterns.[27] Minneapolis exhibits four times the rate of ICU use as Miami. As in other areas of health care delivery, these differences do not seem to be explained by differences in underlying health status or ultimate outcomes of treatment.

The implication of this reality is that the Medicare program needs to take variation more seriously as a tool, and geography more seriously as an administrative and reform matter. Even in Medicare's administrative practices, significant variations can be observed. For example, the Institute of Medicine observed that claims for a common laboratory test were denied 7 percent of the time in one state versus 68 percent of the time in another state, apparently due to differences in interpretations of standards.

In this book, geographic variation will be a recurring theme in such diverse areas of Medicare policy as managed care design and end-of-life care. Variation is the *signal* of administrative opportunity. It is not a foregone conclusion that the variations in use, price, clinical practice, or outcomes are inappropriate. However, these variations are a *prima facie* case for serious and systematic attention to service delivery at a regional level. In other words, this level of variation needs explanation and justification; it is likely that it is symptomatic of poor quality and inefficiency in at least some geographies of Medicare delivery. More importantly, the existence and management of this variation can be diagnostic of agency problems to be addressed in Medicare reform. Cognizance of Medicare's geographical variations will serve as one of the motivations for the regional approach to reform that is developed in the final chapter.

Reality 3: Administration of the Medicare Program Is Halting

Herbert Simon proposed the concept of bounded rationality to characterize the limits of organizations to process information.[28] His idea was that organizations, like people, have cognitive limitations, and these limits bound the ability to make rational, evidence-based decisions. The larger the scope and scale of information that needs to be processed, the more the limits on rationality become tested.

In its current construction, Medicare undoubtedly runs up against these boundaries in both its administration and policy making. In administration, the CMS is responsible for setting and administering prices, writing rules and regulations, administering contracts with intermediaries and carriers to pay claims, administering contracts with professional review organizations, cooperating with other agencies to oversee quality and appropriateness of care, collaborating in efforts to regulate fraud and abuse in the system, conducting a program of intramural and extramural research and evaluation, and providing beneficiary and public information, among other duties. All of this work is to take place in a highly dynamic environment of changing political, technological, and market demands. This work has also taken place in an era of divided government, where there has undoubtedly been ambivalence about how intrusive or aggressive the administration of the program is to be in the context of a health care marketplace. As chapter 2 illustrates, this work also takes place in an environment of scarce resources, where it is a badge of honor that the Medicare program spends only 1 to 2 percent of its total expenditures on administrative activities.

An example of the deliberate pace and inevitable politicization of Medicare's existing administrative structures can be seen in the saga of the Medicare competitive pricing demonstration projects.[29] Interest in competitive pricing for Medicare extends back at least to the Tax Equity and Fiscal Responsibility Act of 1982 (TEFRA), when the Congress began considering alternative approaches for establishing payments to Medicare HMOs. Bryan Dowd and colleagues at the University of Minnesota have evaluated and proposed models of competitive pricing approaches since 1989, and their proposals have engendered considerable discussion in policy and academic circles. HCFA itself began work on a competitive pricing demonstration in 1995 and selected Baltimore as a demonstration site in 1996.

Baltimore was selected for a host of market and design reasons: it had a relatively competitive managed care market with modest Medicare enrollment, its existing payments for managed care plans were high (allowing for a fair test of competition within the constraint of budget neutrality), and there were no other demonstration projects underway to confound the results. Political opposition, led by local members of the House and Senate, however, was stiff, leading HCFA to cease implementation of the demonstration during the summer of 1996.

A subsequent effort to mount a competitive demonstration in Denver met with a similar fate. The Denver proposal, using essentially the same design as the Baltimore demonstration, elicited intense opposition from local health plans and their association, was enjoined by the federal court, was taken up by representatives in the House and Senate, and was ultimately halted by legislative language inserted into a disaster relief bill.

The 1997 BBA tried again, authorizing the Secretary of Health and Human Services to conduct a competitive pricing demonstration for managed care plans in four to seven sites. After a productive start on site selection and preliminary work on local implementation in Kansas City, Kansas, and Phoenix, Arizona, the BBA competitive pricing demonstrations once more ran into political turbulence locally and in the Congress. In mid-1999, the advisory committee to the demonstrations voted to delay implementation (as bids were being readied), the Congress voted to ban the demonstrations in proposed patients' rights legislation and, finally, in appropriations legislation the Congress voted to prohibit spending on the demonstrations in fiscal year 2000. In the waning days of the Clinton administration and of negotiations over final budgetary and policy priorities, the competitive pricing demonstrations were left in policy limbo. Whatever gains were made toward implementation, particularly in the Kansas City site, were essentially lost for future efforts to mount the demonstration.

The information to be gathered from competitive pricing demonstrations was vital to better understanding the merits of many recent Medicare reform proposals, running the spectrum from President Clinton's Medicare modernization plan to the Breaux-Frist proposals introduced in the Senate. The demonstrations held out the potential to formulate and examine a "standard benefit plan" in a local market environment, to script prescription drug policy (such as the details of an actual Medicare formulary and coverage) in a competitive context, to test the implementation of a bidding process, to examine the local processes of participation and governance over health reform, to test enrollment management and communications with beneficiaries, to develop information and quality tools, and to evaluate whether overall efficiencies and cost savings can be obtained through competitive behavior.

Instead, one of the principal lessons from this experience is the administrative, political, and legal quagmire that Medicare reform efforts face, at least in a demonstration mode. Ironically, while Congress has criticized HCFA over the years for its inability to implement elements of a competitive regime for Medicare, it was the Congress—more accurately, individual members of Congress—who created roadblocks to implementing even these relatively modest demonstrations, in spite of the congressional will expressed in the 1997 BBA.

The inability to mobilize administrative responses to the rapidly changing health care marketplace and the rapidly evolving practice of medicine is one of the key problems of Medicare reform. In the case of the competitive pricing demonstrations, the Congress has allowed each individual demonstration to be captured by local special interests and their political representatives.[30] From a local perspective, this could be either good or bad, but it necessarily puts the brakes on overall Medicare policy innovation and ultimately ossifies the program. This pace and these obstacles need to be weighed against the pace in the market that can be demonstrated by plans and providers. This contrast is described in the next section.

Reality 4: Providers Are Nimble and Quick

In contrast to the halting pace of governmental administration of Medicare, the scale, scope, and "intelligence" of many health care providers means that they can alter their industrial organization of care to rapidly take advantage of incentives and regulatory changes. Outpatient care can be substituted for inpatient care; payment for one diagnosis-related group (DRG) can be substituted for another; home care can be substituted for skilled nursing care; skilled nursing care can be substituted for inpatient hospital care. Providers of Medicare services have shown themselves to be very adept at responding to the incentives and opportunities provided by programmatic changes in Medicare. Ronald Vogel has described these dynamics of supplier (provider) response in his writing about the microeconomics of Medicare: "Persons on the supply side are medical entrepreneurs. As such, they rationally respond to economic incentives in their efforts to maximize their own profits and incomes (and/or 'quality'). Therefore, if, as happened beginning in fiscal 1984, DRGs were legislatively mandated for acute care hospitals, but not for other kinds of care . . . where 'reasonable' prices would continue to prevail, these entrepreneurs would begin to create and expand other kinds of care in addition to acute care, and to use the output and pricing rules . . . in order to maximize their profits selling joint kinds of care."[31]

One of the best examples of the responsiveness of the provider sector to opportunity in the Medicare program is the expansion and contraction of the home health industry during the 1990s. Prior to 1997, home health was considered one of the most troubling and uncontrolled sources of growth in Medicare; indeed, it was regarded to be a "Pac-Man," eating up increasing portions of the Medicare budget. Between 1990 and 1997, expenditures for Medicare home health grew from $3.7 billion to $17.8 billion, an annual growth rate of 25 percent. As a proportion of all Medicare expenditures, home health grew from 3 percent of expenditures to 9 percent during this period. Growth in the number of providers and overall utilization of home health services fueled this expenditure growth. The number of users of home health care grew from 57 users per 1,000 beneficiaries to 109 users per 1,000 beneficiaries. The average number of visits per beneficiary also doubled, from 36 to 73. The number of providers doubled during this period, mostly as free-standing, for-profit agencies in urban areas.[32]

By any standard, this growth of home health services was impressive, the result of favorable reimbursement, lax oversight of payments to providers (where fraud was regarded to be significant), and tremendous latent demand for services from beneficiaries and acute-care providers anxious to find in-home supports for postacute care. It is important, however, to understand the trigger for this growth, because it provides a window into how nimble and responsive providers can be to seemingly small changes in rules or incentives.

As a result of a lawsuit that challenged HCFA's interpretation of eligibility for home health services, the criteria for home health coverage were changed from "part-time *and* intermittent care" to "part-time *or* intermittent care." As a result of this interpretation and related technical changes, home health providers could now provide more (nonintermittent) visits, with more latitude for nurse and therapist services and less latitude for intermediaries to deny payments.[33] The tremendous growth in providers, users, and rates of use described above was the direct result of these changes.

In response, the BBA of 1997 authorized HCFA to develop a prospective payment system for home health and gave new definitions to the meanings of "intermittent" and "part-time." In the meantime, HCFA implemented an Interim Payment System that put limits on the cost basis for home health providers, which in turn provided incentives for home health agencies to limit costs and visits.[34] Almost instantly, providers exited the market in relatively large numbers, and the number of providers entering also dropped (see fig. 1). From October 1, 1997, to January 1, 1999, there were 1,436 Medicare-certified home health agencies (14 percent) that exited the market. This shift garnered national attention and appeared as a major story on the front page of the *New York Times*, which reported a 45 percent drop in home health spending during the two years following the BBA changes.[35] Since then, a spirited debate has taken place over whether any adverse effects of this withdrawal have occurred, as well as what remedies, if any, are necessary.

This capacity of providers and plans to respond quickly and nimbly to changes in incentives and regulation has powerful implications for the design of Medicare contractual arrangements. The modern Medicare marketplace is moving swiftly, with sophisticated providers in place to take advantage of opportunity, yet ready to leave the Medicare business if the terms of service become less favorable. Thus, entry and exit can be virtually immediate, leaving beneficiaries and other providers without choices. This lesson has been repeated in many areas of Medicare delivery, most recently in plan entries and exits for Medicare managed care in the Medicare+Choice program.

Reality 5: Medicare Is Big and Complicated
        Although the costs of Medicare's size and complexity are impossible to fully document and quantify, anyone familiar with its operations knows that this

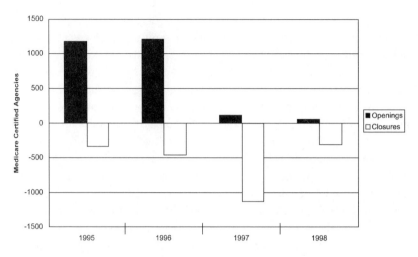

Figure 1. Medicare home health policy response (GAO, May 1999)

is one of the program's defining features.[36] The scale and diversity of Medicare administrative responsibilities are extraordinary: over 6,000 hospitals (1,300 receiving special payment considerations), 830,000 physicians in active patient care, 9,300 home health agencies, 167,000 clinical labs, 3,500 end-stage renal-disease facilities, 2,500 outpatient physical therapy facilities, 700 portable x-ray units, 3,500 rural health clinics, 600 outpatient rehabilitation facilities, 2,600 ambulatory surgical centers, and 2,300 hospices.[37] Medicare's administrators are responsible for the oversight of 56 contractors who process claims in a timely manner, identify errors in claims and inappropriate billing, and pursue fraud investigations with the relevant law enforcement authorities. CMS oversees 11 program "safeguard contractors" who engage in a number of analyses to assure compliance in claims and other functions in the program. CMS also oversees 37 peer-review organizations, which check the validity and medical necessity of claims and quality of provider care. In addition, a number of other contractors provide review and technical assistance on claims administration.

According to the General Accounting Office, CMS, which at the time was still HCFA, is responsible for setting "tens of thousands" of separate rates for the many varieties of providers and jurisdictions under its authority.[38] CMS is also responsible for a host of beneficiary information communications, a responsibility that has grown with the creation of the Medicare+ Choice program.

In addition to these formidable Medicare responsibilities, CMS is also responsible for the federal administration of Medicaid, the oversight of several features of the State Children's Health Insurance Program (SCHIP), and the Health Insurance Portability and Protection Act (HIPPA), as well as a number of national health data and statistical functions. A recent Medicare Payment Advisory Commission (MedPAC) report outlines the formidable regulatory, rulemaking, and claims management responsibilities born by the agency. Estimates of the written regulations vary from 30,000 to 125,000 pages (at the high end including both Medicare and Medicaid). Beyond the formal paper regulations, the MedPAC report documents the layers and layers of regulatory oversight that accompany Medicare, extending into other agencies of the federal government, such as the Office of the Inspector General, as well as private contractors and the peer review organizations. Particular rules require comment and elaboration, all subject to the Federal Administrative Procedures Act. For example, MedPAC describes a process in which three pages of rules defining "provider-based" clinics evolved into one hundred pages of explanation in three separate *Federal Register* notices.[39]

From the perspective of beneficiaries, this massive program and its user interface is often anxiety-provoking, antagonistic, and burdensome in its paperwork and claims processing. A review of Medicare claims processing by the National Academy of Social Insurance found problems in understanding beneficiaries' coverage, delays and confusion over the disposition of claims, and the absence of intermediaries in the system to help reconcile and resolve disputes over claims.[40] Communications about coverage, costs, copayments and deductibles, and judgments from preadmission or preprocedure review are complicated, sometimes misleading, and often out of sync with the timing of doctor and patient decision making about treatment. Richard Margolis, in his critique of the larger system of assistance for older persons, identifies this feature of the Medicare system as its most distressing shortcoming:

> In the end, my picture of Medicare came to resemble that of "the Castle" in Kafka's famous novel. The elderly were like the villagers who live in the valley below. "There's no fixed connection with the Castle," explains the village mayor, "no central exchange that transmits our calls farther. When anybody calls up the Castle from here, the instruments in all the subordinate departments ring, or rather they would ring if practically all the departments—I know this for a certainty—didn't leave their receivers off. . . ." Medicare's failure to either speak clearly or to listen attentively—its essential dumbness and deafness—has kept the elderly in a steady state of nervousness.[41]

A standard trade book for beneficiaries, *Medicare Made Easy*, goes on for a bewildering 331 pages in an attempt to make the program comprehensible.[42] Another trade book, *The Medicare Answer Book,* goes on for 304 pages, introducing topics such as financial planning for Medicare, the interaction with the Medicaid program, and how to select a Medicare+Choice plan.[43] The government's own guide, *Medicare and You 2002,* goes on for 100 pages, 28 of which contain phone numbers for different potential problems and localities.[44] The confusion and misunderstanding that are created by such a complex program structure undermine the intent of many of these provisions: to convey incentives and encourage cost-saving, effective care. It is difficult for beneficiaries to understand basic program features, such as the limits of long-term care coverage, much less the subtleties of economic incentives that are built into coinsurance arrangements. Beneficiaries with dual or multiple coverage—such as Qualified Medicare Beneficiaries, Supplemental Low-Income Medicare Beneficiaries, beneficiaries with private retiree health coverage, or beneficiaries with Medigap plans—face an even more daunting challenge in understanding the program.

Calibrating Reform

An appreciation of these basic realities about the Medicare program and its population—beneficiaries are vulnerable, everything varies by geography, government administration is halting, providers are nimble, and the program is big and complicated—helps place many of the stylized and simple approaches to reform in a more grounded context. Medical savings accounts, Medicare "choice," and other stylized proposals simply do not map to the more complex reality of Medicare as it has evolved. Vulnerable beneficiaries cannot be left to fend for themselves in an unbridled marketplace. A monolithic, underresourced administrative structure in Baltimore (CMS) cannot cope with the geographic variation, communications, need, and complexity that are required to manage Medicare operations in markets as diverse as North Dakota and Southern California. Providers and plans cannot be managed without full appreciation of the strategic and business responses that will attend any change or even lag in Medicare policy. These important realities guide the development of the agency approach taken in this book and motivate many of the reform ideas presented in chapter 7.

In addition to being big and complicated, the Medicare program is now well integrated into the landscape of American health care. Now more than thirty-five years old, Medicare has shaped in important ways the roles and responsibility of professionals, the organizational relationships among providers, and the larger economy of the system. Thus, one has to be exceedingly careful in reengineering Medicare's underlying arrangements.

For example, encouraging new incentive arrangements for physicians to limit treatment has the potential to undermine an important feature of the old contract, namely the trust that was attached to an unambiguous doctor-patient relationship. Reengineering the doctor-patient relationship may bring a corollary responsibility to regulate the profession of medicine: watching over physician incentives, providing new forms of consumer rights, and demanding new disclosure of physician arrangements and practice. Indeed, the government struggled for a decade and a half to create physician incentive rules that would simultaneously encourage cost-saving behavior and new forms of physician organization but not encourage undertreatment of Medicare beneficiaries by "too much."[45] These rules are remarkable in their complexity and demonstrate the difficulties of regulating professional behavior in medicine.

Many of the calls at all levels of government for regulating managed care represent an instinctive reaction to the perception that patients can no longer trust their doctors and other providers. But the alternative, close and aggressive regulation of plans, carries the risk that ultimately plans either will not enter the market or, if they are already providing services, will reduce their coverage or their service areas (or both), or completely withdraw from the market. Because Medicare managed care is a large business, in many cases delivered by large publicly traded companies, the calculus of profits, administrative burden, and legal risk determines the participation of many plans. As the marketplace is rapidly moving forward, Medicare has resorted to a patchwork of regulatory changes, such as the physician incentive rules, that may be reasonable by themselves but do not necessarily implement a larger strategic direction or a public decision calculus for the program. As will be argued throughout this book, there is significant opportunity for improving the design of Medicare's coverage and service delivery by using the tools and frameworks of a contractual approach to reform.

At the same time, one also has to be careful in reengineering these contracts, because the underlying social insurance philosophy of the program (and its associated political support) may ultimately be put at risk. Theda Skocpol is one of the most ardent and articulate exponents of this view:

> Joking aside, my message is directed at all those clashing experts vying for a place on that "Commission to End Medicare as We Know It." My message is, look before you leap. Trained (in most cases) as economists, health care experts are accustomed to arguing in terms of static technical design and rational claims about cost efficiency. But historically grounded moral understandings are much more important for other citizens. And institutional realities are much more relevant

for predicting what will actually occur as plans meet politics, as proposals are evis-
cerated and reworked against congressional and interest-group maneuvers over
reforming Medicare. Remember Ira Magaziner and his friends? They did not pay
much attention to history, institutions, and predictable political processes when
they drew up their ideal health care plan for the Clinton administration to lay before Congress. We all know what happened next.[46]

Many health policy analyses run up against these shoals in the course of
real legislative reform efforts because they avoid explicit and detailed consideration of the relationship of political economy to policy design. The recent experience of the Clinton health care reform effort provides a powerful example
of the influence and sophistication of the stakeholders in halting reform.[47] A
corollary to this observation is that, as a historical matter, the longer it takes to
accomplish large-scale reform of the health care system, the more entrenched
and intransigent will be the enterprises that deliver health care under public
auspices. Medicare is now a mature public program with deeply entrenched
and powerful interests, as diverse as associations representing academic
health centers to organizations that exist to protect beneficiary rights. Savvy
policy analysis must be cognizant of these interests, both their formal functions and their political rationale.

For example, a strange anomaly in the Medicare system of reimbursement is the existence of organizations called intermediaries and carriers,
typically Blue Cross/Blue Shield plans, that process payment requests and
conduct utilization review. Looked at purely from the perspective of design
and efficiency, the intermediary system is puzzling; looked at from the perspective of the political history of Medicare, the creation of intermediaries
provided a convenient and economic way of diverting some of the objections
of third-party insurers who stood to lose a major market with the enactment of
Medicare.[48] To understand intermediaries as simply structural devices—mid-
dlemen who process the Medicare program's paperwork—is to miss their
political raison d'être: to counteract the potential economic losses of the
insurance industry that were heralded by Medicare. The interesting challenge
for policy analysis, however, is to meld these kinds of political realities with
formal reasoning about the properties of good policy design. It is because of
the importance of these institutional and political realities that I will begin the
analysis of the Medicare contract in chapter 2 with a reflection on the history
of the program, its structure, and its political lessons.

Useful reform discussion requires attention to two masters, *real politick*
and the formal (and often technical) aspects of policy design.[49] Looking at
Medicare reform as a problem of contracts provides a vehicle for serving both

masters: raising theoretical questions of design, while being attentive to the realities of Medicare's history, philosophical underpinnings, and political support. Forcing theory onto the problems of Medicare design requires focusing on different questions and different design features than those that surface in the more purely political debate about Medicare. For example, rather than focus on whether or not Medicare is going broke in 2002 or 2010, this approach is more likely to emphasize the information requirements of patients and payers seeking quality in health services, the incentives that the various parties face, the institutional and market context in which Medicare services are delivered, and the strategic responses anticipated from providers and plans.

A Different Kind of Medicare Policy Debate?

A caricature of the popular argument for Medicare reform would go as follows: Medicare cannot sustain its rate of growth, particularly with new promises such as prescription drugs, in the face of the aging of the baby boom generation. Most critics of the program also emphasize the need to control Medicare costs, especially looking into the future, even though historical evidence about the Medicare cost-containment record is mixed and by some accounts mildly positive.[50] The Concord Coalition, for example, makes the following up-front argument for Medicare reform: "Important as Medicare has been, its future is troubled. The program's costs are projected to grow faster than its revenues. When the baby boomers retire, the situation will become much worse unless steps are taken before then to control Medicare spending. This will not be easy. But it is necessary. *The single worst decision our nation could make would be to do nothing*" (Concord Coalition's emphasis).[51]

The specter of the aging of the baby boom generation and the increasing costs of medical care have been the dominant motivations for Medicare reform, especially from a long-term perspective. Despite the hyperbole over Medicare's long-term financing crisis, the reality is that the Congress is simply not in a position to know what Medicare's long-term costs will be or what they should be, especially over the long-term horizons that are contemplated in the trust fund actuaries' seventy-five-year projections. Without having better evidence about and accountability for current services, it is difficult to say whether Medicare is spending too much, too little, or just the right amount.[52]

In the political realm, much of the reform discussion involves the search for a single magic bullet, or a simple financial or organizational fix for Medicare's problems. Managed care, vouchers, or medical savings accounts are seen by certain constituencies as such magic bullets. As policy solutions to the problems of health care delivery for aged and disabled persons, however, these simplistic proposals have mostly rhetorical value; they are not particularly useful for framing the larger and more complicated agenda for legislation and implementation. As anyone familiar with the field knows, the great variety of financial, organizational, and contractual arrangements that exist even under the rubric of "managed care" mean that talk of solving (or exacerbating) Medicare's problems with managed care is by itself virtually meaningless. These rhetorical debates show little appreciation of the complexity of Medicare's coverage or of the political economy of its policy making.

Instead, we need more analysis and debate over the arrangements for managing care—organizational structures, information resources, financial incentives, and so forth—that can move the program and its beneficiaries closer to an emphasis on high quality, responsive, and cost-effective care.

Contract as Metaphor and Toolkit

At a macro level, the Medicare social contract includes promises about care to be provided both now and in the future.[53] Beneficiaries have come to expect a certain level of coverage for hospital and physician coverage, and taxpayers have come to expect to contribute both payroll and general revenue taxes to assure these benefits. It is widely accepted that this contract contains many forms of redistribution, from the well to the sick, from the more affluent to persons with low income and wealth, and from workers to retirees. It is now well understood that the contract has certain limits, such as the lack of coverage for prescription drugs, but it is less well understood that coverage is limited for certain other forms of care, such as rehabilitative services, chronic care, and long-term care.

Beyond these rudimentary understandings, however, the Medicare social contract is extremely vague and increasingly controversial, more a product of its particular political history than a well-articulated policy construct. No widely accepted or even broadly understood notion of the social contract behind Medicare now exists.[54] In an earlier period, Medicare's tie to social insurance provided a kind of rhetorical and symbolic rationale that was sufficient for assuring broad public and congressional support; no more detailed consensus on its purposes and limits as a social contract was necessary. Now, in the face of demographic changes affecting old-age programs, as well as the increasing per capita costs of medical care in old age, a variety of challenges and new interpretations to this ambiguous social contract are emerging. Public opinion polls indicate declining confidence that Medicare will provide sufficient coverage when today's younger workers reach retirement age.

Further clarity and consensus about the nature and extent of the

Medicare social contract are necessary for moving along a significant national reform discussion. To be productive, however, this process of achieving political consensus needs to be framed by narrower and more pragmatic policy questions. The argument and tools developed in this book require that the public interest in particular domains of Medicare policy first needs to be refined and updated. This is largely a political undertaking, but as I will show, the political and administrative institutions for taking on this reform project are challenged. The apparatus in the Congress and in Medicare's administration is not structured or equipped to reformulate Medicare policy on an ongoing basis—to update the social contract—for such a large population and an ever-changing health services enterprise. Defining the contract is not only an exercise of determining what benefits should be included in Medicare coverage, largely the province of political institutions and process, but also creating mechanisms that allow coverage to be updated (prudently) in the face of new technology.

If a more contemporary and definitive concept of the public interest in Medicare is achieved, then the interesting work for policy analysis lies in the design of financing and administrative arrangements that implement these objectives. The Medicare program is already built upon an extremely complicated and fragile structure of contractual arrangements involving the government, intermediaries, providers, and beneficiaries. Some of these contractual elements are explicit, as in the formal agreements for participation between CMS and Medicare+Choice managed care plans, but many of these contracts are implicit, as between doctor and patient or between taxpayers and future beneficiaries. This book treats the problem of reform in Medicare as an exercise in reframing and revising these contractual arrangements, with an emphasis on improving the structure and performance of agency in the system.

Creating an effective Medicare contract requires the structuring of financial and administrative arrangements that allocate risk within the system, provide reimbursement, and manage information so as to send the proper signals among the government, intermediaries, providers, and beneficiaries. A contractual perspective makes possible a change in the mindset of Medicare policy making from passively financing care to actively purchasing care, with emphases on quality, appropriateness, and ultimately outcomes of care. Careful consideration of the administrative arrangements to carry out this contract has too often been neglected in policy discussions.

So how will this analysis help to clarify how principals for the Medicare program can determine coverage, payment, and accountability for new forms of physical therapy for beneficiaries who have suffered stroke, brain injuries, or spinal cord damage—as posed at the beginning of this book? As a preview of the larger story line of the book, the Congress will need structural reform and new forms of analytic support for engaging such specific Medicare coverage questions. In particular, the Congress will need the capacity to undertake technology assessment (broadly considered) to make prudent decisions about coverage, practice, and technology in a timely way. At the level of beneficiaries, new supports for decision making—ranging from information tools to patient advocacy—may be necessary to provide the requisite agency that our complicated Medicare coverage requires. What is interesting about examples such as constrained-induced therapy in rehabilitation services, or the artificial heart example at the high end of medical technology, is that they raise complex ethical, economic, efficacy, and quality-of-life questions, exactly the kinds of questions that will confront Medicare coverage decisions for the foreseeable future. In order to provide the appropriate incentives, oversight, and accountability for services such as rehabilitation care, Medicare's administration, now primarily housed in CMS, will need substantial overhaul. In order for beneficiaries themselves to make informed decisions about coverage, plans, and providers, significant new forms of information and decision support will be necessary. All of these changes involve thinking in fundamentally different ways about the agency relationships in the Medicare program.

A Road Map

What arrangements can we implement to assure that beneficiaries get the care they desire and taxpayers get "value" out of their tax expenditures? Do current arrangements—the CMS, Medicare Hospital Insurance (Part A), Medicare Supplemental Medical Insurance (Part B), and Medicare+Choice (Part C)—represent an effective architecture for Medicare's modern social contract?

Do new forms of Medicare managed care, especially those such as Medicare+Choice which were envisioned in the BBA of 1997 and subsequent amendments, provide an effective vehicle, from a contractual perspective, for society and beneficiaries to achieve value in their purchase of health care? What policy design is necessary to assure that the new inventions of the health care marketplace—managed care plans and integrated delivery systems—actually benefit Medicare enrollees in terms of coverage, quality, and outcomes?

Can new technology be simultaneously encouraged and managed to produce innovation that benefits beneficiaries but at the same time encourages prudent decisions about its costs and deployment? Can Medicare's administrative machinery be organized to evaluate and make decisions about dramatic new technologies, such as the artificial heart? Can public policy and individual decision making be orchestrated—through improved agency—to improve the quality and appropriateness of end-of-life care?

These are the types of Medicare questions that will be addressed in this book, using the toolkit of contracts, agency theory, and institutional reform. The book argues that a pragmatic route to reform involves analysis and development of alternative arrangements for structuring incentives, information, administration, and agency for beneficiaries and providers. In addition to policy makers' historic preoccupation with containing the overall costs of Medicare delivery, especially in hospital and physician payment, arrangements will need to be structured to promote appropriateness of care, quality, and ultimately outcomes for the beneficiary population. Although quality of care has long been on the list of policy priorities for Medicare, the Congress has not yet created the institutions, the incentives, or the informational tools, nor has it allocated the resources, that are necessary for building a significant quality agenda.

Chapter 2 frames the political context of Medicare reform by looking at the origins of the program and the nature of its political influences as revealed in the Medicare Catastrophic Coverage Act repeal, the 1997 Balanced Budget Act (BBA) amendments, the prescription drug debate, and the history of administrative reforms in the program. The outcome of this review of political history is the assertion that future changes in Medicare will be "path dependent," as reformers pick up important elements of Medicare's past structure, institutions, and symbols while they incorporate newer political demands and approaches to health care finance and organization.

Chapter 3 outlines a body of social science theory—agency theory—that provides the basis for considering Medicare reform as an exercise in creating contractual arrangements for the health care of older persons. This chapter asserts that one of the key, and largely neglected, aspects of Medicare policy design is proper *agency*, the incentive and administrative arrangements that determine whether beneficiaries and taxpayers realize their goals in the Medicare contract.

Agency theory per se does not provide a set of answers to how Medicare should be reformed. Instead, it provides a lens for understanding certain aspects of Medicare policy design, emphasizing aspects of representation, information, incentives, and monitoring in the program. At the end of the book, however, this agency framework will also be used to illustrate a particular approach to reform that emphasizes a regional approach to administration, a reliance on certain market institutions and competition, and a so-called purchasing approach to relations with providers.

Chapter 4 examines Medicare managed care policy using the contractual and agency theory framework. First, it asks what implied social contract drives the pursuit of managed care approaches and Medicare+Choice approaches in the program. It then asks the central contractual and agency theory questions about the current managed care regime in Medicare. Do the legal, incentive, informational, and organizational arrangements that undergird Medicare+Choice meet the tests of a good contract for Medicare beneficiaries and the public? What recommendations might we take away from this contractual analysis of Medicare+Choice?

Chapters 5 and 6 provide two case studies for applying this contractual perspective to important contemporary issues of Medicare policy design. The first of these case studies uses artificial heart technology to examine the problem of escalating technology and asks how we can structure arrangements that allow for the uptake of new, cost-worthy technology, but in a prudent way. It concludes that reintroduction of technology assessment in Medicare is necessary, and significant organizational invention in and around the Congress will be required. Chapter 6 examines the problem of caregiving at the end of life and asks how we can structure a contract for a "good death," one that allows for individuals to exert increased control over the means and ends of their care at the end of life.

Chapter 7 returns to the metaproblem of Medicare reform and makes recommendations through the lens of agency theory and the redesign of a Medicare contract. Each of the reform proposals addresses a different level of agency problem identified in the Medicare program. The overall proposed reform program is built upon a regional purchasing approach to Medicare and emphasizes incentive, information, and organizational changes beginning with the Congress and extending all the way down to supports for individual beneficiaries.

Because the Medicare program is so broad and so complex, we should not be deluded into thinking that a single elegant solution—a simple contract—will resolve all of Medicare's pressing issues. Indeed, one of the arguments of the book is that progress on Medicare requires policy debate and analysis of both the macro-social contract and the micro-contractual arrangements that will implement the will of the people and the preferences of beneficiaries. Ultimately, however, for Medicare to be a successful and enduring program, these two contracts—the overarching social contract and the specific, pragmatic arrangements with plans, providers, and beneficiaries—will need to be aligned. In other words, the arrangements that are built into coverage, payment, organization, and information will need to embody the larger social purposes of the Medicare program. New mechanisms to make this match, and improve agency, are necessary.

CHAPTER TWO

Medicare's Politics and the Incomplete Social Contract

Whence It Came

The enactment of Medicare legislation in 1965 reflected the particular political pressures and societal demands of the time. The public wanted increased financial protection for older persons who risked impoverishment from medical expenses in old age. The medical, insurance, and hospital industries wanted protection against the perceived economic control, regulatory incursion, and movement toward "socialized medicine," which was of paramount concern in the 1960s. Congressman Wilbur Mills, the powerful chairman of the House Ways and Means Committee, wanted to limit the exposure of the public fisc to the potentially explosive costs of financing health care for the aged.[1] The political accommodations that reconciled these demands created an architecture for Medicare that had remarkable staying power, lasting virtually unchanged until the Balanced Budget Act (BBA) of 1997. However, this history also created a political economy of interest groups, industries, and symbols that now surround the Medicare program and will have an important influence on its future course. So now Medicare exists in a political environment that is the product of its earlier policy accomplishments: politics creates its own form of policy feedback. Future feasible reform strategies must be cognizant of both this history and its resulting program architecture and politics.

For progressives seeking a comprehensive national health insurance program, the enactment of Medicare in 1965 represented a partial and bittersweet accomplishment. After more than thirty years of halting progress toward universal health care coverage, proponents of national health insurance accepted Medicare as a "loss leader," a foot-in-the-door for larger health care reform. The loss leader concept held that once Medicare established the feasibility of publicly sponsored health coverage, health care coverage would be expanded to the poor and the underinsured. Soon, perhaps as early as 1968, the nation would accept national health insurance for all. Robert Ball, speaking for the original architects of the program, remembers, "We all saw insurance for the elderly as a fallback position, which we advocated solely because it seemed to have the best chance politically. Although the public record contains some explicit denials, we expected Medicare to be a first step towards national health insurance, perhaps with 'Kiddicare' as another step."[2]

The key challenge for Medicare at the time it was enacted was to demonstrate two things: (1) administratively, that a national program of finance and payment could work; and (2) politically, that the doctors, hospitals, and the insurance industry would play. In the early years, the preoccupation of Medicare's architects was with participation of the medical profession. After the protracted opposition of organized medicine, the framers and administrators feared that providers would undermine the program and deny beneficiaries access to care. At the time Medicare was enacted, there was widespread talk among physicians of a boycott or strike.[3]

As a result, the initial incentives and administration of the program strongly encouraged providers to come forward and provide care almost without regard to the long-term economic consequences. As Wilbur Cohen, another of the original architects of the program, remarked, "The primary objective of 1965–67 was to get off to a good start, to avoid any strike, slowdown, or other uncooperative action."[4]

The existence of Part B, supplemental insurance, can be traced to a maneuver by Wilbur Mills in the House Ways and Means Committee in which he added voluntary supplemental coverage (advocated by the Republicans and the American Medical Association [AMA] as an alternative to Medicare) to the committee bill. Thus was born the "layer cake" of Medicaid for the indigent (based on the old Kerr Mills program), Hospital Insurance (Part A), and Supplemental Medical Insurance (Part B) to pay primarily for physician care. The payment policy for physicians in Part B was modeled after a specific plan in the Federal Employees Health Benefit Program administered by Aetna. Hospitals were given generous capital payments that allowed rapid expansion and improvement in their physical plants.[5]

The selection of private insurance companies, such as Blue Cross plans, as carriers and intermediaries for processing Medicare claims was one of the congressional accommodations to the insurance industry. Paul Starr sees a deeper accommodation to provider interests in this administrative structure, because Blue Cross plans themselves were originally a creation of the hospital industry: "The administration of Medicare was lodged in the private insurance system originally established to suit provider interests. And [as such] the federal government surrendered direct control of the program and its costs."[6] This preoccupation with making the program palatable to physicians, hospitals, and the private insurance industry created an initial skeleton and set of incentives that invited acceptance and, over time, profound inefficiency.

A critical aspect of the public persona of the original Medicare legislation was its tie to Social Security. In the early 1960s, Social Security was widely accepted, both philosophically, as a social insurance solution to income security in old age, and administratively, as an efficient and well-run public program. Robert Ball even admits that some of the references to Social Security in the political debate over Medicare were "subliminal."[7] Medicare's tie to Social Security was partially accomplished through the use of payroll tax financing and trust funds, the parallel structure of eligibility to Old Age and Survivors Insurance, and the creation of an "earned right" to benefits without means testing.[8] The conceptual tie to Social Security also had important implications for the original structure and evolution of Medicare administrative arrangements, beginning with the Bureau of Health Insurance housed in the Social Security Administration.[9]

Patashnik and Zelizer have argued that the social insurance concept of trust fund financing for Part A and Part B was also a device orchestrated largely by Wilbur Mills to keep the costs of Medicare from growing beyond the capacity of earmarked funds to support the program, as well as to protect the retirement income side of Social Security from the later incursion of financing demands from escalating health costs. They see in this arrangement the heavy and sophisticated hand of Chairman Mills, establishing a form of fiscal discipline for the long term of the program.

This structure and tie to Social Security was nurtured over twenty-five years by an astute and committed cadre of analysts, managers, and political operatives who believed in a particular ideology and philosophy of social insurance.[10] Wilbur Cohen, Robert Ball, Arthur Altmeyer, Elizabeth Wickenden, and Nelson Cruikshank controlled the terms of debate over Social

Security and Medicare to such a degree that a serious challenge to the core principles of the program was never mounted. Ironically, by keeping the cards of the program so close to their vest, the "apparatus," as Cohen affectionately referred to this group, also neglected to cultivate a long-term and broad understanding of the social contract that was implied in Medicare. Unfortunately for the political and administrative legacy of the program, the "apparatus," however, has no modern-day progenitor, leaving a relatively open field—ideologically and philosophically—for new Medicare concepts, such as vouchers and medical savings accounts, as well as for pure budgetary politics.

Nonetheless, the conceptual and political tie to social insurance retains considerable power even in recent discussions of Medicare reform. For example, the National Academy of Social Insurance in its recent review of Medicare policy options places heavy emphasis on the classic social insurance elements—compulsory participation, government sponsorship, contributory finance, eligibility based on prior contributions, benefits prescribed in law, benefits not directly related to contributions, and separate accounting and long-range financial planning—as building blocks for the future design of Medicare.[11]

On top of this original accommodation to insurance and provider interests, Medicare's design has evolved episodically. In 1972, coverage was extended to the disabled (those receiving Social Security cash benefits) and to patients with end-stage renal disease. Home health coverage was expanded in 1980, and the deductible for Part B Supplemental Medical Insurance was added. In 1983, hospice coverage was added, and the Prospective Payment System (PPS) for hospital reimbursement was established. Rather than pay hospitals on the basis of their costs of care, PPS provided a single, prospectively determined payment based on the diagnosis-related group (DRG) of the patient's primary diagnosis. In 1985, most state and local government workers were made eligible for Medicare coverage. Also in 1985 and again in 1986, new rules made Medicare a secondary payer for workers, including disabled workers, who could rely on primary coverage by their employers. Payment for mental health services, outpatient services, and allied health providers in rural areas was liberalized in 1987.

In 1989, a major reform of physician payment, based on a resource-based relative value scale (RBRVS), was enacted. This new Medicare fee schedule represented a significant departure from Medicare's traditional method of physician payment, which was based on "customary, prevailing, and reasonable charges." In 1990, new rules were enacted for so-called Medigap policies, which were private supplemental insurance plans that cover copayments, deductibles, and other services such as long-term care or prescription drugs. In 1993, several financing changes increased the wages subject to payroll taxes and lowered the Part A premiums. These 1993 amendments also pegged Part B beneficiary premiums at 25 percent of program costs, with the remaining 75 percent to be financed by general revenues. Legislation was passed in 1995 that encouraged the expansion of the Medicare Select option, a preferred provider organization (PPO)-based form of supplemental coverage that had been available in a limited form in fourteen states. In 1997, a number of changes in Medicare payment policy and the plan options available to beneficiaries were enacted under the BBA (see discussion below). These changes forestalled the immediate depletion of the Part A trust fund and delegated the larger debate about Medicare's future to a commission later to be named the National Bipartisan Commission on the Future of Medicare.

While each of these reforms was significant in the small politics of the Medicare program, in the big picture they amount to tinkering within the broad parameters of a program structure still rooted in the early 1960s. What continues to be remarkable about this history is the degree of staying power of the original accommodations. Many political scientists see this staying power as dramatic evidence of conservatism, antistatism (in welfare state terms), and incrementalism in American politics broadly.[12]

This durability, however, also created a problem of identity and policy design for Medicare in the late 1990s. The concept of Medicare as a relatively passive payer of health care claims, not "exercising any supervision or control over the practice of medicine, or the manner in which medical services are provided,"[13] was realized to a remarkable extent over its more than thirty-five-year history. The National Academy of Social Insurance study panel concluded, after a review of Medicare's record of cost containment, that "the records of private-sector insurers and Medicare suggest that, for better or worse, the original legislative intent—that Medicare not dominate or substantially interfere with or constrain the private health care system or insurance markets—was largely achieved."[14] The administration of the program, built on the foundation of indemnity insurance and the political authority of physicians and hospitals, is now largely out of phase with developments in the health care marketplace.

Medicare's original social and private insurance concepts, as well as the political accommodations of 1965, created a structural legacy that is hard to overcome, even in the modern world of managed care that emerged in the 1990s. Medicare's history also left ambiguity and a lack of consensus about its basic social contract. For example, recent Medicare debate, including the deliberations of the National Bipartisan Commission on the Future of Medicare, has been largely framed by two different camps with distinctive ideologies, marketplace rationales, and constituencies—yet both could find justification for their positions in Medicare history and policy design. In general, each camp was defined by (1) a belief that the Medicare contract should represent a commitment to a *defined set of benefits* (i.e., certain services universally guaranteed), or (2) a belief that the Medicare contract should represent a social commitment to a *defined contribution* or subsidy from the government that beneficiaries may use to go out into the health care marketplace to purchase insurance and services.

The legacy of the 1965 solution is everywhere in the current operation of the program: in its language; in its structure of copayments, deductibles, and limits; and in its use of carriers and intermediaries to carry out billing and claims processing. For most beneficiaries, the contemporary Medicare program stubbornly adheres to a 1960s concept of health care that divides services into Hospital Insurance (Part A) and Physicians Services (Part B) with fee-for-service prices administratively determined. The program struggles to define policies for managed care, chronic care, home care, allied health services, and other forms of care that do not fit neatly into Part A or Part B. The creation of a Medicare Part C, discussed below, represents a first significant effort to incorporate alternative delivery systems into Medicare. However, integrated systems of care that attempt to assure that services are continuous—say across the boundaries of acute, chronic, and long-term care—simply do not fit into the incentives and organization of traditional Medicare.

Historically, payment has been the tail that wags the dog in health care and the object of most policy attention in Medicare reform.[15] One of the big lessons of the health services research field is that consumers and providers show impressive responses to economic incentives conveyed in Medicare's payment systems. Seemingly small increments in the prices that individuals pay and providers receive for care have significant consequences for the amount of care received and provided. Changes in the form of payment (such as the movement to prospective payment systems for hospitals) stimulate dramatically new organizations of care. Changes in the economic incentives for physician services have significant effects on the amount of care that they prescribe, so far without discernible effects on health outcomes. Producing efficiencies and cost savings through innovation in payment systems has been the major goal of legislative changes in Medicare from 1983 to the present.

The bifurcation of Medicare into Parts A and B has been enormously consequential for the politics of the program, for the ways in which data are collected and analyzed, and for the ways in which Medicare's future is considered. The movement of some home health spending from Part A to Part B under the 1997 BBA (thereby hiding the budgetary consequences that would be evident in the Part A trust fund) is an example of the kind of political games-manship that this structure promotes. Historically, separate reports have been issued by the trustees who oversee the two sides of Medicare's finances, and they often draw differing conclusions about its actuarial soundness. The illu-sions created by these trust funds affect the politics of and policy making for Medicare and are also significant in the inner workings of the Congress. Until 1997 separate commissions, the Prospective Payment Assessment Commis-sion (ProPAC) and the Physician Payment Review Commission (PPRC) over-saw the respective issues of reimbursement policy for Part A and Part B, issuing separate reports to Congress. The BBA of 1997 merged the two com-missions into MedPAC, the Medicare Payment Advisory Commission. How-ever, the analytic and political legacy from the old hospital payment/physician payment traditions was maintained: the analyses and reports of MedPAC con-tinue to be highly compartmentalized, with relatively little attention to cross-cutting issues or innovative approaches to reform.

More important, this legacy creates mixed political sponsorship and in-terests in Medicare financing and delivery, thus providing a complicated struc-ture of agency relationships. Medicare's financing includes "contributions" into the trust funds by workers paying payroll taxes, "premiums" from en-rolled beneficiaries, copayments and deductibles from those who actually use covered services, and funds from general revenue. The larger public, then, has a financial stake in Medicare delivery because it pays for current care of beneficiaries (via the mechanism of the trust funds), and it supports the pro-gram through general taxes. Conceptually (as I will discuss more formally in chapter 3), this means that the public, meaning the taxpaying public as repre-sented in the Congress, becomes one of the principals in the Medicare con-tract.

Individual beneficiaries have a personal stake in the accessibility and quality of Medicare-sponsored services in the same way as any beneficiary of a private insurance plan. Thus, individual beneficiaries are also principals in the Medicare contract—they treat their health plans and providers as would any individuals overseeing their own contract or arrangements for care.

This bilateral interest in the financial and medical consequences of Medicare services defines the fundamental problem of Medicare policy de-sign: it is neither a pure public transfer program (or "entitlement" in the cur-rent parlance), nor is it an individual insurance plan. In the contemporary politics of Medicare reform, simplistic sound bites—"an earned right," "an entitlement"—distort and polarize consideration of what is a complex con-struction of public finance, insurance coverage, and health care purchasing, one that involves two major principals.

Medicare was born with a fundamental ambiguity in its core policy de-sign: it was not pure social insurance, in the sense of the European Bismarck tradition, nor was it a pure assistance program, though the Medicaid program added significant welfare and redistributive features. It was not comprehen-sive insurance, because key elements of coverage, such as prescription drug coverage, were left out. It was not a conventional insurance pool, because Part B drew significant revenues from general taxation, not the payment of insur-ance premiums. It was not active health care purchasing, because the legisla-tion explicitly forbade the program from trying to influence the practice of medicine. Looking back on this political history, Theodore Marmor concludes that Medicare's structure had "a political explanation, not a philosophical ra-tionale."[16]

Modern Medicare Politics I: The Catastrophic Coverage Act

Modern Medicare and its politics have evolved from the structural blueprint created by the politics of 1965. Large-scale interest groups, such as the Ameri-can Association of Retired Persons (AARP), either did not exist or were not a factor at the outset of the program. However, any program of the size and resource demands of Medicare creates its own constituencies and politics, as Carroll Estes's *The Aging Enterprise* demonstrated years ago.[17] The external po-litical environment for Medicare, and for social insurance more broadly, has evolved as well. In order to understand the nature of the implicit contempo-rary Medicare social contract, it is necessary to examine some of its most re-cent political history.

The most dramatic evidence of the nature and boundaries of the Medicare social contract comes from the 1988–90 passage and subsequent repeal of the Medicare Catastrophic Coverage Act. In effect, this experience serves as a modern political experiment on the status of the Medicare social contract, its constituent support, and the prospects for further expansion or reform. The Catastrophic Coverage Act was actually envisioned by some of its architects as a test case in modern financing of social insurance, especially in the era of scarce budgetary resources and intergenerational politics. If suc-cessful, they believed that it would provide the model for expanding long-term care coverage and making other improvements to Medicare.[18]

The Medicare Catastrophic Coverage Act grew out of increasing recogni-tion during the 1980s that Medicare was falling behind, if not failing, in its mis-sion to provide protection against the heavy financial burdens of illness in old age. The most common illustration given during the time was that the out-of-pocket burden for medical care was greater (as a percentage of income) in the late 1980s than it had been in 1965 at the time Medicare was enacted. These out-of-pocket expenses were a function of copayments and deductibles for care; uncovered prescription drugs; and uncovered dental, vision, and long-term care services. Upward of 70 percent of beneficiaries layered private Medigap or employer plans on top of their Medicare coverage, giving them varying degrees of protection. President Reagan appointed a commission under the leadership of former Secretary of Health and Human Services Otis Bowen to examine the sources of catastrophic expenses and make recommendations to the Congress. After considering the breadth of the coverage gaps created by Medicare's patch-work benefit design, the Bowen Commission recommended a relatively simple plan that would set a $2,000 limit on out-of-pocket liabilities for beneficiaries, to be financed by an annual $59 premium on all beneficiaries.

The legislative debate over Catastrophic Coverage took place during a period of serious fiscal constraint. The escalating deficits of the early 1980s were apparent, and there was bipartisan support for a balanced budget amendment. Within Medicare, the implementation of the Prospective Pay-ment System (in 1983–84) and the announcement of a new Medicare fee schedule for physician services were seen as necessary but not sufficient mechanisms to control both the costs and budgetary exposure of the program. The marching orders of the administration were for any expansion of cover-age to be *self-financed* by beneficiaries; no new general taxes or general revenue expenditures would be permitted to finance new coverage.

As the legislation was debated by the Congress, the original Bowen pro-posal was modified by varying degrees in the House and Senate to increase the protection for low-income aged beneficiaries, to modestly expand long-term care benefits, and to liberalize the asset and income tests for Medicaid nursing home coverage. The House also added a high-deductible prescription drug benefit. As the House expanded the scope of coverage to be provided in the Catastrophic Coverage Act, so too did the costs increase, running higher than the Bowen Commission's original estimate of a $59 premium.

The bill that the Congress eventually passed was a complex and patchy reconciliation of the House's interest in substantial coverage, especially for low-income beneficiaries, and the Senate's concerns about limiting costs and redistribution. Inpatient hospital coverage was expanded and simplified to re-quire only one deductible and unlimited days in any given year. The period of coverage for nursing home care was increased, and the requirement for a prior hospital stay in order to qualify for skilled nursing coverage was elimi-nated. Hospice benefits were extended, Part B coinsurance was capped, and mammography and respite care benefits were instituted. Drug benefits were to be phased in, beginning in 1990 with in-home intravenous and immuno-

suppressive drugs and expanded one year later to cover all outpatient prescription drugs and insulin.

The financing of the Medicare Catastrophic Coverage Act was based on
income tax payments of beneficiaries. In 1989, payments were scheduled to be
$22.50 for every $150 in federal income tax liability, up to a maximum $800
per individual. Initially, the surtax represented a 15 percent marginal tax rate
up to incomes of $40,000 for individuals, $70,000 for couples. The surtax in
1989 preceded the availability of the drug benefits in 1991 and was scheduled
to increase sharply in the early years, growing to 28 percent by 1993. This
financing scheme departed sharply from former principles and politics of
Medicare expansion, which had either added benefits without revealing their
true tax incidence or at least spread the burden over both beneficiaries and all
taxpayers.

Explanations for the demise and repeal of the Catastrophic Coverage Act
vary, but central to any account is this direct linkage of financing to benefits
and the collateral reaction and backlash of Medicare beneficiaries themselves.[19] Many beneficiaries saw the new coverage as costly, once again incomplete, and competitive with their own private Medigap policies. Many more
affluent beneficiaries resented the progressive nature of the financing scheme,
in effect having to pay for the benefits of low-income beneficiaries who did not
have to pay the tax. Some spectacular media coverage—most notably Congressman Daniel Rostenkowski, chairman of the House Ways and Means
Committee, being chased down the street by an incensed group of senior citizens in his own district—fueled the perception that the burden of expanded
coverage was being perpetrated against the will of many beneficiaries.[20]

More scholarly analyses of the demise of the Catastrophic Coverage Act
tell a mixed and more complicated story, with still further implications for understanding the status of the contemporary Medicare social contract. First,
and not surprisingly, reaction to the Catastrophic Coverage Act was deeply
divided and sorted in a diffuse way by class, age, and ideology.[21] Information
problems in Medicare generally, and in the Catastrophic Coverage Act specifically, fueled much of the fear and opposition to the bill. As is widely apparent from survey data, many beneficiaries do not understand the broad
parameters of their coverage, such as the absence of extended nursing home
coverage, much less the details of their coinsurance, deductibles, or limits on
days of care.[22] A survey by Thomas Rice and colleagues at the height of the
Catastrophic Coverage Act debate produced on average only 2.4 correct answers to 8 basic factual questions about the bill.[23] Fewer than 40 percent of
those sampled were even aware that the legislation offered coverage for prescription drugs. Ignorance of benefits and confusion over coverage were com-

pounded by the complicated interaction of Medigap policies, retiree health coverage, and Medicaid dual eligibility. The reality that Medicare is big and complicated confounded and undermined the interpretation of the catastrophic legislation.

Whatever the underlying misconceptions or misunderstandings of the financing philosophy and mechanisms that governed the development of the Catastrophic Coverage proposal, its final structure of financing represented a significant statement in the evolution of Medicare from its social insurance roots.[24] Not only was it a politically implicit requirement that the Catastrophic Coverage Act be forward funded, but its revenue base was to be restricted to older persons themselves. This targeting of revenues and benefits to users, in turn, unleashed a quite narrow and self-interested reaction to the potential costs and benefits of the proposal to subgroups of the elderly and disabled. Thus, the test for many beneficiaries and their advocates became, "Will I receive benefits that offset the new premiums that I am expected to pay (this year)?" This is a much different test than is applied to insurance coverage in pools, much less to legislative debate over the broader notions of social insurance that underlie Medicare's original passage.

Marilyn Moon calls the repeal of the Catastrophic Coverage Act a "watershed" in the evolution of Medicare as a social insurance arrangement. In political terms, it was a rejection of the idea that benefits for those unable to afford them could be financed out of taxes paid by others. This rejection was even stronger than first appears, because it did not even raise the contemporary political challenge of intergenerational subsidies to Medicare. The Catastrophic Coverage Act proposed to (mostly) cover benefits for older (low-income) beneficiaries from supplementary "premiums" levied on higher-income beneficiaries. The lesson of the Catastrophic Coverage Act is that a new principle of financing and coverage for Medicare has been tried and rejected. Nothing that has happened since the repeal of the Catastrophic Coverage Act gives reason to believe that the fiscal and political tests for Medicare reform have changed. Structurally and financially, this political experience further reinforced the traditional roles and boundaries of Medicare's two principals, public taxpayers and individual beneficiaries.

Modern Medicare Politics II: The 1997 Balanced Budget Act, the 1999 Balanced Budget Refinement Act, and 2000 Benefits Improvement Act

The Balanced Budget Act (BBA) of 1997 grew directly out of the 1995–96 efforts of the Republican-controlled Congress to enact the "Contract with America," simultaneously reducing Medicare expenditures, creating budgetary relief, and introducing a number of elements of managed care, choice, and competition into the program. The original proposal, the Medicare Preservation Act, sought to reduce Medicare spending by $270 billion over a seven-year period and another 14 percent over the subsequent seven-year period.[25] The bill was marked up by the Ways and Means Committee in the House in less than a week; the initial hearings were scheduled to be completed in a day; and it passed with virtually no bipartisan support. President Clinton vetoed the bill, brandishing the pen used by Lyndon Johnson to sign the original Medicare legislation in 1965.

Many of the elements of the ill-fated Medicare Preservation Act were brought back for the 1996–97 session, this time to be the subject of serious horse trading over a broad array of budgetary and policy priorities. This time, the Congress was preoccupied with delaying the "bankruptcy" of the Part A trust fund, which was forecast for as early as 2001. The proposed BBA changes were projected to save $116 billion over five years. Individual members of the Congress and several interest groups used this opportunity (and the cover of the budget process) to introduce many new options with the intention of expanding the range of choice in plans and provider types for beneficiaries. Payment rates for many different provider types were reduced, and the development of new prospective payment methodologies for several new classes of providers was mandated. The BBA also made substantial changes in the incentives and rules for graduate medical education. The responsibilities and structure of the Health Care Financing Administration (HCFA) remained essentially the same, as did the organization of Medicare contracting. Information resources for beneficiaries changed only modestly. A number of demonstration projects—competitive bidding, coordinated care, and the use of third-party enrollment brokers—were also authorized as a means to build the groundwork for a more competitive, market-oriented model of Medicare in the future. Finally, a commission was authorized—later to be known as the National Bipartisan Commission on the Future of Medicare (or the Breaux-Thomas Commission) to consider more fundamental changes to Medicare and to make recommendations assuring the long-term fiscal viability of Medicare in light of the aging of the baby boomers.

The BBA created a new class of Medicare options under the Medicare+Choice initiative, also known as Medicare Part C. The introduction of choice as a defining feature of the program represented a shift in the philosophy and design of the program, one that received relatively little public debate. Medicare+Choice allows beneficiaries to select among four plan types:

- Coordinated care plans such as traditional HMOs, PPOs, and other managed care arrangements that are licensed under state law as risk-bearing entities eligible to provide health insurance coverage.

- Plans offered by new provider sponsored organizations (PSOs). These organizations are composed of hospitals, physician groups, or combinations thereof, and they bear a substantial risk for providing the covered services.
- A limited number of plans that are based on medical savings accounts and high-deductible coverage. A maximum of 390,000 beneficiaries are allowed to enroll in the plans (not including low-income beneficiaries). Deductibles may range up to $6,000.
- Private fee-for-service plans that do not place providers at risk for the beneficiaries' use of health care services and do not restrict beneficiaries' choices.

The politics underlying the Medicare + Choice initiative were complex and reveal the diversity of interests that can be marshaled in opposition to the existing Medicare structure. Theodore Marmor sees similarities in the pace and thoughtfulness of the 1965 enactment and the BBA 1997 reforms: "This was not a well-thought out, considered reform of a popular program needing adjustment. What happened in 1997 was, like the original enactment in 1965, a rather pressured, highly uncertain set of policies, adaptations to a transformed political environment."[26]

Republican leadership in the Congress embraced medical savings accounts and other instruments of choice because they fit an ideological concept of Medicare that encourages individual price sensitivity and more freedom of choice for beneficiaries, fewer restrictions on providers in the market, and, theoretically, less intrusion by government. Among the interest groups, the AMA had long lobbied for more flexibility in Medicare's payment methods, with greater latitude for physicians to engage in alternative organizational arrangements, to balance bill patients, or to engage in wholly private contracts outside of Medicare's regulations. Psychiatrists also lobbied hard for the right to contract privately with Medicare patients.

Also at work in the BBA legislative process, especially as it was embedded in larger budgetary politics, is the reality that geographical and district concerns figured prominently in both the design of amendments and the particular positions that members adopted. Because Medicare represents such a large conduit of federal funds, providers and vendors line up with their representatives to assure that a district's or state's "fair share" of Medicare dollars are secured when there are changes to the program. A representative or senator with an influential constituency of academic medical centers looks at

Medicare payment reform through the lens of these providers, their associations, and their lobbyists. The New York State delegation looked carefully at the implications for teaching hospitals. Managed care plans in relatively low-payment counties lobbied that Medicare payment policy disadvantages them relative to other plans in higher payment counties. Politically, all of this can be interpreted in essentially pork-barrel terms: a particular representative and district aim to achieve an "equitable" share of federal funds, whatever the cost or reimbursement rationale might be for the Medicare payment reform.

This form of political calculus was on display in the BBA and in the subsequent Balanced Budget Refinement Act of 1999 (BBRA) and the Medicare, Medicaid, and SCHIP (State Children's Health Insurance Program) Benefits Improvement Act of 2000 (BIPA) reforms. For example, in order to dampen the apparent disadvantage that managed care plans felt under the old payment formula, managed care payment changes were introduced to shrink the variation in payment from place to place. Most important, a floor was established to bring up the payment for managed care plans that were receiving the lowest per-capita reimbursement. Because their reimbursement was now disconnected from the fee-for-service cost experience of beneficiaries in their particular counties, plans that received new, raised-floor payments experienced a windfall increase in their payments with no corresponding obligations or requirements for service. Moreover, plans that were not in areas receiving the enhanced payment "floors" received only small increases in payments, all in the name of compressing the payment distribution from place to place. As Marmor had remarked on an earlier era of Medicare policy, the change had "a political explanation, not a philosophical rationale."[27]

Subsequent updates to the BBA were enacted in the BBRA and the BIPA legislation. Interestingly, the BBRA established bonus payments for Medicare+Choice plans that located in counties with no existing Medicare plans. In the context of a budget surplus and the rapid withdrawal of Medicare+Choice managed care plans, BIPA raised floor payments for certain counties, raised the minimum increase in managed care payments from 2 percent to 3 percent, and further extended the bonus payments for plans to locate in uncovered areas.[28] The combination of these budget amendments to Medicare raised the projected payments to providers over time and tinkered with the incentives, particularly to Medicare+Choice plans, but did not fundamentally change structure, philosophy, or governance of the program. More importantly, they represented incremental path movements for Medicare policy that were primarily motivated by the political need to respond to provider outcry and the threat of further plan and provider withdrawal from the Medicare program.

Lodging much of the contemporary Medicare reform politics within the politics of the budget process reveals both the institutional context of reform and its self-reinforcing character. The role of institutions and the structural features of the political process have been well studied in the area of health policy generally, but the modern era of Medicare policy dramatically illustrates the importance of budgeting politics in shaping reform.[29] Medicare reform as an exercise in budget reconciliation politics submerges questions of principle and design out of sight of public access and involvement and has provided a set of "rules of engagement" for industry lobbyists and Medicare advocates. In particular, the budget process places an emphasis on payment policy and geographical fairness questions (the "stuff" of budgetary wrangling) over more substantive and programmatic concerns in Medicare. Jack Hoadley summarizes the effect of legislating Medicare policy within the framework and constraints of the budget reconciliation process, in this case reacting to the passage of the Medicare Resource Based Relative Value Scale Physician Payment System in the Omnibus Reconciliation Act (OBRA), 1989: "The use of budget reconciliation as the main way to pass health legislation has significant implications for policy making and the legislative process. It has quickened the pace of deliberations, moved much of it behind doors, imposed tight budget constraints on the set of alternatives, curbed outside influence, and altered the relationship between the executive and legislative branches."[30]

Medicare Politics III: The National Bipartisan Commission on the Future of Medicare

While not resulting in any formal legislation, the deliberations and product of the National Bipartisan Commission on the Future of Medicare are instructive for what they reveal about the state of the Medicare social contract and the sharp divisions in interpretation that now exist.[31] The commission, charged by President Clinton to formulate a bipartisan and consensus position on financing and benefits for Medicare, instead put on display contrasting interpretations of the policy "problem" Medicare reform was supposed to address and the philosophy of social insurance that should undergird reform, as well as the range of potential solutions. For example, different members of the commission simultaneously promoted proposals to raise the eligibility age for Medicare (from 65 to 67) and lower the age of eligibility for Medicare. A group of commission members promoted a defined-*benefits* approach to Medicare (arguing traditional social insurance principles), while other members argued that Medicare should move to a defined-*contribution* approach as a way to resolve its long-term financing shortfalls. In the end, the commission failed to achieve a consensus or a required majority vote on the proposal of its chairmen, Senator John Breaux (D) and Representative Bill Thomas (R). The 10 to 7 vote was one vote short of the required supermajority necessary to bring the recommendation of the commission forward to the Congress.

The Breaux-Thomas proposal, based on a concept of providing "premium support," is interesting in its own right because it reveals an important direction of political pressure to reform Medicare, as well as a major line of critique of the current structure and philosophy of the program. In many ways, the premium-support proposal extends a line of reform begun in the BBA of 1997, encouraging competition, beneficiary choice, alternative delivery systems, and insurance products for beneficiaries. Implicitly, these initiatives are converting the government obligation for coverage to a fixed contribution as opposed to a set package of benefits.

Under Breaux-Thomas, traditional fee-for-service Medicare would continue but largely as a fallback option for beneficiaries who are unable or unwilling to find other options in the marketplace. Traditional Medicare would be modified to include a high-option plan, providing prescription drug coverage and stop-loss protection, in addition to a standard plan with revised copayments and deductibles. Any benefit changes would need to be approved by Congress and financially self-sustaining. Under the premium-support alternative, private plans would be required to provide a standard package of benefits plus other coverage, up to some (unspecified) actuarial limit over the level made available in traditional Medicare. At a minimum, plans would be required to offer a high-option alternative, including prescription drug coverage.

The government would provide a subsidy for the purchase of private plans, proposed to be 88 percent of the national weighted plan price for a plan with standard options. For plans that charge less, beneficiaries would pay no premiums; for plans that charge more, beneficiaries would share the cost with the government, up to a limit of 100 percent of the weighted average plan price. Beneficiaries would be responsible for paying the incremental costs of any plans that charge premiums above this specified amount. The government would pay the entire premium for high-option plans for low-income beneficiaries (up to 135 percent of the poverty line), so long as that plan did not cost more than 85 percent of the weighted national average of plans. The actual amount paid to a plan would be adjusted for geography and risk, including the health status of the beneficiary.

What is important is that this new premium-support model included an entirely new administrative structure and national bidding process for plans. While administration of traditional Medicare would continue to be the responsibility of an HCFA-like entity, premium support would be administered by a new quasi-governmental Medicare board that would act something like a benefits office, overseeing open enrollment periods, providing information on plans to beneficiaries, negotiating premiums, and setting payments (including risk adjustment).

While not resulting in a consensus recommendation or successful legislation, the Breaux-Thomas proposal has had significant influence in shaping the terms of the subsequent debate about Medicare reform, furthering its movement along the path of competitive and market-oriented approaches to coverage and pricing and introducing consideration of new administrative structures for the program. Although advocates for a defined-benefit approach to Medicare fought the premium-support approach bitterly, the proposal actually mixes elements of defined-benefit and defined-contribution approaches. Essentially, the Breaux-Thomas proposal moved the center of gravity in discussions of Medicare reform back toward a financing model. If the premium-support model takes hold politically, the essence of the reform debate will center on the nature and size of the subsidy to be provided for old-age health care, rather than the nature of benefits and coverage.

Medicare Politics IV: The Administrative Politics of Medicare

The Health Care Financing Administration (HCFA), and now the Centers for Medicare and Medicaid Services (CMS), have long been a target of criticism and a source of executive and congressional concern in the administration of Medicare. On the one hand, the program has been lauded for its low administrative overhead; on the other hand, critics have cited the inability of its administration to implement a modern regime of information, quality improvement, and accountability for health care expenditures. HCFA has run a relatively lean bureaucracy, employing a staff of only about 4,500 before the reorganization to the CMS in 2001. In 1991, an Academy of Public Administration expert panel warned that the lack of internal administrative resources would result in continued and significant adverse consequences for the performance of the program, consequences that could not be readily solved by outsourcing more and more of Medicare's basic administrative functions. A 1999 open letter to the Congress from a panel of health services experts cited HCFA's lack of resources and administrative authority as a major source of the program's performance problems.[32]

Until recently, Medicare's administration did not garner serious executive or congressional attention. Originally, administration of the program was lodged in a diffuse set of offices in the Social Security Administration, along with an advisory council, the Health Insurance Benefits Advisory Council, then formalized in the Health Insurance Bureau. In retrospect, the implementation of Medicare was a remarkable achievement, given the lack of infrastructure and administrative resources at the time.[33]

HCFA itself was created in 1977 by Secretary Joseph Califano, who was concerned about the diffuse structure of administration of Medicare and Medicaid, particularly the lack of coherence in cost-containment efforts for these two programs.[34] Califano wished to lay the groundwork for administration of a national health insurance program and designed HCFA's scope of authority accordingly. For conservatives wary of expanding the federal role in coverage and management of the national health system, this original ambition for HCFA may have served as a form of political scarlet letter, always a reason to question and challenge the administrative authority of the agency.

Lawrence Brown's analysis of the early history of Medicare's administrative arrangements saw three eras: one in which the administrative game plan was to accommodate providers; a second in which initiatives such as control over capital expenditures and professional review organizations provided a kind of decentralized administrative apparatus; and a third in which the program's administration took on a more centralized and "corporate" character, designed to exert more activist control over the terms of payment and delivery, primarily with the leverage provided by the technical control of payment methods such as DRGs.[35] Writing from the perspective of 1985, Brown anticipated more administrative authority (for HCFA) coming out of the implementation of reimbursement tools such as DRGs than has ultimately come to pass.

Throughout its history, HCFA had relatively little input into policy development and shared its administrative and enforcement functions with other units of government. In policy making, HCFA shared the advisory function to the Secretary of Health and Human Services, the administration, and the Congress with others: the Assistant Secretary for Planning and Evaluation, the White House staff, and other policy advisors in the administration; the Medicare commissions; committee staff; and other advisory bodies such as the Government Accounting Office and Congressional Budget Office on the Hill. The responsibility of the Office of the Inspector General for fraud and abuse, instituted in 1979, further diminished HCFA's authority over the accountability of the program. With enactment of the Health Insurance Portability and Protection Act (HIPPA), and the Clinton administration's emphasis on controlling Medicare fraud and abuse, the Justice Department and the Federal Bureau of Investigation (FBI) assumed a more prominent role in Medicare enforcement, especially from the perspective of providers. As will be seen in the last chapter, CMS's lack of hegemony over the policy and administrative turf of Medicare means that the executive branch is severely limited in changing program features in response to public, beneficiary, or market demands. Important for the analysis of this book is the fact that CMS provides relatively weak agency for the executive branch, perhaps by design of the Congress. There is little doubt that Medicare's weak and unstable administrative arrangements are, in large measure, the product of larger political ambivalence about the role and power that administration per se should enjoy, and the wary suspicions of legislators, providers, and beneficiaries. Brown summarizes this predicament for Medicare administration:

> the difficult but unavoidable task of balancing provider preferences with public accountability has been particularly perplexing for Medicare administrators. Unable to articulate clearly the positions of administrations that have been both unsure of their own objectives and suspicious of the allegiance and intentions of the bureaucracy, officials have often stood by as Congress redefined their tasks, sometimes without their consent or participation. Condemned to wrangling over the details of reimbursement variables set forth in laws that are at once rigid and ambiguous, detailed and porous, they have implemented legislation concocted precisely to protect beneficiary and provider alike from the "excessive bureaucratic discretion" so feared in the United States. Government–group relations have adjusted to these facts of political culture and structure.[36]

With its limited available resources, HCFA labored to keep up with day-to-day administrative demands, as well as respond to the myriad changes in Medicare policy and management mandated by congressional action. In its last year, HCFA was responsible for the oversight of over 900 million claims, roughly $240 billion dollars in federal spending, and accountability for services for about 40 million beneficiaries. Almost every year, Congress mandated significant changes in the program that required administrative implementation, most often through the budget reconciliation process. For example, the 1997 BBA authorized approximately 240 changes in the Medicare program, many raising complex technical reimbursement issues, as well as 110 changes in the Medicaid program.[37] The BBRA added another 133 provisions for HCFA implementation.[38]

From time to time, HCFA (and now CMS) has also been buffeted by exogenous shocks in health care administration, not policy, that required substantial effort and detoured the agency from its ongoing work. For example, retooling computer systems to assure Y2K compliance in 1999 consumed significant financial and human resources, causing many of the agency's ongoing and discretionary projects to be put aside. Often, the agency simply cannot keep up with the technological and administrative demands of managing health systems. For example, a major effort to modernize and centralize Medicare's information and transactions processing system launched in the early 1990s failed because of a series of management problems, leaving the agency with an antiquated and inadequate system at the end of the decade.[39]

Evidence of the precarious political circumstance of HCFA is everywhere. HCFA was directed by seventeen administrators in its twenty-three-year history, an average tenure of only 1.4 years.[40] Acting administrators led the agency 10 percent of the time over this history. Recent signs of administrative vulnerability surfaced in the deliberations of the National Bipartisan Commission (where it was proposed that many of HCFA's functions be replaced by a national Medicare Board), in proposals for managing a Medicare prescription drug benefit (where numerous alternatives to HCFA administration have been proposed), and in the early administrative reorganization of the Bush administration. The creation of the new CMS, one of the early initiatives of Secretary Tommy Thompson, provides still a new administrative structure but no significant new resources, authority, or discretion for Medicare administration. In addition, the Congress has initiated hearings on Medicare governance, the National Academy of Social Insurance has formed a Management and Governance study group, and bold new administrative proposals are appearing in the literature.[41]

Thus, Medicare grew up with a weak and now vulnerable administrative structure. A result of being in the middle of divided government, in the middle of strong ideological differences about the scale and market orientation of federal health policy as a whole, and in the middle of a contentious battle over resources between providers and the Congress, HCFA lived an administrative life of lean resources, transitory leadership, little political support, and an unstable agenda. At its worst, HCFA endured criticism that borders more on personal than administrative. Barbara Cooper and Bruce Vladeck, former administrators, labeled this phenomenon "HCFA bashing" in the Congress and hold it as an independent element accountable for some of the political reaction to the competitive-pricing demonstrations and other proposals before the Congress.[42]

Because Medicare's administration has not received systematic policy attention and purposeful reform, it too reflects the patchwork of pragmatic political compromise and episodic attention that characterizes the structure of the program more generally. MedPAC illustrates this result in Medicare's administrative structure for paying claims: "Although the entire rationale and method of payment has changed, the mechanism for paying claims—relying on local contractors—has not. The original rationale for using local contractors was that they could determine local UCR [usual, customary, and reasonable] charges and audit the costs of local providers. Neither of those determinations is now used under the national PPSs, yet the claims payment mechanism has been preserved. A basic contradiction now exists between the payment mechanism and the payment system."[43] Thus, the agency relationships seen in the administration of the Medicare program—for example, the delegation of claims administration to local contractors who act as agents of CMS, the national administrator—again have their basis in the political history of the program and the critical accommodations that have been made along the way. This example of continued (regional and private) delegation of claims administration is important in two respects: it illustrates again one of the important reasons why "everything varies by geography" in Medicare; and it provides a political foundation for revisiting the concept of regional administration of the program later in this book.

Medicare in the Present

Viewed in the context of its legislative history, Medicare succeeded in establishing its primary mission—institutionalizing access to physician and hospital care for the aged and disabled—but failed in its role as a loss leader for national health insurance. Instead of paving the way for larger health care reform, the economic and political experience of Medicare probably chilled the movement for significant reform of national health policy. Further expansion of the Medicare benefit plan stalled when the Medicare Catastrophic Coverage Act was repealed. When national health care reform was debated in 1993, virtually no consideration was given to what might have been the obvious solution: expanding Medicare coverage to fund other uncovered or undercovered groups in the population. Indeed, the Clinton Administration, with images of the Catastrophic Coverage Act repeal still fresh in its mind, left Medicare reform off the table, fearing that serious consideration of Medicare might incite the senior lobby to oppose large-scale national health reform.[44] The 1997 BBA amendments accomplished significant, though still incremental, change in the underlying social contract of the program. The Medicare+Choice program attempted to broaden the managed care options available and put new responsibilities upon beneficiaries to be prudent shoppers for plans. In the details, the BBA introduced pilot versions of new options for coverage and administration, such as medical savings accounts and private fee-for-service plans, that suggest new forms of agency and divisions of responsibility for beneficiaries, private providers, and the government.

In ideological terms, Medicare still stands at the crossroads of the American welfare state. Conservatives see Medicare as the consummate problem of entitlement in the federal budget, a kind of Pac-Man capable of gobbling up all fiscal resources, especially as the baby boom generation ages.[45] Liberals see Medicare as an unfinished vision of the Great Society, a program that provides only partial (and eroding) financial protection of the aged poor and that fails to enable access to long-term care and other services. The disappearance of the "apparatus" that guided the early evolution of Social Security and Medicare has created highly volatile politics: the proponents of generational equity are pitted against the advocates for traditional Medicare. Age-based voting patterns and interest groups do not provide unambiguous support for particular Medicare policy approaches. Indeed, as the Catastrophic Coverage Act and the literature on politics and aging demonstrate, there is considerable heterogeneity in the voting patterns and substantive political views of older persons.[46] There appears to be very little productive political middle ground for reform. A critical assessment of the history and politics of Medicare leads one to be skeptical of a wholesale change in philosophy, such as the adoption of a defined contribution or voucher model of financing and coverage.

A Kaiser/Harvard/Harris survey of public attitudes on Medicare provides evidence of a modest, underlying split in attitudes toward Medicare across generations. Looking ahead, 60 percent of the population responded that they believed that "the Medicare program should remain as it is today, with a fixed set of benefits and the government providing individuals with a single insurance card." However, 35 percent responded that Medicare should provide a voucher or fixed payment so that individuals could purchase their own private insurance. The public was exactly split on the question of whether "most" Medicare beneficiaries should be enrolled in managed care. Not surprisingly, strong generational differences characterized both the perceptions of Medicare's problems and the desirability of alternative solutions. Among eighteen- to forty-year-olds, 44 percent believed that Congress should completely redesign Medicare, and 40 percent responded that Congress should "replace Medicare with vouchers to buy private insurance."[47] Despite these generational differences in support for Medicare and attitudes toward particular design features, the aggregate story in public opinion data is that this program is enormously popular, both with older voters and the public at large.[48]

More than three decades after its creation, Medicare is a remarkably incomplete and, in many respects, administratively antiquated program. Medicare never completely solved the coverage issue, as the ill-fated Catastrophic Coverage Act and subsequent efforts to pass prescription drug coverage so visibly demonstrated. It never seriously addressed long-term care. It never completely solved the problems of access for vulnerable beneficiaries, as several studies by the Physician Payment Review Commission suggest.[49] It never extensively incorporated data, health services research, and technology assessment into its infrastructure and policies for purchasing health care. And it never adapted to the changing market structure of health care, where new provider organizations and purchasing arrangements, in an atmosphere of intense competition, have grown up alongside conventional fee-for-service arrangements.

Most proponents of continuing Medicare in roughly its current form over both the short and long runs accept that incremental changes are necessary. First, as reflected in many of the proposals debated in the late 1990s, Medicare is under enormous pressure to both reduce and increase its rates of payments to providers. Simply reducing payment rates across the board provides the public with the illusion of saving money without reducing either benefits or service levels. Ratcheting down reimbursement is also politically attractive because it provides the appearance of saving money without exposing the costs or trade-offs of those actions. For many states, reducing and slowing Medicaid payment rates has been a long-standing strategy of coping with real fiscal constraints: state legislatures are unwilling or unable to raise revenues and politically unable to make hard choices about what coverage or eligibility should be reduced. In reality, the erosion of Medicaid rates over time did produce real problems in access, with many physicians opting out of the system altogether. Similarly reducing Medicare payments across the board for hospitals, physicians, and other providers without changing the benefit mix or the ability of providers to compete will invite selective reductions in access, quality, or intensity. Alternatively it will invite cost shifting and price discrimination among other payers who do not exact the lowest competitive prices.

Therefore, the threat of significant reductions in Medicare payments, assuming no other changes in Medicare policy, raise the specter of the quality and access problems that have been observable in many state Medicaid programs.[50] Predictably, a backlash has occurred in recent budget debates as HMOs, academic health centers, home health agencies, and other organized provider groups have effectively lobbied the Congress on payment increases. Both the BBRA and BIPA made payment accommodations for the academic health centers, HMOs, and other provider groups that claimed they had been harmed by the 1997 budget cuts. When the payment adjustments failed to show marked changes in plan behavior (in fact, plan withdrawals continued apace), members of the Congress immediately put the industry back on notice. The reaction of Congressman Pete Stark of California is illustrative: "We were flimflammed by the HMOs. . . . We were induced to support the legislation after being told that the extra money would be used for extra benefits or lower copayments."[51]

The interests of the provider sector, especially in the realm of Medicare payment policy, are a defining feature of its modern politics. In addition to its primary mission of financing care for older persons and disabled persons, Medicare has also become the policy instrument for financing graduate medical education, supporting institutions that disproportionately service the medically indigent, and funding sole providers of care in rural areas. The complexity of the transfers that arise from all of these multiple financing arrangements is daunting. The infusion of so many transfers and subsidies into Medicare's reimbursement system also complicates the politics of Medicare reform. The political economy that surrounds Medicare includes academic medical centers, specialty societies, pharmaceutical companies, and hospitals—in addition to the large organized senior interest groups such as AARP that garner so much attention. These influences on congressional oversight of the Medicare program—its ability to serve as an effective agent for the public—will be considered again in chapter 7.

Despite the search for comprehensive structural fixes to Medicare's problems, reform will in all likelihood not be an apocalyptic event. Understood in a historical context, Medicare was born not in the social moment of the Great Society but rather as unfinished business of the New Deal. Finally in 1965 it was accepted as a bounded entitlement for the elderly with the tacit consent of the professions and industry of medicine. Since 1965, when the plan came into existence, the Congress has carefully nurtured both of these political constituencies and has made halting movements (such as the payment changes in the 1997 BBA) from its structural accommodation with the profession and the industry. In the end, however, this political record gives us no coherent, and certainly no complete, concept of the modern Medicare social contract. Instead, we are left to deduce the implicit social contract in the context of debates about particular Medicare reforms: premium support, prescription drugs, end-of-life care, and patients' rights, among others.

The Implications of Medicare Politics for Policy

For policy analysts, the fundamental insight that can be garnered from a careful review and understanding of Medicare's origins and subsequent politics is an appreciation of its "path dependence."[52] In general, analysts who emphasize the path dependence of policy believe that historical evolution of institutions and relationships among governmental agencies have important and enduring effects on the possibilities for expansion and reform of social programs. Institutions shape the nature of interest group involvement and pressure. Bureau-cratic agencies exert their own authority over policy development. Each succes-sive round of reform is grounded in the institutions, programs, and interest group involvements that were established in previous rounds of policy develop-ment. By this view, politics and policy have a Markov-chain character.

The evolution of Medicare's politics presented in this chapter has pre-cisely this path-dependent character. The architecture of the program (e.g., Part A and Part B), its bureaucracy (e.g., CMS), the institutions that surround it (e.g., the Medicare commissions), and the interest groups that apply pres-sure (e.g., academic medical centers) all define the possibilities and likely tra-jectory for reform in a political sense. The trajectory has elements of tradition, such as Medicare's attachment to social insurance principles and symbolic at-tachment to Social Security, as well as bands of feasible change, defined by the exigencies of the political moment.

This is especially apparent in the administrative reform of the program. Lawrence Brown's analysis of the early administrative history of Medicare em-phasizes the necessary connections between aspirations for administrative re-form, and the exigencies of political history and moment:

> the organizational character of a public agency is never sui generis and self-contained. Rather it blends both continuity and change, the precise mix reflecting the role of the agency and its programs in the larger political environment—the mission and constraints assigned them by executives, legislators, and courts; their place in the federal system; their strength vis-à-vis private-sector groups. Administrative, organizational, and policy variables, then, shuttle back and forth along an analytical continuum; how one plans the itinerary and the stops along the way depends on the objectives.
>
> Issues of administrative reform in Medicare present just such a moving target. One cannot offer practical suggestions on questions of intra- and inter-agency design without sensitivity to the program's administrative character and evolution in the two decades since it began. Such sensitivity in turn demands that Medicare and its administrative history be examined in their policy setting, one in which political leaders have been determined both to preserve continuity and to promote change, and have often been uncertain how to proceed.[53]

For the purposes of this analysis, consider this history as providing the following signposts on the path for Medicare's policy development:

- From the outset, Medicare divided the world into discrete forms of coverage, Parts A and B. These distinctions have had lasting consequences for the politics and types of reforms that are feasible, in part because an industry and an institutionally bound form of politics grew up around these categorical forms of coverage. It follows that the feasible policy space for Medicare will be significantly shaped by the economic interests of Medicare's many vendors, intermediaries, and suppliers of service. One cannot contemplate the feasible set of Medicare reforms without reference to the professional and economic interests of physicians and other medical professionals, such as hospitals, the insurance and managed care industry, the long-term care industry, the pharmaceutical and medical devices industry, and governors and states. One also cannot contemplate Medicare reform without understanding the important geographical context of resource allocation. Medicare reform is all about states and counties. This is the lesson of Medicare's original enactment, the annual budget debates, and most recently the debate over the Medicare prescription drug benefit.

- Beneficiaries (and their children) have become used to certain forms and extents of Medicare coverage, the Medicare entitlement. Taking away benefits will be extremely difficult politically. Adding new benefits, particularly benefits that will increase the projected costs of the program as it takes on the baby boom cohort, will also be difficult. Here the protectors of the fisc, as entrenched in Medicare politics and design as Wilbur Mills's first "layer cake," come home to roost. This is the lesson of the original structure of Medicare, the history of Medicare expansions, the Catastrophic Coverage Act repeal, the more recent National Bipartisan Commission deliberations, and the prescription drug debate.

- Medicare's administrative machinery—CMS, the structure of intermediaries and carriers, the involvement of agencies as diverse as the Department of Justice—results from the profound ambivalence of the Congress in delegating strong authority to an administrative agent, as well as the pragmatic political accommodations that characterize the program more generally. This is the lesson of creating and retaining intermediaries for claims administration, the relatively low historical funding for Medicare administration, HCFA's own political history, and the division of responsibility and authority for Medicare administration across Federal agencies. The many disconnects between administrative form and function provide the opportunity for applying the tools of a principal-agent framework; and to ask whether the structure of delegation and administration is set up to carry out the contemporary interests of the public-as-principal and beneficiaries-as-principals in Medicare services.

- Along this path, some new elements of reform have received some initial vetting and recent political consideration. Market and competitive tools, such as alternative organizations for managed care delivery, competitive bidding, and performance rebates, have been considered and attempted, to varying degrees of fruition. Restructuring and modernizing administrative arrangements, leading to a post-CMS structure for Medicare administration, is clearly in the wind.

The notion that Medicare policy has a form of path dependence provides an important framework for thinking about a set of plausible and feasible reforms. While this suggests that Medicare reform will always have an incremental character, it is not an argument in itself for incrementalism. The more telling implication is that certain philosophies, symbols, and structures will undoubtedly be carried forward as the Medicare program evolves, while new ones are grafted on. Of the recent innovations in Medicare policy design, "choice," administrative "modernization," and some (partial) instruments of competitive behavior for plans and providers are likely to be carried forward in politically salient versions of reform proposals.

The first-order project in Medicare reform will be sorting out its contemporary mission, its coverage, and the elemental statements of its social contract. This is the work of Medicare's political debate. Its architecture, formed out of 1950s and 1960s conceptions of indemnity insurance and medical practice, is clearly outdated. Its interface with beneficiaries is too primitive and complicated for the goals of informed choice and appropriate care to be achieved. Its role as a purchaser in a market representing the interests of taxpayers is shifting. Although managed care emerged in the 1990s as the vehicle through which Medicare would change this role, this agenda is in jeopardy in light of the controversy over managed care in general and the withdrawal of Medicare plans specifically.

In chapter 3, I suspend consideration of the politics of Medicare for the moment and develop a formal conceptual approach to policy design in Medicare. To anticipate this theory, the social contract can be thought of as an instrument of both private demand for health coverage and a social demand for certain aspects and outcomes of medical care. The social demand is not as simple as an interest in subsidizing the premium for beneficiary coverage, nor is it a simple and slavish commitment to certain forms of acute hospital coverage that were appropriate circa 1965. The social demand for Medicare coverage involves preferences for certain categories and outcomes of care, of course mediated through congressional pressure and administrative decision making.

Creating administrative and financing arrangements that serve these multiple masters is the challenge of policy design for Medicare. This is why we see the simultaneous pull for flexibility and innovation in the "choice" and prescription drug agenda, while at the same time we see stubborn commitment to certain principles and elements of coverage (especially for low-income beneficiaries) in virtually all reform proposals. However one views the merits of the specific proposals, such as those produced by the National Bipartisan Commission on the Future of Medicare, its political process and recommendations reflect still another attempt to reconcile significantly different interpretations of the Medicare social contract. However, the proposals themselves always need to be seen as reactions and responses to the legacy of Medicare's rich political history.

Medicare is still not an efficient purchaser. . . . Medicare largely remains a passive bill payer, exercising little meaningful control over the volume of services used.
—David Walker, Comptroller of the United States, September 22, 1999

CHAPTER THREE

Agency and Medicare Policy Design

The Role of Agency Theory in Policy Analysis

Policy analysis and policy debate of Medicare reform has gone on largely in the absence of a framework for understanding the issues of administrative design and reform. Despite some sophisticated analyses since the inception of the program in 1965, the debate over its future lacks a conceptual road map. The policy debate has a profoundly ad hoc character.

Chapter 2 demonstrated that Medicare's existing arrangements came out of its political history, to a large extent from the market circumstances and political accommodations of the 1960s. This history has produced a set of benefit entitlements, payment systems, and administrative arrangements that have political and technical lineage. Setting aside its political history for the moment, this chapter looks at the reform of these arrangements through the lens of a particular social science literature, the so-called principal-agent or agency theory literature. It asks how incentive, organizational, and informational arrangements can be designed to improve the performance and outcomes of the program given this political context.

Good policy design is often about achieving the "second best," with one eye trained on what is theoretically optimal. The good fortune of a growing economy, favorable demographics, and a supportive political environment have forestalled many of the difficult policy design questions for Medicare until now. However, the compound effect of shifting demographics, increasing medical costs, and competing claims for scarce public resources will inevitably call the question of what the public is "purchasing" in its demand for Medicare services. This is an important policy question to be resolved irrespective of the particular political winds of the moment. For the public, it is important to get "value" in what might be thought of as a $241 billion procurement program: (1) on efficiency grounds, (2) to provide maximum health benefits, and (3) to encourage long-term political support of the program.

As chapter 2 demonstrated, one leg of Medicare's policy design follows from its original roots in traditional indemnity insurance. From the perspective of the beneficiary, Medicare has many of the elements of a private insurance policy—much of the same language of premiums, deductibles, and copayments; interactions with private intermediaries and providers; and, since the Balanced Budget Act (BBA) of 1997, emphasis on consumer choice in plans. The Medicare program provides the auspices of their care, determining access, quality, cost sharing, and the broad accountability of their providers. All of this is to say that in original concept and current implementation, Medicare is at least in part a vehicle for the aged and disabled to exercise their private, individual choices over forms of health insurance coverage and the selection and behavior of providers.

Mark Pauly has demonstrated, however, that Medicare also embodies a public—what he calls a "community"—demand for health services provided to the elderly, the disabled, and individuals with end-stage renal disease, which requires its own standing in assuring access, quality, and cost-effectiveness of health services.[1] While the public demand for health services for disabled persons and the aged has many sources and boundaries, it is important that the Congress act as the agent of the public in determining the scope and generosity of Medicare benefits, as well as the particular incentives, regulations, and requirements passed on to plans and providers. Chapter 2 identified some of the political explanations for the form of many of Medicare's administrative arrangements.

Thus, the Medicare program is a unique construction of social policy that mingles private and public, individual and collective, demands for health services. In order to reconcile these potentially divergent interests in Medicare-sponsored services, there must exist a system of joint incentives, information, and accountability between the public payers and private users of the service, on the one hand, and the providers of services on the other. The way in which the joint demand for Medicare services is reconciled is through the incentive, organizational, and informational arrangements that are built into the program. Medicare managed care, for example, combines financing/organizational/informational arrangements intended (in policy terms) to reconcile the public interest in cost containment with private interests in prescription drugs and other objectives in plan choice.

The heuristic that brings agency theory together with the policy problem of Medicare reform is the exercise of writing a "good contract." One can think of such a contract as involving a change in orientation from a program that mostly finances health care to a program that purchases health care in such a way that the interests of individual beneficiaries and the public are more effectively met. This is an exquisitely difficult problem of agency, involving the design of incentives, the structuring of information, and the organization of program administration. Later in the book, I examine how Medicare might write a contract for a "good death" for beneficiaries, how it can write a better contract for managed care for beneficiaries, and how it can incorporate new technology into benefits in ways that strike a balance between public and private interests.

It is not necessary to invoke the narrow legal or philosophical interpretation of contracts for an agency theory perspective to have considerable conceptual and analytic power. In health care, a considerable body of literature has evolved that examines the nature of contractual arrangements, whether explicit or implicit, between doctors and patients; between third-party payers and providers; and more recently between intermediaries, such as managed care plans and HMOs, and doctors. It is also not necessary to invoke a contractarian philosophical argument, based upon Rawlsian notions of distributive justice, to develop the thread of policy argument that agency theory suggests. The use of the contractual metaphor can be fruitfully exploited even in the absence of explicit legal documentation, as Charles Fried's analysis of the moral basis of contract law elegantly demonstrates.[2] In what follows, agency theory provides a framework, a lens, and a toolkit for Medicare policy analysis.

Agency

The key element in making the joint private and public demands for health services operational under Medicare is the design of *agency,* the intermediate structure of incentives, organization, and information that assures the desired goals are carried out in practice.[3] Agents carry out the demands of *principals,* who typically order and pay for the service. The definition of a principal is "one who employs another to act for him or her subject to his or her general control and instruction: the person from whom an agent's responsibility derives." In a simple agency relationship between a single principal and an agent, an individual or organization is delegated to act on behalf of the principal. An agent is supposed to do what the principal wants to have done. A perfect agent performs exactly as if the principal were acting, except that the principal does not have sufficient information, time, or other capabilities to perform the service in question.

To the extent that the agent's performance departs from what the principal would have done in a similar position, there is an agency loss, or agency cost, associated with substituting the agent for either a direct transaction or carrying out the activity oneself. Interesting problems emerge when the objectives of the agent diverge from those of the principal; when there are conflicts of interest; when the agent is more or less risk averse than the principal; when it is difficult to monitor the behavior of the agent; when the principal and agent face markedly different access to relevant information (information asymmetries); or when the agent faces disincentives to do the right thing or incentives to shirk or even to be overzealous.

We are most familiar with agents as intermediaries in the world of real estate, insurance, and finance. These agents are necessary when information is "costly," when it is impossible for individuals to know everything necessary to make an informed choice without extensive investments in education, information, and monitoring. We use financial agents because it is extremely costly for individuals to gather all the information necessary about investment opportunities to make an informed choice about all the elements of an optimal portfolio.

Numerous complications can get in the way of our financial agent performing the role perfectly. When agents are not independent, a potential conflict of interest arises: the agent may stand to gain by selling you a product in which he or she has a financial interest.[4] Indeed, the existence of the Securities and Exchange Commission is motivated exactly by this potential for agency failure. The involvement of accounting firms in Enron and other financial consulting arrangements, where they stand to gain financially by questionable auditing practices, illustrates this lack of independence, and thus an agency failure. Alternatively, because the principal cannot monitor the behavior of the agent completely, it is possible that the agent may shirk his or her responsibility for investigating the full range of investment possibilities. How is an investor to know if an agent has researched and analyzed all of the possible investment vehicles?

In firms, the general problem of agency involves getting managers (the agents) to act in the interests of shareholders (the principals) when much of the manager's behavior cannot be observed, at least without high cost. The least-cost contract (which avoids the requirement for all behavior to be observed) aligns the incentives of the agent with the principal, often in the form of incentive compensation arrangements, stock options, or other instruments of profit sharing. Thus, even in this simple case of contracting with an investment counselor, the problems of structuring an effective agency relationship are potentially significant.

Economists have developed a rich and rigorous theoretical literature about agency that explores in a formal way problems of designing efficient contracts in the face of moral hazard.[5] The theoretical literature focuses on the design of efficient contracts under different assumptions about risk, under different conditions of observability, and under alternative game-theoretic conditions, such as whether or not contracts are multiperiod, can be renegotiated, or involve multiple principals or agents. In this literature, assumptions are carefully stated and axioms are derived deductively, usually formally and mathematically. Applied studies in the economics literature have examined the phenomena of sharecropping, employer-employee relationships, and regulation of oil spills, defense procurement, and steam-electric power plant design.[6]

One of the general implications of this literature for health care is that contracts (and their related payment and information systems) will necessarily be enormously complex and incomplete: just taking account of the variability created by elements of risk-aversion, informational deficits and asymmetries, transactions costs, and whether or not the contract is repeated implies tremendous complexity in the design of contracts and the arrangements for agents. In the real world, however, this variability and complexity of contracts is not evident, especially not in health services. The resolution of this gap between the theoretical and the applied world of contract design must certainly lie in the variety of informal or implicit influences on the contracts that are feasible in real practice: the existence of professional ethics, professional norms, and the role of interest groups; the set of political and organizational propensities for rules; and the available technology for monitoring. For example, in the context of Medicare, the bounded rationality of its administrative organizations and the inherent legislative and procedural constraints on the Medicare administration (described in chapter 2) limit the complexity and responsiveness of the contractual arrangements that can be employed.

Ultimately, this means that effective control over Medicare services will be an amalgam of traditional contracting and incentives, as well as organizational and other nonfinancial influences over practice. In fact, some theorists

have recognized that the analysis and design of these complementary arrangements (to reimbursement policy) may represent the frontier in the application
of an agency perspective. As Kenneth Arrow has noted,

> further extensions are needed to capture some aspects of reality, for there is a
> whole world of rewards and penalties that take social rather than monetary forms.
> Professional responsibility is clearly enforced in good measure by a system of
> ethics, internalized during the education process and enforced in some measure
> by formal punishments and more broadly by reputations. Ultimately, these social
> systems have economic consequences but they are not the immediate ones of cur-
> rent principal agent models. All of these limiting elements—cost of communica-
> tion, variety and vagueness of monitoring, and socially mediated rewards—go
> beyond the usual boundaries of economic analysis. It may ultimately be one of
> the greatest accomplishments of the principal agent literature to provide some
> structure for the much-sought goal of integrating these elements with the impres-
> sive structure of economic analysis.[7]

Indeed, much of the recent development of the agency literature has fo-
cused on the interaction of organizational and incentive arrangements. Insights from this work have extended the literature for relatively simple models
of compensation and reward for objective performance to more complex for-
mulations that take into account the realities of multiple-task environments
(of which medicine is an ideal example), repeated games, subjective assessments, and contracts across firm boundaries or between organizations.[8]
Organizational theorists have been more concerned with the design of
governance and administration that solves the agency problem by inducing
behavior among agents that carries out the wishes of the principal. Seen in
this context, agency is something to be exploited, not maligned.[9] Harrison
White has observed that "although economists may speak of the 'agency problem,' agency is in fact a solution, a neat kind of social plumbing. The problem
is the ancient and ineluctable one of how to attain and maintain control in order to carry out definite, yet varying, purposes."[10] White sees agency relationships in much richer, textured terms, in complicated webs of relationships
that have differing strategic and operational implications. For example, as relationships evolve and agents become more sophisticated, roles can become
reversed and principals can come under the control of the agents, a situation
familiar to students of the defense industry. So too, the agency relationships
and implications analyzed in this book are broader than a strict reading of economic theory allows, yet this exercise applies the insights and perspective
from agency theory to a real policy design problem. I will point out versions of

White's insight—agents become principals in this complex hierarchy of organization and administration—as I work through the layers of agency relations in Medicare.

Political scientists have extended this theory to understanding the conditions under which public bureaucracy responds to legislative intent. Here the translation is from contractual and agency relations that explain *firms in markets,* to contractual and agency relations that explain the functions and performance of *administrative units charged with carrying out public purposes.*[11] This literature suggests that the same general analytic apparatus can be utilized—bureaucracy as an organizational approach to contractual problems, incomplete and asymmetric information, and incentives—for financing, provision, and purchase of goods and services. The challenge in making these extensions is to establish goals and performance measures that are appropriate alternatives to the financial metrics (e.g., profit and loss) of firms operating in markets. Health care applications of an agency approach provide rich opportunities for making these extensions through quality measurement, utilization measurement, organizational report cards, and outcomes research.

Each of these perspectives on agency in the social sciences provides some purchase for policy analysis of Medicare. The economics tradition motivates questions about the incentive arrangements in payment systems and contracting, the control of moral hazard in insurance arrangements, and the role of transactions costs in evaluating alternative institutional arrangements. The organizational tradition motivates questions about scale, scope, networks, and control under different structural and environmental circumstances. The political science tradition motivates questions about the degree of control, autonomy, and discretion to be achieved under different arrangements of legislative, executive, and bureaucratic authority.

Agency in Medicine

In medicine, a principal-agent relationship occurs between doctors and patients. In fact, the doctor-patient relationship is treated in both the ethics literature and the economics literature as a paradigmatic example of agency.[12] In an agency interpretation of the doctor-patient relationship, patients are assumed to choose physicians who will carry out their wishes, and physicians are assumed to honor the preferences of patients in order to retain their business. A doctor performs as a perfect agent if he or she decides on a course of treatment *exactly* as the patient would decide, if only the patient had incurred the costs of going through medical school and residency and thus had the same knowledge base as the physician. In a model of pure agency, the doctor represents the patient's interests directly and in an unbiased way. Both parties are utility maximizing and will only enter into a contract if there is mutual benefit. Long-term relationships between doctors and patients serve an important search and information function: the patient monitors the quality and responsiveness of the doctor and retains his or her services so long as they appear to be delivering above average quality.[13] In an era of primary care gatekeepers, the role of primary care doctors as not only clinicians, but as referral agents, provides further rationale for a long-term relationship because the patient can then gather more data on the quality of the services rendered, and the physician can exploit more specific information about the preferences and characteristics of the patient.[14]

Mark Schlesinger has provided the most complete analysis of emerging agency conflicts in medicine (in the context of managed competition proposals) and their potential implications for the doctor-patient relationship:

> Not only does managed competition not reduce the importance of patient-provider trust; it actually increases its salience while threatening to undermine its existence. By introducing health plans, managed competition adds to the roles that physicians must play as agents, in this case helping patients to deal with their plans. . . . They must trust their providers not only to have strong clinical skills, but also to be effective negotiators on their behalf. . . . In addition, patients rely on physicians as an unbiased source of information about the strengths and weaknesses of health plans in which they are enrolled. . . .
>
> Because conventional managed competition plans provide no regulatory oversight on the relations between patients and providers, or providers and plans, they offer no protection in this area. Worse yet, the very processes intended to foster consumer accountability at the plan level are likely to undermine trust between patients and health professionals.[15]

Schlesinger promotes the need for creating "countervailing agency" to enhance the "fidelity" of the patient-provider relationship, while at the same time creating mechanisms for representing the societal interest in health care decisions.

J. Gregory Dees has argued that merely framing problems in principal-agent terms runs the risk of suppressing key ethical issues in contracting. In particular, he worries that the form of the theory and its constructs leads to (1) ignoring the obligations of the principal to the agent (in this problem, the responsibility of the patient or the state to the physician); (2) encouraging excessive distrust and disrespect of the agents; (3) overlooking ethical constraints on problems, such as fairness considerations; and (4) missing solutions that include ethical norms.[16] Similarly, David Mechanic, in an extensive review of the role of and threat to trust in medicine, sees many of the new financial and organizational developments in health services as reinforcing more general trends in society that erode trust, public confidence, and faith in both individual physicians and medical institutions.[17]

One of the professed defining characteristics of the profession of medicine is its ethical foundation and, in particular, its commitment to a doctor-patient relationship that assumes trust, beneficence on the part of the physician, and patient autonomy. An enormous literature in medicine proclaims the benefits of this presumed relationship, and much of the angst about the evolution of modern systems of health care stems from a belief that a functional bond between doctors and patients is being broken. Much of the literature in medicine and ethics presumes a disposition among physicians to sacrifice on behalf of the patient, to place the interests of the patient above all others, and to be unencumbered by conflicts of interest—economic or otherwise—that might get in the way of a pure commitment to the best interests of the patient. A long-standing and continuous relationship between the doctor and the patient is perceived to inculcate information about the patient's preferences and condition in the doctor's decision making, provide the patient with repeated observations about the doctor's performance and inclinations, and create an expectation of mutual loyalty and reward. In the terms of agency theory, this relationship has elements of a repeated game, in which both the doctor and patient learn to behave with an eye toward their future encounters, not only the present. Trust creates a form of commitment in the relationship and treatment decisions that would require complex contracting arrangements to replicate.

Several aspects of the emerging organization and finance of health services are seen as threatening to this prototypical doctor-patient relationship. First, the widespread use of risk-based payment systems places direct incentives on physicians to limit care. With capitation, where physicians receive a fixed payment per member per month, the fewer services that are ordered, the more surplus the physician or the physician's group retains. For doctors and ethicists, two problems accompany this transference of risk to physicians: doctors may indeed compromise their care decisions, or patients may no longer trust their decisions and thus engage in behaviors that compromise their care. For example, some ethicists believe that the increased involvement of physicians in equity arrangements in the provision of care means that their financial interest in referrals can compromise their fidelity to patients.[18]

The interesting question, for which there is no empirical evidence, is the degree to which trust, believed by many physicians to be a defining characteristic of the doctor-patient relationship, serves as an efficient solution to the agency problems of asymmetry of information, alignment of interests, and monitoring of behavior. A change in the traditional concept of a doctor-patient relationship may require markedly different organizations of practice, with much more attention to the structure of incentives, the reporting of practice and outcomes, and the availability of due process when results are questioned. While there is no empirical evidence of the value that trust plays in the cost, quality, and outcomes of medical practice, it may still be important to consider the potential role of norms, values, and professional ethics in the structuring of agency. For example, if the doctor-patient relationship has value in the trust, communication, and information that is conveyed, then it is worth considering whether contracts and reimbursement should reward continuity, longevity, and intensity of communications and relationships between doctors and patients. This topic will be revisited in chapter 5, in the context of end-of-life care.

Agency in Medicare

Medicare operates under levels of agency relationships that begin with the Congress and extend all the way down to the individual beneficiary and his or her doctor-patient relationship. Figure 2 presents the short list of agency relationships at work in current Medicare policy and identifies the places where at least two principals exist.

The degree to which Congress functions as a proper or effective agent of the public can be interpreted through the lens of the program's history as well as in structural political terms. Certainly a major line of criticism of Medicare policy is directed at congressional policy making, as in the apparent inability of Congress to tackle issues such as long-term care policy or prescription drug coverage, despite expressed public interest in these issues. Addressing the general question of whether the Congress serves as an effective agent of the public interest is a large topic, beyond the scope of this book.

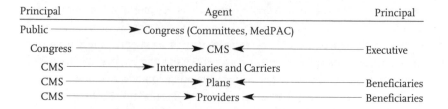

Principal	Agent	Principal
Public	———▶ Congress (Committees, MedPAC)	
Congress	——————▶ CMS ◀——————	Executive
CMS	———————▶ Intermediaries and Carriers	
CMS	———————▶ Plans ◀——————	Beneficiaries
CMS	———————▶ Providers ◀——————	Beneficiaries

Figure 2. Multiple agency in Medicare

Congress establishes the broad contours of the program, delegating on-going authority to carry out its mandate to the Centers for Medicare and Medicaid Services (CMS), an arm of the executive branch. Because CMS operates as an agency in the Department of Health and Human Services, it is also accountable to the president and secretary. Even at this level, a conflicted structure of agency exists, in which the "intent" of Congress may not always be carried out by CMS. The agency relationship of greatest interest emanates from CMS itself and extends to the providers. CMS acts as a principal in many health care transactions, with hospitals, physicians, community health centers, nursing homes, home health agencies, hospices, durable medical equipment suppliers, ambulance service providers, Medicare+Choice providers, and other health care providers serving as agents providing services to patients—all under the authority and payment of the federal government.

Within the health care system, layers upon layers of complex agency relationships also exist within intermediary and provider systems. Here, multiple principals attempt to exercise their will over individual medical encounters. The state, operating through Medicaid and Medicare, has an interest in access, cost, and quality of care but has incomplete mechanisms (payment, incentives, regulation, administrative oversight) to express that interest. Other payers, operating principally through retiree health plans and Medigap policies, also have an interest in the conduct of care, but their involvement in care decisions is relatively limited.

At the level of beneficiaries, other interested parties, including family members, loved ones, and at times legal guardians, enter into health care decision making and often behave like principals. Finally, there are the patients themselves, prototypical principals in an agency framework but often without the information, resources, or capacity to execute an effective contract with their doctors or other health care providers.

In practice, agency problems appear in decision making about health services in both personal and organizational contexts. Individual beneficiaries make use of many resources—spouses, other family members, organizations—in making decisions about plans, providers, and whether or not to have particular health services provided. For example, a beneficiary going through the process of selecting a Medicare managed care plan may rely on the advice or even decision making of others or may even pay for counseling. Once a form of coverage is selected, then new agency relationships, flowing through the organizations that make payments and assure quality and accountability of services (such as Medicare+Choice plans), condition the actual use of service under different Medicare alternatives.

Figure 3 illustrates the most simplified version of the structure of

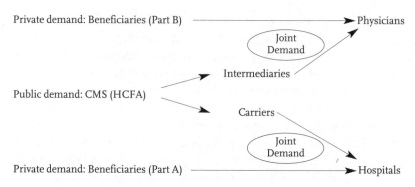

Figure 3. The structure of agency in traditional Medicare

agency that has characterized Medicare provision under traditional Medicare fee-for-service coverage. In traditional Medicare, the agency relationships flow from the structure of Part A and Part B financing and administration. Part A is financed from payroll taxes on current workers that are accumulated in a trust fund and paid out through intermediaries under contract with CMS. Part B is financed through a combination of premiums and general revenue taxes that are paid out to providers through carriers also under contract with CMS.

This basic structure of public finance for Medicare reveals how health services for older and disabled persons are actually *demanded* by two parties, each with specific interests in the quantity, costs, type, and quality of care. The private and public demands for this care are translated through alternative forms of agency—the intermediate structures of payment, information, administration, and oversight—that discipline health care transactions.

The degree to which these two are joint demands is evident in other details of payment policy, administration of the program, and regulation. Co-payments and deductibles are examples of payment mechanisms that are intended to—and, if designed properly, will—align the incentives of the public sponsor and the individual beneficiary around each individual episode of care. In Part A, both beneficiaries and CMS make payments for individual services: beneficiaries through deductibles and CMS through provider payments. For example, a beneficiary pays a deductible of $792 per benefit period, and the program pays the hospital an additional amount (based on diagnosis-related groups or DRGs). In Part B, beneficiaries are responsible for a copayment of typically 20 percent for each service rendered. In other words, each service has two payers involved in the transaction and, thus, each is entitled to act as a principal, in the most formal economic sense, if not in political terms. Despite the importance of aligning Medicare's cost-sharing arrangements in hospital and physician payment, in practice these arrangements are not well calibrated to the financial circumstances or supplemental coverage of beneficiaries, and do not necessarily function to encourage cost-effective care.[19]

Another example of the joint responsibility over care can be found in mechanisms for enforcement of quality and the prevention of fraud or abuse. A significant amount of payment enforcement is triggered by beneficiary reports to the Medicare contractors, the Inspector General, the FBI, and other administrative contacts. These reports are often the result of beneficiaries' reading their Explanation of Medicare Benefits, which describes the services that were billed to Medicare and discovering that either mistakes were made or fraud may have been perpetrated.[20] With the expansion of Medicare fraud and abuse enforcement, the involvement of third parties such as the Inspector General and the Justice Department in investigating and enforcing the propriety of Medicare reimbursed services, especially billing practices, has escalated. From the perspective of agency theory, these activities represent a monitoring and sanctioning function: if the service is carried out in accordance with the principal's expectations for payment, coding, medical necessity, and so on, then a secondary process of oversight and enforcement would not be required. The scale and cost of these enforcement efforts are an indication of the perceived agency loss in Medicare.

From an agency perspective, the overarching reform problem for Medicare is the design of "reasonably efficient" and enforceable contracts for health care among the many parties to a Medicare patient encounter. These contracts are difficult because information is asymmetric (doctors and other providers will know more about the particular circumstances of any given case than either patients or the public organization paying for care) and much of the relevant behavior will be always be unobservable.

How do we know that there are agency problems in Medicare and elsewhere in the health care system? Following Pauly, an optimal solution to the Medicare problem would establish a least-cost solution that would provide as much appropriate health care as individuals would demand (if they were properly informed), coupled with the amount that society is demanding for them under the aegis of the Medicare program.[21] Both patient and the state (Congress, CMS) would express demands to agents, and these agents would provide health services that precisely respond to the wishes of the principals. This problem becomes complicated when the expressions of the principals and the behavior of the agents diverge, but the extent of this problem is unknown.

Because there is no way to specify *ex ante* the solution to Medicare delivery that would be generated by an optimally functioning system, it is impossible to specify the exact magnitude and nature of the agency loss. It is important to note that this loss includes both the transactions and administrative costs associated with a poorly functioning agency structure, as well as the welfare losses accruing to patients and taxpayers from a system that provides either more or less care than what would be demanded in a "first-best," or theoretically perfect, world. While it is impossible to specify an optimally functioning system, a heuristic illustrates the potential losses associated with the current configuration.

Imagine a system in which physicians, hospitals, or health plans played the role of perfect dual agents of public and private demand for health services. These providers could be rewarded either through contracts that paid for the relevant outcome or on the basis of observing their behavior precisely and costlessly. The multibillion dollar administrative machinery that attends Medicare and the rest of the health care system could be dismantled in favor of a simple check-writing program. The current preoccupation with finding and punishing fraud and abuse in Medicare would go away. Because information is readily available to both private and public demanders of care, patients would be assured that they were receiving the "right" amount of care, no more and no less than was indicated by both the clinical evidence with respect to outcomes from treatment and a set of mutually agreed upon community standards. The tort system might or might not be a functional part of the solution because the deterrence and compliance functions of tort actions could also be embodied in the compensation system. In this mythical world, patients and payers would also not be held hostage to gaming in a system that attempts to take advantage of where reimbursement is available, not where care can be provided most efficiently and effectively.

Evidence that the Medicare-sponsored system departs from this ideal will be presented in subsequent chapters, but a roadmap to these findings can be previewed here. First, there is considerable evidence that a significant portion of services provided to Medicare beneficiaries are not medically indicated (nor did they meet more stringent cost-benefit tests). For example, the well-known RAND results on appropriateness of care indicate that between 3 and 60 percent of procedures in an elderly population were not clinically indicated, meaning that they were not justified by reference to the best available medical literature.[22] There is evidence of both overprovision and underprovision in Medicare. Second, the tremendous variations in rates of service and quality of care from market to market in Medicare suggest that discretion is playing a large role in treatment decisions, without evidence that outcomes are appreciably affected.[23] The existence of this variation does not inform the question of exactly what rate of use is appropriate, but it does provide indirect evidence that in some places Medicare and beneficiaries are paying for more or less service than is necessary. Third, in various arenas of Medicare purchasing, other payers are receiving more favorable prices, despite Medicare's undeniable market power. Finally, evidence from oversight of Medicare's administration suggests that CMS's management of purchasing is inadequate.[24]

Kathleen Eisenhardt asserts that "agency theory is most relevant in situations where contracting problems are difficult . . . situations in which there is (a) substantial goal conflict between principals and agents, such as where agent opportunism is likely . . . (b) sufficient outcome uncertainty to trigger the risk implications of the theory . . . , and (c) unprogrammed or team-oriented jobs in which evaluation of behaviors is difficult. By keying on these contexts, researchers can use agency theory where it provides the most leverage and where the theory can be most rigorously tested."[25] Further, Eisenhardt suggests that agency theory can be most productively employed in cases where contracts have elements of both behavior and outcome incentives and where rewards are multiple and mixed. Health care delivery in general, and Medicare specifically, dramatically meets these tests.

Contracts in Agency Theory

The normative standard for an agency relationship is the result that would occur under an optimal contract. Two kinds of optimal contracts are possible, depending upon the conditions of information or risk taking among principals and agents. In broad terms, the principal can choose to structure the agent's compensation on the basis of outcomes or on the basis of monitoring the process. An outcome-based contract would reward the provider when a cure or other observable medical result occurs after treatment. By extension, under this "pay-if-cured" contract, the physician would not be paid if the patient does not get better, however getting better has been defined *ex ante*.

Alternatively, when a principal can monitor the behavior of an agent completely and without cost, an optimal contract will be one that observes the agent's actions directly and rewards them accordingly.[26] We assume that the agent enters into the contract freely, that the principal has a choice of agents, and that moral hazard is not present. Almost always, however, monitoring behavior is costly, and as a practical matter many of the actions of the agent will go unobserved. The entire enterprise of utilization management in health care can be thought of as a vehicle to monitor and condition the behavior of providers in the face of moral hazard. Under utilization review and management, physicians require authorization, a form of permission, to proceed. Even when prior authorization is not required, a vast enterprise within the health system, among payers and in the regulatory arena, monitors the decisions of providers to assure that only "appropriate" care is provided. Despite the size and growing sophistication of this enterprise, the inability to monitor behavior perfectly presents the agent with the opportunity to be negligent, incompetent, or overzealous. The principal will not always be able to determine the appropriateness or quality of the effort. The respective problems with outcome- and process-based contracts are summarized below.

Outcome-Based Solutions

The most significant problem with implementing our outcome-based contract in health care is that it asks the agent to bear the full risk of the contract in a world of considerable uncertainty, a world where the outcome most often cannot be directly attributed to the behavior of the agent. If the agent is risk averse—worried about such things as the uncertainty of personal income and its vulnerability to random or uncontrollable medical circumstances of patients—then he or she will likely balk at participating in this outcome-based contract.

When outcomes are observable (and agents are not risk averse), optimal contracts can be obtained by conditioning the reward on a relevant outcome, such as a cure, rate of return, or other observable result. Writing outcome-based contracts has the effect of correlating the interests of the agent directly to those of the principal. Providers might still be reluctant to participate in an outcome-based scheme if they are risk averse and cannot insure against the possibility that patients may suffer bad outcomes.[27] Where uncertainty, and not agent behavior, is the dominant predictor of outcomes, as most would argue occurs in health care, then rewarding outcomes is not an effective solution to the problem of agency.[28] For example, if physicians are risk averse, then a strict-liability, outcome-based standard may induce doctors to be overcautious or leave practice all together.[29]

Just as behavior is often not observable, or at least is very costly to observe, so outcomes are difficult to observe, measure, and document. If outcomes are binary, such as winning a game or losing, the principal has little difficulty discerning whether the outcome has occurred, and the problem of compensation is trivial. Some observers of health care argue that clinical practice can be decomposed into procedures that have binary and observable outcomes with little uncertainty and those that do not. An uncomplicated fracture in an adolescent should have one outcome if the clinical intervention is properly carried out: we should be able to observe the bone heal (in an X-ray) in a predictable period of time. In the more common and complicated case where there are numerous outcomes, the trigger can be specified in advance and a distribution of compensation amounts could be established.

Outcome-based contracts are extremely rare in health services and virtually nonexistent between individual doctors and patients. Incentive-based or outcome-based contracts in health services would most likely happen where the results are directly observable, the uncertainty is low, and actions of the agent (the physician) are the primary determinant of outcome. Some forms of cosmetic surgery have this form: the likelihood of success is extremely high, responsibility for the success or failure of the surgery lies largely in the hands of the surgeon, and the standards of outcome are definable and knowable in advance. Indeed, many plastic surgeons now show before-and-after composite pictures—sometimes computer generated—to patients to aid in their informed consent before surgery.

Agreements between fertility clinics and patients represent the most dramatic forms of outcome-based contracts so far in medicine. In part, these contracts have emerged because conventional insurance coverage does not apply to many fertility treatments.[30] For example, Pacific Fertility Clinics, a chain based on the West Coast, offered patients a 90 percent rebate if the patient failed to become pregnant or miscarried. Reproductive Health Associates in St. Paul, Minnesota, offered to refund all expenses after $2,000 if the patient did not become pregnant in an eighteen-month course of treatment. The agreements involve higher fees than if patients simply paid the typical expenses involved in fertility treatments, yet limit the financial exposure of the patient in the event that the treatment is unsuccessful.

Concerns that have already been raised over these fertility contracts provide a summary of the ethical, administrative, and informational problems of using outcome-based compensation in health care. As a careful reading of the incentives would suggest, clinics carefully select patients so as to find candidates with the highest likelihood of success. Clinics restrict participation of older women, those with definable infertility problems, or those who might select older donors. Observers worry that physicians and clinics, whose compensation depends on the women actually becoming pregnant, may be too zealous in their fertility treatments, to the point where some women may be put at risk. Considerable controversy rages about the propriety of certain features of these contracts. Interestingly, although pregnancy would seem to be an easily definable "outcome" for such a contract, the treatment of late-term miscarriages as either "successes" or "failures" is the kind of contracting issue that turns out to be significant in determining compensation.

Outcome-based reimbursement is rarely used, but it is much discussed in particular areas of health services policy. The major problem with applying outcome-based reimbursement to health services is the probabilistic nature of illness and therapy. Great uncertainty is associated with most health care interventions; the role of the surgeon is often not unlike the role of the gambler, except that the agent's behavior has some influence on the odds of cure, survival, or maintenance.[31] In theory, reimbursement could be designed to cope with this uncertainty, so long as indemnity-like instruments could be developed to distribute the expected monetary value of successful outcomes. Although some illnesses have clearly identifiable symptoms that can be quantified and measured with objective metrics, such as body temperature and diastolic blood pressure, many do not have clear indications, symptomatology, or outcomes. In the end, the complexity and transactions costs of writing and observing outcome-based contracts at the individual level for a Medicare population argue against their widespread adoption, at least until the state of the art in outcomes research has significantly advanced.

Process-Based Contracts

Alternatively, a contract that monitors the behavior or process of the agent could be designed if the agent cannot be held directly accountable for outcomes. If the contract is with a financial agent or broker, one could imagine directly observing the agent's research, asking for documentation about the research, or gathering second opinions or advice about the quality of the agent's investment selections.

Much of the recent movement in health care to develop information systems, technologies of utilization review, and mechanisms for quality assurance can be seen as an attempt by principals to move along a continuum toward more direct monitoring of agent behavior. As Eisenhardt has demonstrated, the degree to which tasks are "programmable" will determine the feasibility of behavior-based contracts.[32] Purchasers and managed care plans are now demanding critical pathways or structured practice guidelines as one of the requirements for their contracts. These tools represent an attempt to make the delivery of health care more programmable.

Clark Havighurst's provocative proposal to build health care reform around the design and enforcement of more sophisticated private contracts is heavily influenced by the potential of practice guidelines to be incorporated into contractual instruments for health care coverage. Indeed, his model guidelines would provide much of the basis for competition among plans and would define the relationship between payers and providers:

> What is visualized is, in effect, a pluralistic marketplace of ideas in which there is room to differ over complex issues. In such a market, organized health plans would be in a position, for the first time, to offer consumers a chance to write their own tickets in ordering medical care. By selecting guidelines that best articu-

late their desired clinical policies and by referencing those guidelines in their contracts with subscribers, health plans could explicitly differentiate themselves from each other regarding the style of medical care that they provide. Their respective prices would then reflect the precise obligations that each plan assumes. Once consumers could choose among a variety of plans with different general policies about benefit-cost trade-offs and other matters, the market for health services should finally be able to allocate scarce resources according to the preferences of (appropriately subsidized) consumers.[33]

In Havighurst's model, the agency relationship is clear—the private consumer is the principal and the competitive plan is the agent—and based on the programmability of medical practice in guidelines. Whether guidelines can be stated with the requisite specificity and accountability is an important question for this model, as is the ability of older and disabled beneficiaries to engage in the kind of informed shopping that Havighurst envisions.[34] In practice, the dissemination and use of practice guidelines in health services has not lived up to the promises of the outcomes movement of the 1980s and early 1990s. At this stage in the evolution of health services, we appear not to have the will, the scientific basis, or the organizational capacity to implement a strong version of guideline-driven medical care. Guidelines have had limited implementation in health systems, let alone in the contractual arrangements between payers and providers.

For many, but not all, of Medicare's reimbursable services, guidelines could indicate appropriate services. Whether or not guidelines are enforced in strict terms by intermediaries and carriers is a more subtle question of administrative and clinical judgment.

Challenges to Structuring Agency in Medicare

In Medicare, the central agency question can be stated as follows: How do we delegate the task of providing medical care for the aged and the disabled so we know that the care is appropriate, that it is delivered efficiently, and that it is of satisfactory quality? The contribution of agency theory is that it provides a framework for answering this question, useful insights into why solutions are not achieved, and some useful guidance about how we might proceed to develop alternative structures. Agency theory also provides a framework for examining issues of strategic and operational control in Medicare policy. For example, the statement that a physician is an agent of the patient implies a particular conception of medical practice with powerful implications for the flow of information, the design of reimbursement, and the monitoring of

practice.[35] As discussed earlier, it also implies ethical and professional requirements. Health services in general, and the Medicare program in particular, raise particularly difficult issues of structuring agency and writing optimal
contracts. The next section of this chapter reviews these classic challenges:
managing dual or multiple interests in care, managing strategic behavior, and
managing moral hazard.

Resolving Interests in Medicare-Sponsored Care: Multiple Principals

One of the major assertions of this analysis is that there are (at least) two
principals in a Medicare-sponsored medical encounter.[36] The first insight
brought by an agency perspective on Medicare services is that the public demand for particular health services may or may not correspond to the private
demand. Two extreme cases illustrate the contrast between private and public
demand: (1) A patient may wish to have an elective cosmetic surgery which
would improve her or his quality of life, but society may not wish to pay for this
surgery because it is does not prolong life, reduce suffering, or alter the course
of an illness or disease.[37] (2) On the other hand, society may wish to pay for
certain tests, screening procedures, or vaccinations because their associated
illnesses generate significant externalities (spillover effects to others in society), even though these interventions would not have been demanded by patients with their own dollars. Indeed, these interventions with a public good
character are often provided free of charge in public health programs. These
are the easy cases in which the public and private interests are easy to discern
and readily bounded. Most health care, however, falls into a broad middle
band, in which the public and private interests in care are more ambiguous,
the marginal benefit of treatment may be uncertain or achievable at high
costs, and information about effectiveness is lacking. If an individual has an
acute illness that needs hospitalization to be resolved, then generally both society and the individual have a common interest in purchasing hospital care
that is effective, efficiently produced, and of high quality.

The state, operating through Medicare and administratively through
CMS, asks physicians, hospitals, nursing homes, home health agencies, hospices, and other purveyors of medical care to act as the agents of taxpayers. Because the government pays for the service, it has an interest in the quality and
outcome of the service.[38] The government's interest in care may or may not be
independent of those of the patient in question. At the same time, the patient
sees the physician (or other provider) as his or her own agent and expects this
provider to act in his or her singular best interest. Physicians operating in
some managed care companies, in some managed health plans with strong
incentive arrangements, and in some vertically integrated health care organi-

zations may perceive that they are embedded in still more complex agency arrangements.

This particular situation of multiple principals and multiple agents turns each medical encounter into a game (in the formal sense) within which the state may or may not be demanding the same behavior from the provider as the patient or the plan. The problem is that the provider will not necessarily be able to serve simultaneously as the servant of these multiple masters. This problem of dual interests has caused much conflict in the administration of utilization management, especially in managed care.

The table below illustrates the possible contrasts of interests with two principals involved in Medicare-sponsored services. The thought experiment in this table considers whether a service should be provided (paid for) if both principals were fully informed. In later chapters, I will examine in more detail where the agency breakdown occurs in each of these cases, but for now it is sufficient to recognize that interests in these particular forms of Medicare-sponsored service are not always compatible, either across the two principals, or between the principal and the agent. In the case of end-of-life care, for example, chapter 7 will argue that there is remarkable agreement about what kinds of care should be available to beneficiaries, but agents in health care delivery are unable or unwilling to provide appropriate palliative care in many instances for complex reasons.

Quadrant I of table 1 represents the easy case, in which the interests presumably converge. Examples include medically necessary care that is clinically indicated and efficiently provided. Both the public and the beneficiary would demand such care. Other examples include specific health promotion or preventative activities that are demanded by both the public and individual beneficiaries. Eliminating the deductibles and coinsurance for diabetes outpatient self-management or colorectal cancer screening are examples of services (both proposed in the Medicare Wellness Act) that belong in this quadrant. Many beneficiaries would utilize these services if there was not a financial barrier, and covering them makes sense from an economic and so-

Multiple Interests in Medicare-Sponsored Care

	Medicare Principal (CMS)	
	Yes	No
Informed beneficiary: Yes	I Most Medicare services?	II First-generation technology
Informed beneficiary: No	II Utilization management in managed care	IV Intensive end-of-life care

cial perspective. There is at least the possibility that the interests in services between the private and public agents are collateral in the majority of health care
encounters. However, one would be aware of the extent of agreement only if
moral hazard were eliminated or at least reduced (see discussion below), if patients were better informed about the effectiveness of care, and if liability
arrangements were functioning satisfactorily.

The more interesting problems occur in quadrants II, III, and IV, where
types of Medicare services are provided, but either individual beneficiaries or
the state—or both—do not necessarily value that service. Quadrant II represents cases where expensive, first-generation technology may be demanded by
beneficiaries but not necessarily be viewed as a prudent expenditure by the
public principals. An example is a first-generation high-technology medical
procedure or intervention with extremely high cost and low expected quality
and years of life. Chapter 5 explores one of these cases, the potential adoption
of artificial heart technology. Here the expectation is that patients with end-
stage heart disease (and no other options) will be demanders of the early technology, but the public will be negatively disposed, given the anticipated high
cost compared to quality-adjusted life years gained.

In quadrant III, care that is recommended by a physician, desired by the
patient, but restricted under managed care arrangements is probably a relatively small but extremely controversial set. Even in managed, non-Medicare,
commercial indemnity plans, the denial of payment for recommended services has become a major source of concern for physicians, a major cause for
grievances by covered enrollees, and one of the major motivations for patients' rights legislation. Typically, these disagreements arise over interpretations of whether denied care is experimental or not, or clinically indicated or
not. Within managed care plans, an implicit denial of care (or a referral) that is
recommended by the primary care physician can occur without the beneficiary ever being aware that a certain treatment was an option.

Suppose that the state and beneficiaries actually share an interest in for-
going care (quadrant IV)? Suppose that many beneficiaries prefer conservative, palliative end-of-life care but instead find themselves in intensive, acute,
and hospital-based care. This occurs in a situation where there is not sufficient
information or communication; where the physician-agent may misunderstand or for other reasons not implement the beneficiary's preferences; or for
reasons of defensive medicine, standards of practice, or interpretations of
medical ethics, where the physician's decision may diverge from the underlying preferences of the payer and the beneficiary. The reason we do not know
how many medical encounters fall into the fourth quadrant is that the con-
veyance of this type of medical information is so limited. It is possible that a

significant amount of medical care has this property: left to themselves and fully informed, patients and the public sponsor of care (Medicare) would reject a certain quantity of care that otherwise would be provided by their agents. In chapter 5, data from the SUPPORT study on end-of-life care will suggest that a significant number of patients do not receive the care they desire or presumably what the public, as the other principal for Medicare, desires. This is why, among other reasons, this particular domain of care is so interesting from an agency theory perspective.

If there is a suspicion that membership in quadrants II, III, or IV is large, a strong policy argument can be made for redirecting incentives and making public investments in information, utilization management, organization, and the development of new instruments of decision making, such as advance directives. Each of these quadrants represents candidates for improved agency.

Managing Strategic Behavior

Several forms of strategic behavior are of concern in Medicare policy. Strategic risk selection among health plans, especially in the absence of effective instruments of risk adjustment, is the primary threat to both access to Medicare managed care plans and efficiency in contracting. So long as plans (and even providers) can select favorable risks, the Medicare program cannot assure that its adjusted payments are not producing surpluses for these plans or providers. Even partially solving this problem will require better instruments of risk adjustment, as well as organizational invention to provide discipline over the behavior of plans and their associated providers.[39]

Strategic and selective supply of services for Medicare beneficiaries occurs as providers shift services for the aged and disabled to take advantage of the most favorable reimbursement. Thus, substitutions of service occur among hospitals, physicians and other health professionals, skilled nursing facilities, and home health agencies. For example, hospitals responded to relatively favorable subacute reimbursement in the 1980s and early 1990s by building step-down long-term care units, then shifting patients across levels of care (often down the hall from their acute beds), without regard to the larger overall efficiency of these substitutions.[40]

Each of these providers requires specialized approaches in order to extract efficient and appropriate delivery, and the Medicare program has been trying to catch up by implementing prospective payment systems in successive areas of health care delivery: psychiatric care, specialized hospitals, nursing homes, and home health. However, what has been mostly absent from Medicare's approach to each of these domains of health care is an appreciation of the degree to which all of these activities are interrelated, both in practice and increasingly in terms of corporate structure; and with that appreciation, an overall contracting approach that encourages care to be provided in the most efficient modality and setting. Medicare is still extremely compartmentalized in its payment policies, leading to inefficiencies in capital investments and service provision and to the costs of adjustment to continually changing payment regimes. From an agency theory perspective, the problem is that the contracts with these agents (e.g., hospitals) are incomplete, allowing the agents to exploit other contracts—in this case other reimbursement systems— to their own advantage. This problem motivates the discussion of social health maintenance organizations (chapters 4 and 7) and other models for creating more comprehensive and integrated approaches to care.

There is an oft-used imagery that illustrates the behavioral response of providers to fragmented policy approaches in health and long-term care. The health care industry is like a balloon: if you punch it in one place, it pops out somewhere else. When hospital utilization is clamped through a combination of reimbursement and utilization controls, increased utilization of skilled nursing and ambulatory services often results. When nursing home supply and reimbursement is constrained (and reimbursement for home care is available), increasing provision and utilization of home care often results. In effect, to contain costs and manage the utilization of the system, a larger girdle needs to be employed; partial fixes will merely cause substitutions of demand elsewhere in the system. The distortions in the delivery of care that result from providers' gaming of the system do not necessarily increase the efficiency of delivery. It is now becoming apparent, for example, that some outpatient procedures, undertaken under the strong hand of reimbursement and utilization controls, are actually more costly to perform in ambulatory settings than on an inpatient basis.

Managing Moral Hazard

Moral hazard arises when financial rewards of insurance or other forms of third-party health care coverage encourage either excess demand by consumers or excess supply by providers.[41] Under cost-based and fee-for-service reimbursement, contracts with providers obviously contained enormous incentives to overprovide care. Cost-based reimbursement arrangements in Medicare came to be known as "blank-check medicine," where the rewards for a service were directly based on the volume and costs of that service. Here the incentive was obviously perverse: the more costly the provision and the greater the quantity, the greater the reward, irrespective of the need or the benefits of the service.

In cases where outcomes are not observable and the costs of monitoring behavior are high, there is the potential for the agent to underprovide, over-provide, or inappropriately provide care. Even in the absence of such an invitation for excess as that provided by cost-based reimbursement, providers have numerous opportunities to overprovide health services. One of the ongoing debates in health economics has to do with the ability of physicians to induce demand. The fear is that because doctors have such control over the information that determines health care use, they have the power to serve as both the supplier and demander of health services.

However, a number of interpretations are possible, including the possibility that what is perceived to be physician-induced overprovision of health services may in fact reflect the preferences of patients. First, there may be something analogous to a bias in judgment, that more medical care is better, driving patients' expectations about the quality of medical care.[42] Second, patients may demand an inappropriate level of medical care because they distrust their agents, especially in an era of cost containment. Third, physicians may have been socialized to practice styles, either in schooling or groups, where decisions are made without regard to costs and where extravagance goes unchallenged. Fourth, concern about liability may lead physicians to order too many tests and procedures in order to insure against the risk of future tort actions, behavior known as "defensive medicine."[43] Indeed, an NBER analysis of defensive medicine suggests that this practice may produce significant inefficiency in the system.[44]

It is important to note, however, that this defensive stance does not involve only the behavior of physicians. Nursing homes impose architectural standards, dietary restrictions, and extensive regulation of personal behavior that increase the costs of care, all in the name of limiting the risk of sanctions by regulators and payers or exposure to tort actions. The end result of this cycle of protection and response is rules that shape the nature of institutional life for many older persons and result in a significant loss of autonomy and welfare.

Carol A. Heimer, in her analysis of problems in controlling moral hazard in insurance, characterizes the problem of managing moral hazard as one of controlling "reactive risk."[45] In her conceptualization, fixed risk (risk which would be present whether insurance is present or not) needs to be separated from reactive risk, which will only surface as a response to economic incentives in insurance and other arrangements. Four general strategic principles govern the management of reactive risk:

(1) reactivity varies inversely with distance between the policyholder and the person who controls losses, as well as with the degree of volitional control over the

loss-producing action, and contractual arrangements must vary accordingly; (2)
policyholders can be made to behave like prudent uninsured owners by making
them participate in losses and gains; (3) control of important loss-prevention activities can be placed in the hands of other parties when it is difficult to motivate
policyholders; and (4) frequent renegotiation of insurance contracts is necessary
to guarantee that the value of property is reflected in the policy so policyholders
will not be motivated to cause losses to collect insurance money.[46]

Each of these strategies can have direct implications for the design of
those aspects of the Medicare contract that are intended to deal with moral
hazard.

- The "distance" in the relationships between principals and agents
  has not been a subject of serious policy inquiry, though many of the
  major stylized reform proposals are explicit attempts to alter the
  locus of control and thus the distance between principals and the
  agent who makes medical decisions. Managed care plans also have
  the effect of changing the distance between principals and agents.
  The ideas for creating a regional approach to Medicare budgeting
  and administration at the end of this book are in part motivated by
  the desire to shrink the distance between principals and agents.
- The structure of copayments and deductibles is specifically designed to make Medicare enrollees participate in the losses associated with episodes of care, to "test" the demands of the patient for
  care, to reduce the opportunities for moral hazard, and to help force
  some convergence between the demands of patients and the state.
  Medical savings account proposals for Medicare provide beneficiaries the opportunity to share in gains and losses and thereby coun-
  tervail the potential for moral hazard. Similarly, at an organizational
  level, the structuring of the Medicare managed care contracting
  process around the calculation of an adjusted community rate
  (ACR) was in theory an effort to require HMOs to "give back" any
  savings that accrue to the plan in the form of increased benefits, and
  thus permit beneficiaries to participate in gains.

Many proposals for Medicare reform build on aspects of this theory. Unfortunately, the contemporary structure of copayments and deductibles, when
combined with other elements of the contractual structure, has little potential
to perform this function and only succeeds in creating some adverse distribu-
tional outcomes.[47] Roughly 70 percent of Medicare recipients have Medigap

protection, and while there is some diversity in these plans, many eliminate the first-dollar liability that Medicare patients face. In other words, the price functions that deductibles and copayments could possibly serve in disciplining the use of medical resources are virtually eliminated by secondary coverage that picks up these costs. In addition to those who do have private Medigap coverage, many low-income older persons are also covered by Medicaid, again effectively shielding them from the price of their medical care.

An Agency Toolkit for Medicare Reform

Agency theory provides both a language and a set of lenses for examining the design problem of Medicare reform. The idea of writing an efficient and enforceable contract can be applied to large-scale problems of Medicare design, such as the design of Medicare managed care arrangements, as well as specific issues of payment and oversight, such as the design of coverage and reimbursement in the hospice benefit. The basic conceptual preoccupations of agency theory (information, risk, incentives, transactions costs, governance, and organizational arrangements) provide a consistent and formal set of analytic touchstones for conceptualizing reform. This framework provides some insights into why the current contract appears so complicated and why the new initiatives in health services administration—utilization management, outcomes research, and the desire to make managed care organizations perform a major role in the system—have such underlying logic.

A Contractual Perspective

Imagine the goal of Medicare is to purchase health care that produces optimal outcomes for older persons and the disabled. How then should this contract be structured? Can outcome features be specified and rewarded? Who are the principals? Who are the agents? As shown in figure 2, the simplest depiction of Medicare's structure, the program embodies a number of principals and a number of agents, layered from the setting of broad policy goals to the street-level delivery of medical care (between a doctor and a patient). Can an outcome contract be written? If not, are there forms of process contracts that encourage appropriate, efficient, and even innovative approaches among providers?

A contractual perspective is, among other things, a change of mindset for the Medicare program. A contractual perspective for Medicare requires that the Congress, and ultimately the administrative entities that are created, be more purposeful in defining the processes and outcomes of care, structuring information, constructing incentives, and creating organizational solutions (especially for administration) that have the potential for implementing Medicare's agency functions.

A Preoccupation with Structures of Information

The major informational problem that shapes contracting for health care is its asymmetry: the agent (e.g., the provider) is the controller of important evidence about both the level and quality of effort provided and, in many cases, about the outcomes themselves. It would be extraordinarily costly to undertake truly independent monitoring of all physician or facility behavior, and reimbursement systems have typically relied on the veracity of agents in reporting.[48] As the phenomenon of "DRG creep" suggests, however, when rewards are tied to reporting in situations where information is asymmetric, there will be opportunities for strategic behavior of a different sort, for misrepresenting the behavior or outcomes of the agent's actions. When DRGs were initially implemented, epidemiologists and health service researchers noticed that the actual coding of medical procedures changed—"creeping" into higher reimbursed categories—as a result of the new payment system.

Medicare largely carries out its information role through national administration, with functions of claims processing and some utilization review delegated to intermediaries and carriers; quality review is delegated to quality improvement organizations, state agencies, and to a lesser extent the Joint Commission on Accreditation of Healthcare Organizations (JCAHO) and the National Committee for Quality Assurance (NCQA). Historically, versions of peer review and utilization screens have been the major devices to review quality and uncover misreporting of clinical practice. More recently, the surge in Medicare fraud and abuse enforcement in the late 1990s represented a reaction to concerns about the reliance on physicians, hospitals, and plans to accurately report diagnosis and claims data. Despite some recent steps toward modernization, CMS's own information resources have not kept pace with the demands of the program, the requirements for analysis and management, and the possibilities of new information technology.[49]

Aside from the recent emphasis on fraud and abuse, the Medicare program maintains a relatively passive attitude with respect to the behavior and quality of provider activities, expecting problems to be revealed mostly through the complaints and choices exercised by beneficiaries themselves. For example, considerable discretion and variation occurs among the intermediaries and carriers who pay Medicare claims. A 1995 General Accounting Office (GAO) analysis of the use of medical screens for high cost/high use Medicare procedures revealed that ten of the seventeen contractors lacked screens for echocardiography (the most costly Medicare diagnostic test), and eleven had no screens for colonoscopy, despite the urging of the Inspector General in 1991 to scrutinize these claims. The GAO estimates large savings if only screening practices were uniformly applied, with no increase in the aggressiveness of review.[50] Complaints about Medicare's procurement are long-standing but ironically have been accompanied by reductions, not increases, in the resources available for administration of contracts. Payments to contractors to review claims have declined in real terms from 74 cents per claim to 48 cents per claim since 1989. The GAO reports that only 3 percent of Part A claims received "more than superficial screening" before payment.

For all the analysis of beneficiary information wants and needs and the requirements for information on quality and outcomes of Medicare services, the state of Medicare information resources to guide purchasing is extremely primitive. An agency perspective emphasizes the information agenda for reference and motivates a search for cost-effective instruments of performance monitoring. However, a larger implication of the agency literature on the role of information in promoting and enhancing performance is that such a strategy must be crafted with some sophistication and breadth to avoid the often counterproductive reactions to simple pay-for-observed-performance schemes.[51]

An Emphasis on Incentive Arrangements

As David Smith has demonstrated, payment policy has been the historic preoccupation of Medicare policy makers for virtually the program's entire history.[52] The Congress, especially as it has been influenced by the work of the Medicare commissions, ProPAC, the PPRC, and MedPAC, has emphasized the design of reimbursement policy in its reform efforts for Medicare. In particular, the congressional search for a prospective payment system that would hold Medicare expenditures in check migrated from hospital payment policy, to physician payment policy, to long-term care and specialty providers. Despite this preoccupation with payment policy, Medicare's incentive arrangements remain extremely blunt. Prices are still centrally administered, rates are slow to change, the connections between value and payment are weak, if not nonexistent, and relationships of payments to the circumstances of individual markets for service are tenuous.

A Search for Organizational Invention

At the broadest level of generality, the control of Medicare delivery can be solved by "hierarchy," meaning a combination of organization and administration that places decisions of agents under the direction of principals, or through "markets," in which relatively unbridled transactions take the place of organization. A growing body of theory, pioneered by the work of Oliver Williamson,[53] is articulating the conditions under which alternative organizational forms of control and governance are appropriate. While this literature for public organization is still in its infancy, the prospect of defining a new organization for the administration of Medicare services is suddenly very real.

Recently, specific concerns about Medicare's administrative arrangements, and especially the structure and organization of HCFA, have surfaced in the public debate about reform. The 1999 Breaux-Frist proposal for Medicare reform called for the creation of a new Medicare board for governance of the program and the movement of numerous functions, such as administration of prescription drug coverage, outside of HCFA.[54] Lynn Etheredge proposed the elimination of HCFA altogether, replacing it by a set of new public arrangements for Medicare that include different structures for congressional oversight (a Joint Health Committee) and revised federal health programs administration that would emphasize health care quality and outcomes for the Medicare population.[55] An agency approach will help with the analysis of these and other alternative administrative structures.

Conclusions: Toward an Agency Approach to the Design of Medicare Policy

In the concept of Medicare design developed in this chapter, the structure of agency is both important and complex. Not only are mechanisms needed to empower older and disabled beneficiaries to gain access to and use health services appropriately (given their own preferences) but also to reconcile the joint demand for services by individuals and the public. Beneficiaries require better agency in order to make the complex decisions that are envisioned by current Medicare arrangements, such as choosing health plans in Medicare+Choice. Beneficiaries and their families facing cognitive or other challenges require much more sophisticated agency than exists virtually anywhere in our health system. Beneficiaries and families navigating Alzheimer's disease, for example, confront a confusing and bewildering patchwork of coverage, services, and informal supports that are an unfortunate match with the nature of the disease itself.

Administratively, Medicare's structure of agency is the product of its political history, as described in chapter 2. The existence of CMS, the intermediaries, the carriers, and other institutional features of Medicare represent both structural and political responses to the problem of administering such a large federal program as it evolves over time. The interesting policy project ahead of us, however, is how to be inventive in the way Medicare solves its agency problems within new structures of governance and administration that are flexible, responsive, and tailored to the market circumstances of the modern program.

The next three chapters provide "case studies" of the way in which an agency approach can be utilized to analyze contracting arrangements in particular domains of Medicare—managed care delivery, decisions about the adoption of technology, and medical decisions at the end of life. These case studies play off of a powerful structural dilemma (illustrated in the table on page 73) that is lurking in the background of much of the current dissatisfaction with the performance of Medicare policy: at least two principals (and often multiple agents) exert their interests in each Medicare-sponsored encounter. The conclusion of this analysis is that new incentive, organizational, and information arrangements must be designed in order to execute the Medicare contract. Medicare must create new structures of agency that represent the interests of the public in the health care of older and disabled persons yet still allow the exercise of private demand over health care. In the final chapter, an approach to Medicare reform will be structured around the agency relationships described in figure 2.

Most physicians and hospitals no longer aspire to the dual role of agent for society and for the individual patient, for managing costs as well as quality. Physicians want to be on the side of their patients, advocating for more resources and better quality, rather than taking on the social responsibility for comparing costs and benefits in a complex and volatile environment.

—James Robinson, "The End of Managed Care"

CHAPTER FOUR

Medicare Managed Care

Medicare's Dance with Managed Care

Managed care has been touted as the solution to Medicare's cost and financing problems on the one hand and as a villainous threat to the doctor-patient relationship, beneficiary's quality of care, and the coverage traditionally afforded by the program on the other. Increasingly, the escalation of the rhetoric about managed care has made it difficult to conduct rational deliberations about its role, design, and regulation in Medicare. Politicians have been under intense pressure to regulate managed care plans, dampen the incentives for cost savings to providers, and add layers of accountability and due process to treatment decisions. In the wake of consumer backlash, plan withdrawals, and the financial difficulties of the industry, some analysts have wondered if we have reached the end of managed care. James Robinson concludes that "the managed care system has achieved considerable economic success, but has proven itself a cultural and political failure."[1]

Fueling the drive for governmental regulation of managed care is a fundamental logical inconsistency: the public and the payers of health care would like to exploit the potential cost-saving features and inherent incentives of managed care models while, at the same time, seeking to micromanage the mechanisms by which plans control their use of resources. For managed care to work in Medicare, there will need to be some larger accommodations made with the organizational and economic realities of this form of delivery. We may decide as a society that we do not wish to live with these accommodations, but better to be explicit prospectively about the nature of the contract—its goals, financing, payment mechanisms, information, and regulation—and accept or reject it. If Medicare managed care comes to represent nothing but reductions in care, with the attendant anecdotes, grievances, and litigation, then this regime of organizing and financing care will have led a stormy political life and ultimately will have realized little positive impact. If Medicare managed care comes to represent a budgetary game between government and plans over what level of annual increase in payment will be tolerable, then we can anticipate a future of unstable, declining plan participation, with collateral adverse effects on beneficiaries.

"Success" for Medicare managed care in most policy discussions seems to imply (1) higher enrollment (soon) of Medicare beneficiaries in managed care options, (2) moderation of premium growth, and (3) preservation of at least the current levels of access and satisfaction that have been achieved in traditional Medicare. Tentative answers to whether or not managed care will be successful in meeting the first two tests can be offered now. Managed care's longer term effects on quality, access, and outcomes for Medicare beneficiaries are a matter of much greater speculation, but many of the issues can at least be identified. Even more uncertain will be the fit between managed care models of organization and finance, and the health care needs of Medicare's specialized populations: the disabled, end-stage renal disease (ESRD) beneficiaries, beneficiaries with chronic conditions, and the very poor elderly. Herein lies the key question for the future of Medicare managed care: Can this mode be adapted to provide more effective agency and delivery of care for Medicare's most vulnerable beneficiaries?

As with other aspects of Medicare policy, managed care offerings and enrollments have emerged with a distinctive geographical footprint. As late as the end of 1998, only five states accounted for 57 percent of the total enrollment in Medicare+Choice plans: Florida, California, New York, Pennsylvania, and Texas. Six states had no Medicare+Choice offerings: Alaska, Mississippi, Montana, South Dakota, Vermont, and Wyoming. Across the states with Medicare+Choice plans, the ability to choose among plans and the distribution of supplementary benefits, such as prescription drug benefits, varied widely. In addition to new managed care organization and practices, there are variations in the relations with the provider community and in the familiarity and acceptance of managed care by beneficiaries. These differences were demonstrated in case studies done for the Kaiser Family Foundation by Mathematica, where markets were matched by their Medicare payment levels and studied in depth for their variation in market characteristics, plan characteristics, and beneficiary knowledge and attitudes.[2] These findings have important implications for the recommendations at the end of this book, where the argument for regional financing and administration of Medicare managed care is presented.

So far, the public policy aspirations for Medicare managed care have been quite modest. The case for Medicare managed care has been largely built on relatively small enrollment growth projections and relatively low expectations of cost reduction emanating from gently encouraging beneficiaries into conventional managed care products. The evidence on cost savings, quality differences, and outcomes of managed care in general is surprisingly spotty and inconclusive for all of the momentum behind these arrangements both in public policy and the private marketplace. The evidence regarding Medicare managed care is even weaker.[3] Studies of managed care have had an extremely difficult time controlling for selection bias in the risk pools. Evaluations of managed care also are handicapped by serious problems of comparability of data, timeliness, and the representativeness of enrolled populations.

In this discussion, as in other analyses of managed care, the usual caveats apply: so many varieties of organization, enrolled populations, and incentives fall under the rhetoric of managed care that it is easy to misstate its characteristics and to have a false sense of precision about the effects of managed care. Up until the 1997 amendments, Medicare managed care operated under some specific contractual rules that allowed some level of generalization about the experience. With the implementation of the new Medicare+Choice options, the ability to make meaningful statements about the broad experience of beneficiaries under managed care became further complicated.

The plan for this chapter is as follows: First, I present the logic and theory of how managed care approaches the organization and financing of care for the aged and disabled. Second, I summarize the evolution of Medicare managed care, including the principal concerns and criticisms. Third, I describe the structure of agency in models of Medicare managed care. Fourth, I summarize the legal and regulatory backdrop, a significant issue in establishing agency responsibility and accountability with health plans. Fifth, I analyze several of the challenges of designing a Medicare contract and structuring agency: for example, the design of incentives and payment, the development of better risk adjustment, the implementation of quality and performance monitoring, and the creation of new mechanisms for beneficiary agency. Finally, as a precursor to the broader policy strategy for Medicare proposed at the end of the book, I review the elements of a model Medicare managed contract. The payoff to reforming Medicare managed care arrangements can ultimately be a transformation of care management and delivery arrangements, especially for beneficiaries facing chronic and long-term care needs. Unfortunately, Medicare's current agency arrangements are far from able to pull off this transformation.

A Theory of Managed Care

Managed care systems seek to change the organization of health care, its financing, and the incentives facing providers and enrollees. Instead of rewarding providers who do more and charge more, as in fee-for-service medicine, managed care systems attempt to discipline care so that only necessary, appropriate, and cost-effective services are provided. This discipline is provided in part by capitation payments (a fixed budget per person for a defined period of time); other risk-based forms of financial incentives to providers (such as bonus payments to physicians for low levels of hospitalization or relatively few referrals to specialists); and the use of so-called utilization management techniques (the oversight or explicit approval for services by a third party).

Unlike unmanaged fee-for-service care, managed care arrangements shift the financial risks of health services from the payer to plans and providers. In the classic case, if a provider receives a single capitated payment for providing all contracted medical services in a given period, the provider bears the risk of a costly patient. In practice, mechanisms such as stop-loss provisions and secondary insurance arrangements dampen the financial risks borne by providers. Traditionally, strongly managed care plans rely more on primary care practitioners than on specialists and subspecialists, more on outpatient services than on inpatient hospitalizations, and more on volume discounts and contracting arrangements than on the free exercise of choice and the discretion of doctors and patients.

A major shift in the philosophy, incentives, and unit of delivery occurs in strong managed care arrangements. Unlike fee-for-service medicine, the unit of payment is no longer the individual visit or stay; instead, patients are joined to providers over longer periods of engagement in care. Early proponents of prepaid health, such as Paul Ellwood, imagined that this long-term relationship between enrollee and provider would shift the emphasis of care toward health promotion and prevention. In a long-term financial and caregiving relationship, providers have stronger incentives to find interventions that will preempt costly episodes of care, especially hospitalizations. In effect, these forward externalities become internalized to the risk-bearing plan. Proponents of a managed-competition model of system reform, such as Alain Enthoven, imagined that plans would compete over quality and price of care, with incentives pushed down to both the enrollees and the plans to produce care that is appropriate and cost effective.

If the expected duration of the enrollee's participation in the plan is short or if the plan has little confidence in the ability of health prevention efforts to actually reduce costs, then the investments in these prevention activities will be low. The classic example of this forward incentive effect for prevention is immunization: it is presumably in the interest of a managed care provider to have enrolled members immunized because it will prevent future, more costly episodes of care. However, if significant numbers of enrollees disenroll, or if the plan can free-ride on the herd immunity of the larger population, then the incentives for investing in immunizations will be low. Further, if the plan or its members have a high discount rate—they prefer current consumption or savings to the uncertain prospect of future health benefits—they will also tend to invest little in health prevention activities.

For all of these reasons, even the theoretical expectation for health prevention and promotion in managed care has to be limited. In a Medicare population, relatively short life expectancies in the aged population, relatively high rates of disenrollment, and the relative absence of interventions with known positive benefit/cost evaluations mean that the case for health prevention is even more tenuous than managed care in a commercially insured population.[4] For early proponents of HMOs, one of the great disappointments of the old prepaid group health movement is that health promotion and prevention never really became the defining features of these organizations. In part, this simply reflects the fact that the economic calculus of health promotion often does not favor these interventions in the short run, at least so long as there is significant churning and instability of enrollees in managed care plans.

Because strongly managed care plans are contracted to care for the "whole person" (thus the expression a "covered life") for a given period of time, there is also the opportunity to provide greater coordination of care. Plans that utilize primary care practitioners to oversee care or employ effective versions of case management have the potential to orchestrate care in such a way that patients see the right specialist at the right time, do not experience redundant or inappropriate tests and procedures, and face administratively seamless care decisions.[5]

Some observers expected that large, managed care plans would come to symbolize a "brand name" of health care, reflecting attributes of quality and accessibility that would be difficult to ascertain on an individual physician basis.[6] HMOs in theory deal with information problems in health services delivery by substituting evidence about the performance of the *organization* (information that arguably can be gathered and cognitively processed by individuals) for evidence about the performance of a particular physician. In other words, a consumer could be expected to learn something of the "quality" of an HMO and select a physician within the HMO (believing that a quality organization will monitor and police the individual physician's practice) at relatively low cost.[7]

The individual consumer would trust that the plan generalizes this quality of care across its participating doctors and hospitals. Consistent with the theory, individuals who face the highest informational costs in selecting and monitoring a physician, the young and the mobile, would be most likely to opt for an HMO model of delivery. Individuals with long-standing relationships with physicians and providers (many Medicare beneficiaries), and thus with relatively good information about their expected individual performance, would be least likely to be influenced by the brand marketing of new health plans.

Just as one would expect a certain standard of quality, responsiveness, and amenities at Nieman Marcus (and another at Wal-Mart), so too would one expect large health care plans to differentiate and reflect certain dimensions of quality and service easily identified by consumers and patients. Thus, in the absence of information about the quality of individual physicians, patients have access to the next best thing: information about the (perceived) quality of the overall system that has credentialed and certified its physicians and other providers. Many of the national managed care vendors and many of the early national health systems attempted to develop both internal standardization and external name recognition to support brand name marketing of their products. Examples of this approach included Columbia Hospital Corporation, Humana, United Health Care, and Kaiser Permanente. Regional health systems such as Henry Ford Health System, Intermountain Health, and the Advocate system have also attempted to establish brand name identity for their integrated delivery systems. These systems want patients to search for their hospitals and physician groups when they choose health plans and subsequently providers.[8]

In theory, large managed care plans also have the ability to dramatically simplify the interface between the patient and the provider. When individual claims no longer matter, patients can use services without the legendary burden of claims and paperwork that have become one of the hallmarks of American health care delivery. Of course, managed care plans often substitute some new administrative burdens for the old: patients are often responsible for obtaining prior approval for services from specialists or out-of-plan providers in order for claims to be paid.

Finally, with the organization and information management that is possible in strong managed care arrangements, numerous health care transaction costs could be driven down.[9] Through economies of scale and scope of information, large managed care plans have the potential to offer new levels of standardization, accountability, and disclosure that are impossible in a system of disparate providers and fee-for-service payment. Because large plans have the ability to monitor and reward physicians, they also have the potential to implement practice guidelines and evaluate practice patterns in a systematic way. The advent of report cards, such as the Health Employee Data Information Set (HEDIS) sponsored by the National Committee for Quality Assurance (NCQA), means that plans have the ability to monitor and report their own performance on indicators such as access measures, extent of preventative care, and satisfaction. Of course, organizational report cards have not lived up to their advance billing in health care. As applications in other industries have demonstrated, politics, organizational resistance, and the economics of information have conspired to slow down and, in some cases, halt development of these tools and their dissemination to the public.[10]

The Evolution of Medicare Managed Care

Before the 1997 Balanced Budget Act (BBA) amendments, Medicare allowed beneficiaries to enroll in managed care options under several different arrangements. Originally, under the 1965 Medicare legislation, beneficiaries could enroll in prepaid health plans for Part B services only, but only a small number of beneficiaries and plans ever made use of this option. In the 1972 legislation and in further amendments under the Tax Equity and Fiscal Responsibility Act (TEFRA) in 1982, beneficiaries were given the option of participating in cost contracts that paid plans an initial amount based on the forecasted expenses of their enrollees, with a final payment that compensated plans for any expenses over and above that forecasted amount. Enrollees in cost contracts were also allowed to see providers outside of the network. Out-of-network providers were paid under Medicare's traditional fee-for-service reimbursement.[11] A third option, also authorized in the 1982 TEFRA legislation, allowed HMOs to enter into Medicare risk contracts that paid a fixed amount per beneficiary for all covered services. To encourage beneficiaries to enroll, virtually all risk plans provided some form of supplemental benefits, such as prescription drug coverage or coverage of cost-sharing expenses. In exchange, beneficiaries were required to see providers in their network and abide by the clinical and coverage decisions made by their plan. Beginning in 1995, Medicare began to offer a point-of-service managed care option to a small number of beneficiaries. This option allows beneficiaries to enroll in a plan that offers all Medicare covered services, but also the option to opt out of the plan to use specialized services or providers. The features of these early point-of-service plans varied tremendously.

Medicare has also sponsored demonstration projects offering managed care to special populations. Four social health maintenance organizations (S/HMOs) offering acute and long-term care services enrolled over 22,000 beneficiaries in 1994. S/HMO providers receive the same payment rates as fee-for-service care plus higher payments for enrollees who are eligible for nursing home care but receive care in the community instead. Medicare *Select* is a preferred provider option made available to beneficiaries in fifteen states. Insurers choosing to participate offer lower Medigap premiums to beneficiaries if they use a certain network of providers. Participating insurers are required to assure beneficiary access and care quality as well as to disclose information about use restrictions and the cost and availability of other Medigap options.

Prior to the 1997 BBA, Medicare's scheme for paying its risk contractors was deceptively simple. In order to achieve a discount over what Medicare would ordinarily pay under fee-for-service arrangements, the program paid 95 percent of the average adjusted per capita cost (AAPCC) in the beneficiary's county. The payment was adjusted for the age, sex, welfare classification, working age status, institutional status, and disability status for the specific pool of enrollees. Each HMO was required to submit a proposal, called an adjusted community rate (ACR) proposal, which estimated and justified its projected expenses for the enrolled population. If the ACR was lower than the expected Medicare AAPCC, funds had to be returned to Medicare, benefits added to the plan, cost sharing lowered for beneficiaries, or the excess put in a "benefits stabilization fund." The plan could also charge beneficiaries for additional services they wished it to cover. The opportunity for plans to make these choices in design resulted in significant variations in plan benefits and copayments. Better benefits without extra premiums tended to be available in areas with higher AAPCCs.

Since the AAPCC formula was based on the cost of providing fee-for-service care, not necessarily well-managed care, it reflected the costs (and perhaps inefficiencies) outside of the Medicare managed care pool for that county. For example, payment adjustments for teaching and disproportionate share hospitals were included in the AAPCC, even though HMOs were not required to use these providers or allocate payment adjustments to them. In some markets, there may have been a significant disparity between the costs and risk pool enrolled in a Medicare plan and the fee-for-service cost experience in a particular county that provides the basis for that plan's managed care payment. The AAPCC payments exhibited considerable variability across counties, including considerable differentials between adjacent counties. This lack of meaningful connection between fee-for-service experience, especially at the county level, and managed care policy goals led to proposals that would decouple the two payment systems.[12] Interestingly, the level of HMO penetration did not seem to be strongly related to the level of the AAPCC. HMOs that lost considerable amounts on Medicare risk contracts believe that the AAPCC underpaid them for the underlying health conditions, comorbidities, and severity of illness in their plans. At the same time, HMOs with either the marketing skill or good luck to enroll a relatively healthy population made considerable margins on their Medicare risk contracts. W. Pete Welch's analysis of the determinants of the Medicare HMO market share suggests that the response to geographic variations in AAPCC was relatively small.[13] In a regression, a large increase in average payment on the order of $100 per month generated an increase of only approximately 3.4 percentage points in Medicare HMO market share. On the other hand, the general HMO market share appeared to be a much more important predictor of Medicare managed care penetration. Indeed, in Welch's analysis, Portland, Oregon—which has one of the lowest price-adjusted AAPCCs among metropolitan areas—was at the top of the distribution of Medicare managed care markets; and New Orleans—which has one of the highest price-adjusted rates—was at the bottom of the distribution.

The 1997 BBA changed the relationship between payments to Medicare+Choice plans and the costs of delivering fee-for-service care at the county level. Under Medicare+Choice, plans are to be paid 95 percent of what the national fee-for-service amount would be for an enrollee, based on fee-for-service experience, with adjustments for local cost differences and federal budget savings over time. These adjustments at the county level are based on the calculation of a standardized county rate, initially calculated from the five-year fee-for-service experience in that county. However, this county-level standardized rate was to be gradually "blended" with the national fee-for-service rate, resulting in a 50/50 blend between the local and national cost experience by 2002. (Payments for graduate medical education were also gradually taken out of this county rate and fully eliminated by 2002.) The national payment rate is based on the previous year's overall per capita fee-for-service expenditures, then adjusted for any predicted changes in provider payments, coverage, or benefits. Finally, the BBA established a floor for payments in counties that previously had low AAPCCs.

Each year plans are paid the maximum of (1) a minimum 2 percent increase; (2) the updated floor amount, based on the national increase in Medicare spending; or (3) the blended amount. Once these maximum payment amounts are calculated for each county, they are adjusted again so that the program as a whole achieves budget neutrality. Despite this complicated payment scheme, the requirement for budget neutrality dominated in 1999 and 2000, meaning that all plans simply received the 2 percent minimum increase.

The 1997 amendments also created a series of new options for beneficiaries under the rubric of Medicare+Choice. Changes to the payment methodology for Medicare HMOs were enacted with the goal of limiting overall Medicare managed care spending but at the same time making Medicare enrollees more attractive to plans in rural areas and markets that have historically had low enrollments. Payments to provider sponsored organizations (PSOs) and preferred provider organizations (PPOs) were authorized again with the expectation that more managed care options would become available and would be attractive to beneficiaries. PSOs were new health plans created by doctors and hospitals to compete with traditional Medicare HMOs founded by prepaid health providers or insurance sponsors. PPO arrangements, like the point-of-service options described above, were designed to allow enrollees to receive care from providers outside of the network list for an additional fee.

The Congress again increased payment levels in 1999 (Balanced Budget Refinement Act—BBRA) and 2000 (Benefits Improvement Act—BIPA) to counteract the withdrawal of plans, encourage the entry of new plans where Medicare+Choice plans were not available, and to discourage further reductions in benefits. The 2000 changes concentrated on raising the base floor payments and the floor payments for larger urban counties. However, an early evaluation of the effects of these payment increases by the GAO has indicated only minimal responses from plans.[14] The coexistence of significant plan withdrawals with pressures on the Congress to raise payments has spurred a vigorous debate about whether Medicare is paying "too much" or "too little" for market participation in the program, given risk selection, pressures for prescription drug coverage, and the alternative of traditional Medicare fee-for-service coverage.[15]

Criticisms and Concerns with the Medicare Managed Care Experience

Numerous problems—some real, some perceived—with Medicare managed care plans surfaced even in its early history. Beginning in 1982, when Medicare allowed enrollment in risk-based HMOs as an alternative to traditional fee-for-service coverage, concerns were raised about marketing and sales practices. Highly publicized abuses and plan failures led to considerable caution in expanding the options or promoting enrollment in Medicare managed care. Early enrollment stalled.

The much-publicized foreclosure of International Medical Centers Inc. (IMC) of Florida, at the time the largest Medicare HMO contractor in the country, put a dark cloud over the entire Medicare HMO initiative in the late 1980s. IMC was operating under a $360 million contract with HCFA, serving 136,000 Medicare beneficiaries. Beginning in May 1987, IMC experienced a series of management crises, including notice of termination of the Medicare contract, declaration of insolvency, receivership, and indictments of the founder and president for conspiracy, obstruction of justice, and other charges. IMC was eventually purchased by the Humana Corporation and its Medicare contracts were transferred. However, the IMC episode raised early and major questions about the ability of the federal government to manage and oversee a large-scale HMO program for Medicare beneficiaries.

Concern about marketing abuses in Medicare managed care, though largely anecdotal, never produced a systematic response.[16] Many plans employ enrollment brokers, often working on commissions. Critics claimed that many brokers were uninformed or practiced deceptive marketing when explaining the options available to beneficiaries. In early 1997, AARP proposed to offer a form of enrollment brokerage—a type of agency—that would have certified selected plans and processed the enrollment of beneficiaries in exchange for a fee. From AARP's perspective, the argument for this service was that legitimate and independent services would be useful alternatives to the underground and often deceptive marketing practices of many plans. Several states have adopted models of independent enrollment brokers for Medicaid managed care because of the potential for abuse by plans that have strong incentives for enrolling often-vulnerable members. However, the AARP proposal was shelved when HCFA suggested that the proposed arrangements with plans would violate Medicare antikickback provisions.

Evidence on disenrollment patterns provides suggestive, but not hard, evidence that many beneficiaries "voted with their feet" year-to-year with their managed care providers and that more vulnerable beneficiaries (e.g., older and sicker) may have experienced greater problems of access and responsiveness from managed care versus fee-for-service providers. During the early experience in Medicare managed care, about 18 percent of participants in Medicare HMOs disenrolled per year. However, analysis of disenrollment rates for cancer patients, one group that may signal the tendency of plans to encourage sicker and higher cost members to disenroll, did not find evidence of selective treatment.[17]

An early analysis of a sample of Medicare enrollees and disenrollees in managed care plans by Mathematica for the Physician Payment Review Commission (PPRC) revealed that the number of reported problems was generally low, the satisfaction with Medicare managed care relatively high, and the provision of selected preventative services (a measure of health promotion) relatively high.[18] Eight percent of respondents had trouble making appointments, 6 percent were not referred to a specialist when they themselves thought such a referral was warranted, and 6 percent felt they had been discharged too early from the hospital. Ninety-six percent of respondents rated their overall health care as either excellent, very good, or good. At the same time, the survey revealed disproportionate problems of access for functionally impaired, old, poor, and chronically ill beneficiaries. The study also raised more subtle questions about access to home care, where 17 percent of respondents reported wanting "more" services than those offered under their plans. The results for Medicare utilization included (1) HMO enrollees had shorter lengths of stay but comparable admission rates to hospitals; (2) HMO enrollees were more likely to visit a physician during the course of a year, but the rate of physician visits went down slightly; (3) HMO enrollees were more likely to use skilled nursing facilities, but the total number of skilled nursing days did not increase; (4) Medicare HMOs appeared to increase the volume of services but reduce their intensity; (5) Medicare HMOs appeared to reduce services the most for the sickest patients, those with the most serious functional limitations, or those who subsequently died; (6) no significant differences were detected in outcomes of inpatient or outpatient care; and (7) satisfaction with the HMOs varied widely and depended on which dimension of satisfaction was being measured (e.g., care processes or out-of-pocket expenditures). About 20 percent of HMO enrollees withdrew from these plans within a year.

As the managed care experience has evolved, the impacts on quality, costs, and access have been extremely difficult to document and evaluate. Generalizations are limited by the selection issues, the lack of comparable data for fee-for-service and managed care populations, the rapid movement of enrollees and changes in plan types, and the relative dearth of research. Robert Miller and Harold Luft's assessments of the managed care literature found mixed results (relative to fee-for-service) for physician visits and outpatient use, enrollee satisfaction, total spending, and quality. HMOs tended to show more consistent results in producing enrollee satisfaction with the financial aspects of their plans and troubling results on quality and satisfaction for enrollees with chronic conditions and diseases.[19]

In its middle history, enrollment in Medicare managed care did not grow significantly, even in markets where HMOs for the non-Medicare population grew rapidly. From 1995 to 1999, enrollment in Medicare risk and choice plans had its most impressive period of growth, from 3.1 million to 6.4 million beneficiaries. Since 1999, however, enrollment has declined, a product of plan withdrawals, significant reductions in coverage, and beneficiary disenrollment.[20] Changes in the cost and coverage of plans undoubtedly contributed to this decline. For example, the percentage of beneficiaries with zero premiums declined from almost 80 percent in 1999 to 45 percent in 2001. Drug coverage declined, benefits declined, premiums increased, and copayments increased during this period. In 1999, forty-three plans chose not to renew their Medicare contracts, and fifty-four remaining plans reduced their service areas. All told, about 407,000 beneficiaries were affected. In 2000, another forty-one contracts were withdrawn and another fifty-four service areas were reduced, affecting an additional 327,000 enrollees. A significant number of beneficiaries lost their access to managed care options as a result of these withdrawals. For example, in 2000, one-quarter of the beneficiaries who lost their Medicare+Choice plan did not have another option available in their locality. About 40 percent of these plans that did not renew or that reduced their service areas were affiliated with four national managed care firms.[21] Again in 2001, another 934,000 beneficiaries lost their managed care coverage as a result of announced contract nonrenewals or service area reductions. In both 2000 and 2001, many beneficiaries forced out of plans experienced a loss of coverage; many experienced confusion about their options and subsequent coverage choices. A disproportionate number were poor and vulnerable.[22] A disproportionate number also lived in rural areas, often without another choice of managed care plan.[23] This trajectory of payment constraints, benefit reductions, increasing beneficiary cost sharing, and plan withdrawals has led to concerns that the story of Medicare managed care will be "enrollees spend more and receive less" as the program moves forward.[24]

With a peak enrollment of only 16 percent of beneficiaries, the decline in managed care participation raises fundamental questions about the future role of managed care approaches for Medicare. However, at the beginning of the George W. Bush administration, Medicare managed care was still in retreat, down to 14 percent coverage of the beneficiary population. Despite plan withdrawals, congressional concern with payment policy, and the clamor for increased patients' rights legislation, Thomas Sculley, the newly appointed administrator of the CMS, announced intentions to double Medicare's enrollment in managed care in a four-year period, up to 30 percent of beneficiaries by 2005.[25]

Despite these ambitions, Marsha Gold's assessment of Medicare+ Choice is discouraging: "By almost any measure, the interim grade for the

M+C program as of the start of 2001 must be graded a 'D' if not an 'F.'"[26] MedPAC itself concluded that beneficiaries had less choice of private plans and less generous benefit packages under Medicare+Choice than with Medicare offerings prior to the program. The commission believes that Medicare+ Choice did not produce cost savings, nor did it redress geographic disparities in plan availability or benefit offerings.[27]

Agency in Medicare Managed Care

Under Medicare managed care arrangements, the key agency relationship is shifted from CMS and the beneficiary to the provider to CMS and the beneficiary to the plan. David Dranove and William White—in one of the first applications of agency theory to interpreting health services design— identified the possible efficiencies in monitoring and information available to consumers and public payers contracting with large HMOs or group practices instead of individual, autonomous physicians.[28] They speculated that brand name identity for managed care plans might become a way for plans to market certain dimensions of quality and for consumers to sort out competitors in a crowded marketplace.

As shown in figure 4, plans such as Medicare managed care organizations become the units accountable for health care delivery, the agents mediating among the government sponsor (e.g., CMS), beneficiaries, and the providers. In both the organization and marketing of managed care plans, performance is regarded to be a function of the management of the plan itself. The government pays an adjusted community rate, and, in certain circumstances, beneficiaries pay premiums and copayments. Thus, managed care plans face the classic situation of dual principals described in chapter 3.

As agents, plans vouch for the quality of care, report data on their overall

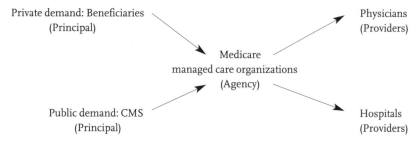

Figure 4. The structure of agency in Medicare managed care

performance, and market themselves to beneficiaries with a brand name identity that is supposed to convey information about their standards of care relative to their competitors'. The early evolution of HCFA's payment policy for
risk contracts, its reporting requirements from plans, if not its definition of its
own legal responsibility for care delivered by HMOs (see the next section), imply the structure of agency illustrated in figure 4.

Until the 1997 BBA, beneficiaries were able to opt out of their plans at
any time, undermining the beneficiary attachment to the plan (and whatever
care-management might be in place) as well as the plan's incentives to provide
prevention, health promotion, or care management. Indeed, the churning of
enrollees in and out of Medicare managed care plans has been a significant
problem. From a public principal's point of view, the lack of any lock-in provisions meant that risk-selection behavior, particularly beneficiaries selecting
into managed care and fee-for-service alternatives, could happen without
checks and balances. Before the BBA, policy makers were reluctant to impose
lock-in provisions, because beneficiaries are often poorly informed and, as a
political matter, lock-in provisions are perceived to be coercive. Especially during an era when managed care has been so controversial and choice has
become the dominant policy theme, there has been little enthusiasm for shep-
herding beneficiaries into longer term managed care contractual arrangements. Indeed, the movement to emphasize choice in Medicare and weaken
the role of managed care plans in the oversight of care means that the potential agency role that plans themselves—as organizations—can play is seriously threatened.

A modest but interesting alternative agency arrangement for Medicare
is evident in the private fee-for-service option made available in Medicare
+Choice. Although only one vendor, Sterling Health, initially stepped forward to offer a private fee-for-service option, it represents a significant departure for the structure of risk and governance in Medicare. Under the private
fee-for-service option, Sterling receives a capitated payment based on the service area of the enrolled beneficiary, but there is no expectation of management of care. Instead the private fee-for-service plan acts like indemnity
insurance, paying out claims to any Medicare provider. To beneficiaries, this
option looks like traditional fee-for-service; to providers, it looks like traditional Medicare without the traditional intermediaries and carriers. However,
the private fee-for-service plan bears the risk of the expenditures, and by extension keeps any surpluses, that may result from claims less than capitated
amounts.

The Sterling Health Care example in Medicare+Choice represents an
extremely interesting development in agency terms, even though it represents

a tiny fraction of Medicare coverage. In effect, this plan is substituting private agency over fee-for-service Medicare delivery for public agency as it has traditionally been administered by CMS and the intermediaries and carriers. From a delivery standpoint, the private fee-for-service plans represent a weak form of agency, taking on risk and administration of claims with the expectation that the agent will capture some of the economic surplus from discounting fee-for-service and providing some efficiencies of claims administration. Nonetheless, these private fee-for-service plans create actual separation in the direct contracting and risk bearing between the public sponsor of the program and the individual provider. At the same time, it is interesting that in the first generation of a private fee-for-service option in Medicare, there is no increase in the accountability expected from the private agent. Nonetheless, the Sterling example, as well as the debate over the locus of control over the Medicare prescription drug benefit, illustrates the significance of potentially new agency relationships in reform.

The Legal and Regulatory Context for Agency in Medicare Managed Care

Medicare's legal concept of its role as a principal is evident in the arguments made in *Shalala v. Grijalva*,[29] heard in the District Court for Arizona, and in subsequent cases. The case was brought by Medicare beneficiaries who were denied services by HMOs and who sought protection and advocacy from Medicare. The Department of Health and Human Services argued that because HMOs are private, nongovernmental entities denials of service do not constitute state action and, therefore, do not trigger a host of due process requirements that would be enforceable by the state.

In other cases cited, the court found that contracting with private providers for the delivery of care did not absolve the state of its responsibilities for overseeing the care of beneficiaries. In two related cases, the tests for determining the responsibility of the state to beneficiaries had included (1) the government pays for the covered services; (2) the government regulates the (HMO) providers, especially regarding coverage decisions; (3) the secretary creates the legal framework, rules, and regulations that govern the activities of the providers; (4) the Secretary of Health and Human Services has the authority to audit, inspect, and terminate HMO contracts; and (5) beneficiaries appeal service denials directly to the secretary, who has the power to overturn the HMO decision.[30]

In *Shalala*, the court defined broad and significant responsibilities for the government in setting and enforcing standards of coverage for beneficiaries in HMOs. The court specified responsibilities for HMOs in educating beneficiaries, as well as for the Secretary of Health and Human Services in promoting and administering a timely hearings and appeals process. For example, the court held that the secretary is responsible for assuring that beneficiaries have access to hearings on coverage decisions that "shall be informal, in-person communication with the decision maker; shall be available upon request for all service denials; shall be timely according to the seriousness of the medical condition implicated by the service denial. Immediate hearing shall be available for acute service denials, specifically where delivery of the service is prevented by the denial."[31] In response to this decision, Health and Human Services announced it would issue new regulations that strengthen the appeal rights of Medicare HMO enrollees.[32]

This case illustrates three aspects of the agency problem that confronts Medicare, especially if it were to rely significantly on the responsibility of managed care providers for overseeing care. First, the courts, in their interpretation of the Medicare statute, the secretary's own regulations, and a number of constitutional claims (most notably the due process clause of the Constitution), found significant responsibilities for public oversight and accountability of Medicare services. The court held that these responsibilities could not simply be delegated to HMOs or other forms of provider/insurance entity. They must be performed by an independent entity, either the administrative arm of the government itself or its agent.[33]

Second, these responsibilities imply institutional arrangements different from those currently available in order to achieve the levels of authority, responsiveness, and access to information that are necessary to carry out these due process requirements. Imagine the agency requirements needed to provide "immediate," often "informal" hearings that would reverse specific denials of coverage at the time a beneficiary is acutely sick in a hospital. Further, the courts imagine that these processes will be conducted with special sensitivities and techniques that take account of the fact that the beneficiaries are at risk, old, or disabled.

Third, the court recognized that the interactions of beneficiaries with HMOs present a number of new substantive requirements for protection, due process, and appeals procedures. For example, the court recognized that appeals processes must confront organizational decisions by HMOs as opposed to the traditional fee-for-service decisions made by individual doctors participating in Medicare. Interestingly (and reflective of the discussion in chapter 2), the appeals processes discussed in this case were a direct adaptation of Part A and Part B rules, not a new regulatory construct intended to take account of the differences posed by managed care delivery.

For their part, HMOs and managed care plans have tried in the courts to distance themselves from strong versions of an agency responsibility for enrollees. In a series of cases testing the malpractice liability of HMOs for negligence or error by providers, managed care plans have asserted that they are not responsible for the actions of providers: they are merely acting as a vehicle of employee benefits, not as a formal organizational instrument of health care provision. In legal terms, these plans have claimed that the Employee Retirement Income Security Act (ERISA) preempts claims against them, because they are merely acting as benefits administrators and are subject to the protections that federal ERISA provisions provide as a matter of law.

For example, in *Jass v. Prudential Health Care Plan, Inc.*,[34] Betty Jass claimed that the denial of rehabilitative care after knee replacement surgery resulted in permanent injury. Although the case raised questions of federal court jurisdiction as well as numerous other technical legal issues, the interesting feature of the case from an agency perspective is that Prudential claimed preemption from state law because it functioned merely as a benefit plan: any agency relationship that existed occurred between Betty Jass and the doctors involved, not the health plan. The plan merely "listed" the particular doctor who served Ms. Jass but did not bear responsibility for the doctor's actions even though the actual denial of care stemmed from a decision by a Prudential Health Care Plan utilization review administrator.

Although these cases present their own legal controversies, they also signal a major policy issue that is not only a by-product of legislative history but, more important, a reflection of the rapid evolution of new structures of insurance, medical managed care plans, and the provision of health care. In effect, these cases reveal that no definitive agency relationship exists for Medicare beneficiaries in this complex world of coverage, medical decision making, quality oversight, and accountability.

Health and Human Services argued in court in 1996 that it is not responsible for the actions of managed care vendors because they are private nongovernmental entities—providing services directly to beneficiaries—and not an extension of state action or responsibility. Managed care plans have argued in court that they are not responsible for the actions of doctors or other providers because they are merely health benefit plans, a conduit for monies going to providers and, therefore, should not be held accountable for the actions that ultimately are taken by providers.

The specific question of whether or not Medicare managed care plans are liable for damages caused by plan decisions has received varying interpretations by the courts (see *Pegram v. Herdrich*, *Pappas v. Asbel*, and *Przybowski v. U.S. Healthcare*).[35] For managed care plans generally, the *Pegram* decision appeared to provide some immunity (through ERISA preemption) for plan-level decisions but made clinical and mixed clinical/coverage decisions made by physicians subject to state law, in effect asserting the dual agency of physicians under the modern incentive arrangement in many plans.[36] For Medicare beneficiaries, the courts have found that the existence of Medicare coverage does not necessarily preempt beneficiaries from seeking relief under state laws. However, given the availability of Medicare grievance mechanisms, the courts are to look closely to ensure that state jurisdiction is appropriate (usually over cases of poor quality and actual personal injury) instead of relying on administrative responses and remedies that might be available through the Medicare program.

In May 2001, the California Supreme Court ruled in *McCall v. PacifiCare* that Medicare beneficiaries could sue in state court for denial of care.[37] George McCall had sued in state court in 1997 for PacifiCare's refusal to allow him to see a specialist, put him on a lung transplant list, or provide other care he believed appropriate. (Ironically, he ultimately received a lung transplant paid for by Medicare after he disenrolled from his HMO.[38]) In October 2001, the U.S. Supreme Court declined to review the California Supreme Court ruling, meaning that for the time being Medicare beneficiaries could continue to bring claims against managed care organizations to California state court.

All of this suggests that, as a legal matter, the agency arrangements—the mechanisms of finance, payment, information gathering and dissemination, and decision making—for Medicare managed care are indeed incomplete and not up-to-date with the structures of responsibility and delivery elsewhere in the market. The governmental sponsors for Medicare (Health and Human Services and CMS) are not designed for and do not claim responsibility for overseeing the quality and appropriateness of care provided by managed care vendors. The courts have left large areas of ambiguity in the legal accountability and mechanisms for redress by beneficiaries in managed care arrangements.

Sara Rosenbaum concludes that this legal experience implies a role for state courts in addressing quality-related harms but probably not a role in coverage and access disputes. Given this potential pothole in legal accountability for Medicare managed care, she urges the Congress to revise its mechanisms for external review of Medicare managed care.[39] The legal contests themselves are evidence of unresolved agency for Medicare managed care. The substance of these legal cases, as well as the positions that public agencies (e.g., CMS) and private plans have taken in fending off accountability and responsibility for care decisions, means that important aspects of agency are indeed missing in the design of Medicare's administration.

If the plans are to adopt this broader role of accountability for the health and social supports of their covered Medicare beneficiaries, then a parallel evolution in legal interpretations of accountability and liability for practice will be required. The balance that will be required is a mixture of independence and protection for plans to innovate and grow; the implicit or explicit setting of standards of practice that give beneficiaries legitimate expectations for performance of plans; the creation of well-functioning grievance mechanisms, whether judicial or not; and perhaps most important, an expectation of disclosure about coverage, services, and quality that gives beneficiaries and their agents valid bases for making plan choices.[40]

Toward a Model Medicare Managed Care Contract

Medicare's managed care plans already submit a contract under a prescribed set of rules.[41] These rules specify benefits to be provided, beneficiary and provider protections, reporting requirements, grievance procedures, expectations for renewals of the contract, and so forth. However, despite these details, Medicare's managed care program and contractual requirements lack a clear, coherent, and purposeful set of objectives. Just as payment for Medicare managed care was derivative of fee-for-service payment in a county, so the larger framework of contracting is derivative of traditional Medicare fee-for-service, not a new concept of health care purchasing, quality, and outcomes. As managed care approaches were politically brokered and changed, budgetary priorities, geographical considerations, and an emphasis on choice took over. Any coherent overarching objective and philosophy that may have existed for the HMOs was lost. Medicare managed care became a pastiche of plan types, disconnected budgetary and reimbursement concepts, and payment concerns.

What kind of Medicare managed care will further the objective of limiting the growth of per capita costs and increasing the appropriateness of care? A strong Medicare managed care regime, borrowing from the principles of a managed competition approach, would mandate (perhaps through some phase-in) that all beneficiaries enroll in a closed risk-based health plan. Each plan would compete for Medicare enrollees by offering the most attractive combinations of price, benefits, quality, and so-called amenities. Enrollees would be aware of the performance of these plans through accessible and standardized reports that include objective measures of utilization, outcomes, and satisfaction, as well as the marketing efforts of the individual plans. Plans would be required to participate in open enrollment, provide a minimum specified package of benefits, and satisfy a set of external standards for quality. In exchange, each plan would be paid a risk-adjusted payment that provides an actuarially fair compensation for the expected cost of that class of enrollee.

Such a scenario can be expected to produce a kind of competitive solution and is close to what was envisioned by the proponents of a managed competition approach. This strong version of a Medicare managed care solution requires plans and contracts with sufficient scale to overcome risk adjustment and selection problems, generate efficiencies of clinical practice, manage doctors, and produce valid measures of performance for the purposes of purchasing and accountability. This form of Medicare managed care would look much more like industrial production and less like individual boutique medicine. It would be highly standardized. It is remarkable how far from this standard the current Medicare managed care program is.

A useful place to begin reconstructing a Medicare managed care agenda is to return to the roots of prepaid health care and the HMO movement, with its attendant emphasis on population health, prevention, and an alignment of incentives for patients and providers to produce least cost, effective health services. The concept of Medicare managed care that follows from the contractual perspective in this book is *the purchase of agreed-upon health care for a population of beneficiaries, accounting for outcomes, at prepaid rates, for a unit period of time.* From an agency theory perspective, this contract requires clarity in the principal-agent relationship, clarity in the accountability and performance expectations of the plan, clarity and fairness in payment and risk bearing, and clarity in the reporting of information to enrollees and the public sponsor. Because this Medicare application of managed care involves many vulnerable enrollees, often with chronic conditions, the creation of individual beneficiary agency—the support of beneficiaries in making plan and health care decisions—becomes a central problem to be solved in the implementation of this model.

Specified Coverage, Process, and Outcomes

An important missing ingredient from the modern Medicare managed care regime has been assertive specification of the health program that is desired from providers. Many elements of this program can be specified in advance, but again the political process will have much to say about priorities and content. Despite the mixed history of outcomes research, report cards, and purchasing arrangements, it is possible to design a contract that incorporates both the public interest in particular health processes and outcomes and beneficiaries' interests in accessibility, satisfaction with service, and coverage. The theory presented in chapter 3 would have Medicare concentrate on writing outcomes-based contracts when possible and process-based contracts when clinical and supportive activities are programmable.

An initial list would include the obvious major health and social support threats to the aged and disabled population. Most of these are known, and even reflected in Medicare's current quality and information agenda, but have not been seriously promoted as the goals of purchasing in managed care arrangements. Neither have contracting arrangements been developed that reward plans for excelling and providing quality information about their care in selected domains of service. The initial list could build directly on HEDIS and Medicare quality priorities: health prevention and promotion (e.g., access to preventative services); quality cardiac care, including treatment for congestive heart failure; cancer treatment and screening (e.g., breast cancer screening rates); selected indicators of mental health service; appropriate diabetes care and follow-up; and appropriate end-of-life care (see chapter 5). Significant quality measures, including process-of-care and outcomes in some selected domains of care, would need to be developed for more effective contracting for Medicare managed care. Significant application of practice guidelines, especially in key areas of Medicare clinical concern and potential for disease management, can be part of the contracting process with plans. This is the implication of the theory of monitoring an agent's performance in a process-based approach to contracting.

Perhaps the most significant missed opportunity in Medicare's approach to managed care is the relative absence of systematic approaches to disease management, especially in selected areas of chronic care where the economic and quality-of-life payoffs to an organized program of care management can be substantial.[42] Christopher Tompkins and colleagues have described both the approach and potential payoffs to a Medicare disease management regime for patients with end-stage renal disease.[43] Their approach involves modeling the natural history or life course of the disease, screening and segmenting the population at risk for the purposes of targeting clinical and psychosocial interventions, implementing the proper administrative systems to ensure the necessary behavior change on the part of patients and providers, and supporting disease management through public policy that encourages prevention, efficient delivery, and quality monitoring. A great deal of wisdom about disease management has also grown up in fee-for-service settings through disparate but extremely effective provider initiatives designed to better coordinate care and provide organized forms of care management.

Comprehensive and long-term interventions of the type envisioned in the disease management/care management literature require a level of systems integration and oversight that is characteristic of both stronger contractual guidance of care as well as stronger forms of managed care on the provider side. In theory, the most promising managed care models for solving this agency problem in Medicare are variants of the social health maintenance organizations (S/HMOs) and Program of All-inclusive Care for the Elderly (PACE) demonstrations.[44] S/HMOs not only can shift much of the risk for medical costs to the agent, they also eliminate the opportunity to shift the costs of care to whatever reimbursement is available. Thus, there is no inherent incentive in an S/HMO to transfer a patient to a nursing home or outpatient setting merely to latch onto a new reimbursement source, because the contract spans medical, long-term care, and social service demands for care. S/HMOs help address the potential problem of moral hazard in the utilization of social and home-based services for the long-term care of enrollees. The provider has powerful incentives to find ways to limit the utilization of these services. Thus, the expectation is that effective case management would go hand-in-hand with S/HMO financing and organization.

As theory would suggest, one of the most contentious issues in the implementation of the S/HMO demonstrations has been the allocation of risks between the Medicare and Medicaid plans (the principals) and the providers (the agents). In order for the efficiencies of a capitated system to be realized, the providers must face something approximating full risk; if the agent realizes there will be slippage in the payment for service that accompanies increases in the costs of that service, the incentive to control costs will be loosened. In the case of S/HMOs, the issue was complicated because there was virtually no experience by which principals or agents could forecast the likely utilization and costs of the enrollees. As an indication of the vast uncertainty that accompanied these demonstrations, initially no private reinsurers would offer coverage for the losses associated with either costly individuals or bottom-line losses.

From a design perspective, S/HMOs represent a promising solution to many of the agency problems in Medicare. S/HMOs deal with information problems by aggregating choices over providers and care to the organizational level. Because S/HMOs place a girdle around the heretofore separate domains of ambulatory care, hospital care, skilled nursing care, and home care, they limit the possibilities for gaming separate reimbursement systems.

Five S/HMO models have been implemented and evaluated with mixed results. In the first round of demonstrations, begun in 1985, program evaluation indicated that S/HMO participants generated higher levels of nursing home use and home care use, but lower levels of hospitalization than the comparison group.[45] The demonstrations did not produce the expected higher levels of satisfaction or even the kind of integrated care that was anticipated. A troubling, though much debated, finding was that S/HMO participants had slightly higher mortality rates. Partly in response to these findings, a second generation of S/HMOs, so-called S/HMO IIs, were authorized, though only one out of the six proposed demonstrations was ever fielded.[46] A subsequent review of the combined experience of these demonstrations by Mathematica concludes that there is no evidence that S/HMOs produced better outcomes than the comparisons, cost more than Medicare+Choice plans with comparable case mix, or produced comparable levels of satisfaction to Medicare+Choice plans.[47] Indeed, the evaluation suggested that the payment methodology for S/HMOs amounted to a very expensive approach to producing very standard approaches and outcomes.

Although the overall message from this evaluation literature does not support broad adoption of this model in Medicare+Choice (and the Mathematica team concludes that Congress should not provide S/HMOs as a Medicare+Choice option), the reality is that the relative lack of experience and unmeasured factors in these models precludes any definitive conclusions about their broad applicability, even after all this time. The one S/HMO II plan, Senior Dimensions in Las Vegas and Reno, produced enough positive results in the organization of care and exhibited enough limitations in evaluation design to at least justify further demonstration and evaluation.

Evaluation results from the Program of All-inclusive Care for the Elderly (PACE) provide some further motivation for demonstration and analysis but still not a definitive statement of cost-effectiveness and benefit that full-blown adoption of this model would require. The goal of the PACE approach, modeled after the original On Lok community-based approach for care of the elderly in San Francisco, is to provide comprehensive care for frail and socially complex enrollees, relying on an integrated package of preventative, acute, and long-term care services. These demonstrations combined Medicare and Medicaid financing for this range of service. The original Abt evaluation of outcomes found numerous positive benefits and showed the expected substitution of outpatient and home-based services for inpatient and skilled nursing facility use. The subsequent evaluation of costs and payments suggested either modest savings (from what Medicare and Medicaid would have paid on a capitated basis) or a breakeven result. However, inferences from these evaluations were limited by numerous design and data limitations.[48]

Time

One of the basic problems of managed care contracting is the mismatch between the expectations for efficiencies in care and the time periods of both enrollment and payment. The short-run nature of the incentives and participation in managed care leads to the kinds of strategic behavior on the part of plans that has undermined enrollment and trust in managed care approaches for Medicare. Selection behavior, plan and beneficiary churning, "stinting," plan withdrawals, reductions in coverage, and precipitous changes in service areas are all symptoms of a poorly functioning Medicare contract, where strategic behavior, instead of activities that lead to long-term quality and cost reduction, is the main order of business. The BBA's requirements to lock in beneficiaries for a year provided a controversial but logical first step in aligning the incentives for clinical and programmatic interventions that provide longer term payoffs for beneficiaries.

A much more comprehensive approach, bringing managed care into the kinds of process and outcome contracts described in chapter 3, will be necessary for a fundamental change in plan behavior. A different longitudinal requirement for effective contracting will be stability in payment policy for plans and providers of managed care. In order for stronger versions of managed care to develop—models that include clinical integration of services, especially for chronically ill and disabled beneficiaries; health prevention and promotion approaches; and improved information systems and performance measurement—significant capital investment and organizational development is required. In order for plans to make these investments, both in people and systems, providers, plans, and investors will need confidence that the public sponsors will provide some stability of payment over time. The political backlash against managed care and the withdrawal of plans from the market make the prospect of such an investment unlikely. Absent this investment, it is hard to see a successful trajectory for Medicare managed care.

Risk Adjustment

The most difficult technical issue in Medicare managed care payment policy involves the specification and implementation of risk-adjustment mechanisms. Different classes of patients present varying levels of expected financial risk, or expense, to plans and providers. An older patient, on average, presents a higher risk than a younger patient; an individual with a history of chronic disease presents higher levels of risk to a plan or provider than an enrollee with no history. A patient with high medical expenses in the past year presents an increased risk of medical expenses in the next year. If we knew perfectly all of the predictors of medical expense in the coming year, we could compensate plans and providers for taking on these risks, and we would expect to observe little or no strategic risk-selection behavior.

An early Mathematica Policy Research study concluded that selection of healthier Medicare beneficiaries into HMOs significantly undermined the cost savings that could accrue to Medicare as a result of managed care.[49] HMO enrollees had lower use of health services (than their counterparts in fee-for-service) prior to enrollment, had higher self-reports of their own health status, had fewer limitations in activities of daily living, and had histories of fewer serious illnesses (cancer, heart disease, or stroke). The authors estimated that Medicare risk plans spent 10.5 percent less on enrollees in their plans than would have been spent in fee-for-service arrangements with a comparable population. More recent evidence paints a mixed picture of the effect of selection on Medicare cost savings.

Across a broad range of studies, Medicare HMOs appear to have drawn healthier enrollees than the average pool of fee-for-service enrollees, and enrollment and disenrollment appears to systematically move healthier enrollees into plans and sicker beneficiaries into fee-for-service.[50] The possibility that substantial selection of enrollees may be occurring raises questions about whether the claimed (or even potential) cost and efficiency gains of Medicare HMOs are real. Some evidence suggests that even though Medicare extracts a discount for enrollees in HMOs, it is possible that this discount is less than the expected use and costs of their demand for care when risk is taken into account. In other words, the discount for Medicare risk enrollees may be illusory, and the net effect of Medicare HMOs may be to increase costs to the program.

A considerable amount of research and analysis has gone into the question of appropriate risk adjustment for Medicare contracts.[51] The candidates for risk adjustment of Medicare contracts include the traditional measures of age and sex; self-reported health status; behavioral risk factors, such as smoking or excessive alcohol use; chronic disease; physician estimates or assignments of morbidity; or histories of medical utilization. Potential sources of data for risk adjustment include traditional claims records, encounter data, other administrative records, or specialized surveys. On its face, the standard model for risk adjustment, using just demographic variables, predicts a relatively small proportion of the variance in charges or other measures of expense, typically in the range of 5 to 10 percent.[52] However, when applied to groups, a relatively small number of adjusters can account for a large proportion of the across-group variance.

The data, administrative, and technical requirements of any sophisticated risk adjustment techniques are formidable. Moving from the traditions of claims-based, fee-for-service data, which characterize most of health services delivery and health services research, to get better estimates of true risk under a managed care regime is a major leap. It will be especially difficult to gather data on the costs of outpatient experiences of patients in managed care environments.

Perfect risk adjustment will never be completely feasible or necessarily even desirable. Very high risk groups would require extremely high capitation rates in order to fully compensate providers for taking them on. Truly fair rates for these groups do not currently exist in many real market situations.[53] At its limits, perfect risk adjustment approaches cost-based reimbursement, where providers or insurers are completely compensated for the expenses that different profiles of sickness or utilization present to them. A perfect risk adjustment solution might take away some of the "edge" of a risk-based payment system that encourages providers to engage in cost savings and search for efficiencies, especially for the few high-cost cases.[54] However, in the absence of perfect risk adjustment, protection of beneficiaries against provider behavior that either discriminates or adversely affects their health will continue to a be a major task for appropriately designing and overseeing a Medicare managed care contract.[55]

Under Medicare+Choice, a program to improve risk adjustment using diagnosis cost groups is underway. Numerous other strategies to modify or extend this program to improve risk adjustment are being debated: the use of partial risk adjustment methods, to be supplemented by payments based on actual cost experience; the use of adjusters that account for the functional status of older persons; and the use of outlier adjustments, for example. These methods represent an important technical agenda in Medicare reform. Better risk adjustment is essential to minimize risk-selection behavior by providers and improve the overall fairness of the program. A fair contract that does not induce risk selection or other deleterious, strategic behavior by plans rests on the ability to implement better risk adjustment.

The Congress mandated changes in the risk adjustment formula in the Balanced Budget Refinement Act of 1999 (BBRA) and the Medicare, Medicaid, and SCHIP Benefits Improvement Act of 2000 (BIPA). The most recent changes freeze the current risk adjuster at 10 percent of the plan payment until a new model for risk adjustment is ready to be implemented. CMS expects a new model to be ready in 2004 and then phased in over a subsequent ten-year period. The set of delays and difficulties experienced in the effort to achieve a sophisticated and fair approach to risk adjustment in Medicare payment policy—a critical ingredient in the creation of a fair and effective managed care contract—is an object lesson in the reality that *government administration is halting.*

Information

The management adage "what gets measured, gets done" provides the essential motivation for building a more systematic and useful framework for reporting on plan performance, especially on measures that reflect medical, long-term care, and social supports that are valued by the public and beneficiaries. The information requirements for a successful managed care experience differ from the information usually gathered by a beneficiary before entering into a traditional fee-for-service relationship with a physician or hospital and differ at all levels of decision making, from beneficiary choices about plans up to the federal certification of plans. Since the nature of the contract among beneficiaries, public sponsors, and providers is for a complete package of service over an extended period of time, the purchase of care is broader in scope and longer in duration under managed care. A Medicare beneficiary in traditional fee-for-service can go to the doctor, request a particular service, assess its quality and appropriateness, and then incorporate the information from the experience into the next treatment decision. The classic HMO beneficiary decision, by contrast, focuses on the selection of a plan: when the Medicare lock-in provisions take effect, he or she will be choosing coverage and organization of care (including choice of a physician) for a twelve-month period, based primarily on information about the performance of the overall plan.

The reality of most Medicare managed care arrangements is that the beneficiaries have relationships with individual doctors and relatively weak attachments to the plan as their agent. Many features of emerging managed care systems have attempted to strengthen this agency relationship with the organization, usually the health plan, as agent as opposed to an individual physician agency. Marketing materials emphasize location, affiliated hospitals, convenience, and other attributes of the service that are external to the individual physician. Marketing materials also emphasize coverage features of the plan, such as drug benefits. Reporting mechanisms, such as the Health Employee Data Information Set (HEDIS) standards promoted by the National Committee for Quality Assurance (NCQA) and CMS, reinforce this accountability for service at the level of the plan, not of the individual provider. The creation of a beneficiary-plan relationship, as opposed to a doctor-patient relationship, changes the incentive, risk, monitoring, and enforcement environment for beneficiaries. Nonetheless, the desire for beneficiaries to maintain their choice of personal physician illustrates the power and enduring role of physicians-as-agents.

A series of focus groups conducted for the Kaiser Foundation Medicare project revealed that the primary concern of beneficiaries not enrolled in an HMO was that they would lose their physicians if they enrolled. Secondary concerns included perceived low quality and the potential for hassle and access problems, such as the difficulty in getting through on the telephone. Perhaps just as interesting, the focus groups revealed a great deal of misinformation and lack of understanding of the Medicare managed care options.

Beneficiaries with traditional Medicare did not understand the supplemental benefits that would be available with HMO coverage, did not understand how federal payments would pass through to plans, and did not understand how the need for their Medigap coverage would be affected by HMO coverage. The level of understanding appeared to vary significantly by market: those beneficiaries in markets such as Minneapolis, with a high managed care penetration and longer experiences with HMOs, appeared to have much higher levels of general knowledge about Medicare managed care.[56] The discussions also revealed that high levels of knowledge and even positive attitudes toward Medicare managed care did not necessarily translate into the desire to enroll.

A significant body of research on the information needs and processing of information for health plan decision making has followed the development of the consumer movement in health care. This research raises fundamental questions about the viability of the consumer movement for health care generally, let alone among vulnerable Medicare beneficiaries. In making health plan choices, consumers have demonstrated limited ability to comprehend plan information in the form it is usually presented (e.g., marketing materials and report cards), to provide stable responses in the face of alternative framing of information or in the face of competing evaluations, to cognitively entertain more than a small number of variables or information sources at once, or to forecast health care needs or utilization. Because the decision research literature demonstrates how much information needs and cognitive processing vary from individual to individual, reforms that imagine a strong role for individual health plan and health care decision making will need to incorporate more explicit structures of intermediaries or agents to assure that reasoned decisions can occur.

The most recent regime of quality and information reporting on Medicare managed care began in 1996 with the development of the Medicare Quality Improvement System for Managed Care (QUISMC). These standards built on a set of negotiations and instruments that involved state Medicaid plans, insurance commissioners, representatives of health plans, and the NCQA. Standards and guidelines were further modified to take into account the requirements of the BBA, Medicare+Choice rules, and the BBRA.

Wrapping around the formal QUISMC requirements are a host of other quality assurance organizations, reporting requirements, and rules for plans. The NCQA requires plans to report performance measures under HEDIS that are mostly consistent with Medicare requirements. The Consumer Assessment of Health Plans Study (CAHPS), administered by the Agency for Healthcare Research and Quality, has become the basis for a consumer valuation of plan quality. Along with CMS regional offices, the Medicare+Choice

Quality Review Organizations have responsibility for overseeing a set of quality improvement projects on selected topics with Medicare+Choice plans.

What is the state of the art in reporting quality measures of plan performance? The 2000 HEDIS reports provide public data on numerous measures of plan performance, such as availability of language interpreters, rates of high cost/high occurrence diagnoses, rates of breast cancer screening, follow up after hospitalization for mental illness, rates of comprehensive diabetes care, rates of cholesterol management, use of antidepressant medications, treatment of high blood pressure, disenrollment, provider turnover, financial stability of the plan, physician payment arrangements, mental health utilization, chemical dependency utilization, and characteristics of the providers (e.g., percent of physicians that are board certified).

The reality of these measures is that many are not reported; many are difficult to interpret for clinical, epidemiological, and statistical reasons; and many show tremendous variation across plans and even variation in performance across measures within plans. As an example, these measures provided reports on the percentage of plan members with a diagnosis of acute myocardial infarction who received an ambulatory order for beta blockers on discharge. Out of a possible 302 plans, 107 plans did not have measures reported (primarily for statistical reasons), and 12 were not reported. Of the plans that reported, the use of beta blockers ranged from 34 percent to 100 percent.[57] Just this measure alone reveals the potential value of this form of reporting, as well as the work that still needs to be done.

Agency for Beneficiaries

In order for beneficiaries to successfully participate in selecting and managing Medicare plans and to effectively evaluate plan performance, new approaches must be developed for producing and interpreting health plan information. Development of the information tools for consumers has begun under CAHPS. However, making use of this information will require better understanding of the limitations and influences (such as cultural and experiential influences) on decision making for Medicare beneficiaries, new forms of communication, and new forms of outreach for beneficiaries. At the front end, beneficiaries need support in making initial plan choices. Ultimately, this will require the involvement of organizations and professionals with the capacity to work effectively and impartially with older and disabled persons.

Judith Hibbard and colleagues have emphasized the need for developing a legitimate role for intermediaries to assist consumers in making plan decisions and processing complex information:

Because of the difficulty of the cognitive skills required to use complex performance information, many consumers will be unwilling or unable to incorporate
this information into their choices. Even when the information is carefully pack-
aged and the decision process is incrementally structured, consumers may still
feel overwhelmed and confused. The fact that only 47 percent of the population
either is capable of performing only simple literacy tasks or is illiterate constitutes
a significant barrier. . . . Many of these consumers will explicitly or implicitly rely
on the expertise and choices made by intermediaries (e.g., benefits managers,
purchasing alliances, and advocates). If large numbers of consumers do not use
performance information, decisions at the intermediary level may become the
most consequential ones, both in terms of their influence on the market and in
how they shape the choices made by individuals.

Thus, a dual strategy is needed: one for consumers as end-users, who will
directly use performance information for plan choices; and one for intermediaries, who narrow the choices that consumers make and assist them in decision
making.[58]

Hibbard and colleagues have enumerated the challenges in constructing
beneficiary agency in their extensive work on the requirements for informed
health care decision making.[59] Consumers may have limited capacity and motivation to deal with the information overload that is associated with rational
decision making about complex plan choices. Expert intermediaries themselves may have difficulty in managing the complexity of information that is
involved. In cases in which the expert intermediaries have relationships with
plans or providers, consumers will also be concerned with potential conflicts
of interest, one of the classic problems of structuring agency relationships.

A review by the Institute of Medicine of possible institutional approaches to improving the agency and communication with Medicare beneficiaries examined media (print and electronic); public agencies, such as area
agencies on aging; community and consumer-based organizations; counseling programs; health plans; employers and business groups; health plans; and
a number of nontraditional ideas, such as using libraries and information
kiosks.[60] In the past, private, nonprofit, age-based organizations such as AARP
have considered taking on an intermediary role for beneficiaries. An interesting group of for-profit firms is emerging to provide assistance to caregivers
looking for quality home care and personal care services. CMS has expanded
its advertising, Web presence, and promotion of a 1-800 help line. At present,
however, there is no obvious single model for implementing systematic
beneficiary agency on a national or regional level.

The state of the art in conceptualizing and implementing the information and decision-making support that would be necessary for informed managed care choice is still primitive. The creation of active and appropriate beneficiary communication will take a measure of organizational invention and the creative use of existing resources and supports for beneficiaries. Because these interventions and communications will need to engage vulnerable and elderly patients in making health and life-plan decisions, often with medical complexities and complicated family and social circumstances, the development of this agency capacity for successful managed care will be a substantial policy undertaking in its own right. Some beneficiaries, by virtue of conflicts and disagreements within their families, will present complicated issues of decision making. Some beneficiaries with Alzheimer's disease or other cognitive deficits will require further supports, though as Robert and Rosalie Kane have pointed out, they may still retain the capacity to express their preferences for certain forms of care.[61] Nothing is more central, however, to the viability of exercising "choice" and making legitimate use of information on plan coverage, quality, and performance, than the design of good agency arrangements at the level of a beneficiary's real-life experience.

Conclusions

Standing back from the details, what is so intriguing about the Medicare managed care experience is that the program is at once so near, yet so far, from a progressive and innovative mode of financing and delivery of care that implements principles of a sound contract and effective agency. Conceptually, Medicare is near to having a model of care that (1) envelopes the social and long-term care dimensions of care (such as that modeled in the S/HMO and PACE demonstrations); (2) emphasizes care management and quality initiatives, especially around selected disease areas, such as congestive heart failure; (3) informs beneficiaries about the performance of plans in delivering services of concern to beneficiaries (e.g., access to preventative visits, availability of language interpreters, reporting rates of prostate screening, etc.); and (4) captures efficiencies in organization and delivery through the competitive actions of plans. However, in practice, these features of managed care are often so elusive or incomplete, and the payment and participation in the Medicare+Choice plans so unstable, that there has been no momentum toward or broad acceptance of managed care approaches, either by beneficiaries or the industry. Indeed, Medicare managed care enrollment is declining, not expanding.

Medicare's experience with managed care so far should give pause to those who imagine a wholesale and rapid conversion of the program to Medicare+Choice options or other alternatives to Medicare fee-for-service.

For reasons that are not completely understood, Medicare beneficiaries have not "gotten with the program" of managed care even after a long period of gestation. In many states and markets, structural barriers such as low population density will limit the extent and rapidity of the managed care transition, especially for Medicare beneficiaries. In other places, where both the population and market characteristics are favorable, the fitful development of managed care generally and the policy instability surrounding Medicare models have inhibited the uptake of Medicare+Choice plans.

A great deal of emphasis has been placed on technical refinements of the payment mechanisms as the vehicle for expanding participation in managed care. Until recently, payment for Medicare managed care has been calibrated to payment for fee-for-service health care in counties. This framework carries obvious perverse incentives and inequities from place to place. Changes in payment policy resulting from the 1997 BBA, the 1999 BBRA, and the 2000 BIPA have broken this link somewhat and begun to introduce better risk adjustment into payment, however halting. However, managed care payment is still largely divorced from the "true" cost structure of managed care delivery and the outcomes of service. Administratively determined payment systems can close this gap only so far, and with the priority of geographic fairness in the politics of recent managed care payment reforms, there is little hope of closing this gap under current arrangements. In order to get closer to the ideal of a competitively determined pricing and payment system, considerable experimentation, technical development, and administrative experience must be gathered. This is why the political stalemate over the competitive pricing demonstrations, described in chapter 2, is so consequential.

Better adjustments for differences in risk among plans is undeniably a critical step toward broadening the participation of vendors, providing equity in payment, and assuring access to managed care for beneficiaries who may have histories or signals of high medical costs. The issues involved in reforming payment policy and adjusting for risk in Medicare managed care are conceptually and technically difficult, but essential for eventually designing an effective Medicare managed care contract.

So long as relatively weak organizational models of managed care, such as PSOs, represent simple holding companies for fee-for-service style medicine, then few of the innovations in practice, clinical resource management, and service quality that have been promoted by managed care advocates will occur. So long as managed care products feature weak incentives (internally for physicians), little organizational discipline and loyalty, and liberal options for out-of-network use of services, then the potential for cost savings and behavioral change will be extremely limited.

The behavior and results that have characterized Medicare experience with managed care are predictable from the incentives and pressures that force providers to produce care at low cost. The strategies that have been employed to date flow directly from these incentives: reduce costly inpatient admissions and stays; shift care to least-cost settings; use lower cost personnel (e.g., primary care physicians instead of subspecialists, social workers instead of psychiatrists); substitute pharmaceutical approaches for procedures, evaluation, and therapy; and utilize administrative screens and techniques to challenge the use of certain kinds of services.

Medicare's current initiatives to nationally orchestrate payment levels, beneficiary education, and regulation of managed care plans from a national platform are likely to continue to produce unsatisfactory results. A defining feature of the uptake of Medicare managed care is its local and regional character. A defining characteristic of provider innovation under the broad rubric of managed care has been the use of a variety of incentive arrangements for physicians to reduce costs, improve quality, increase enrollee satisfaction, reduce turnover, and so forth. The ability to microregulate these incentives down at the plan level will be extremely limited and often counterproductive, especially when undertaken from a national perspective. Chapter 7 will argue that this role is best carried out in the context of regional administration of the program, where information and management can be more closely held, and the prospect for active engagement with plans and providers is more likely.

In agency terms, the success of Medicare managed care requires attention to the design and organization of a solution to the two-principal problem at the core of a managed care approach. For Medicare managed care to realize its potential as a vehicle of organizing and paying for systems of care for beneficiaries, considerable effort will need to go into conceptualizing and defining the contract that guides plan behavior. This means the creation of information, outcomes, and monitoring systems that largely do not exist now. CMS, or its administrative successor, must assume the role of a principal in this contract, paying for and demanding performance of a contract for service. Beneficiaries will require a significant upgrading of the supports and information—their own agency—available to them to make effective use of plans. Finally, for managed care to work in Medicare, plans must also assume the role of the formal organizational agent for care, in both the legal and service-delivery senses of that role.

A significant long-term challenge for Medicare managed care will be the development and promotion of new models of payment (incentives), accountability, and support of beneficiary agency that are appropriate to serving geriatric populations with chronic and disabling conditions, limitations on mobility and functioning, and complex bundles of medical and social needs.[62] In many respects, Medicare and Medicaid face similar challenges in adapting managed care to populations with special health care needs. Very few examples of successful managed care for these populations exist. The early optimism behind S/HMO and PACE models has not borne fruit in definitive evaluations, significant market penetration, congressional uptake, or further dissemination of these models. Without this form of innovation, however, Medicare managed care may well fade even further, to be seen as a contentious and largely ineffective effort at cost containment that did not realize its larger potential. At a minimum, these innovations deserve a serious, well-designed, and appropriately resourced research and development effort.

The artificial heart represents medical technology at its most mindless.

—*New York Times* editorial

All too often, health reforms transfer wealth from individuals in their 30s, burdened with heavy taxes and the expenses of raising families, to their more affluent elders with clogged arteries who could have and should have taken better care of their own health.

—Richard Epstein

I realize that death is inevitable, but also I realize that if there is an opportunity to extend it, you take it, and that is what I did.

—Robert Tools, first recipient of a self-contained artificial heart

CHAPTER FIVE

A Medicare Parable: Technology and the Artificial Heart Story

The Role of Technology in Health Reform

Technology growth and technology assessment occupy an uncomfortable place in health policy discussions. The consensus opinion among leading health economists and health policy analysts holds that technology growth is a major culprit in the escalation of medical expenditures.[1] Despite this consensus, it is difficult to pin down the specific sources, quantitative significance, and trajectories of cost-increasing technologies in a way that is useful for policy. Joseph Newhouse has made the principal argument that technology constitutes the most important engine of expenditure growth, but the evidence for his argument is indirect: he believes that technology is the most likely residual explanation for expenditure growth after all other plausible explanations—such as demography, health insurance, practice patterns, prices, and volume—have been taken into account.[2] Because some technologies are cost saving, some induce additional services to be provided to patients, and some raise quality of care, the macro-observation that technology is raising costs does little to help guide case-by-case decision making about what innovations should be adopted and paid for.

Unlike many components of health expenditure growth, such as the aging of the population, medical technology is perceived to be at least somewhat controllable by policy intervention. Yet for all of its consequences, health policy makers and health services managers have used precious few tools for prudently managing technology growth. Medicare shares in this dilemma: the program has been more a captive of technology growth than its master. Beneficiaries confront new technologies at the point of delivery; at the time they are aware of the possibilities of breakthroughs, such as new imaging technology, new medical devices, or new pharmaceuticals that their physicians have prescribed or recommended.

Two schools of thought have dominated the policy discussion about managing the growth of technology in medicine. Some analysts believe technology is something to be prudently controlled, that forethought and technology assessment can be employed to make good choices about which technologies should enter into the health care pipeline and ultimately be paid for. An alternative school of thought believes that medical technology growth is inherently difficult to predict or control, and thus regulation will be futile, or worse, counterproductive. This school believes that no amount of analysis or wisdom will permit regulators to make good choices *ex ante* about which interventions will work, what they will cost, or how they will be received by doctors and patients.

Technology is rapidly changing the nature of medicine and the content of health services delivery. If technology growth has been an important source of cost escalation in health care and Medicare in the past, new scientific advances that will fuel the growth and intensity of health services in the future are already working their way through stages of testing and clinical introduction. Advances in genetic research are leading to many new screening approaches for disease, as well as targeted drug therapies for many diagnoses. In the short run, the ability to screen for a specific disease, however, will be a double-edged sword. Testing will allow for costly detection of certain genetic tendencies without the results giving the full clinical implications of this tendency, much less giving guidance about appropriate and cost-effective interventions to go along with this knowledge. The early experiences with screening for prostate cancer with prostate specific antigen (PSA) and the tentative identification of genetic markers for breast cancer (BCRA) illustrate this dilemma.

Other advances in biology, such as tissue engineering, are opening up fantastic new possibilities for organ replacement and harvesting. Advances in clinical technologies—imaging for diagnosis and new applications for lasers and scopes for procedures, as well as new materials and miniaturization for implants—mean that medicine will be able to be more accurate, less invasive, and more appropriately responsive to challenging clinical presentations.

Technology advance is not the province only of advanced high-tech medical centers—tremendous change in the equipment and devices available for home health care are also in the pipeline. The development of nonmedical appliances, such as robotics for home health applications, have potentially large implications for Medicare and its beneficiary population in addition to some of the fanciest genetic and biotechnology advances. All of these innovations have their costs.

A second general concern about the march of medical technology is the potential access and equity problems that new hardware and new procedures present. The payers of medical care are extremely wary of entitling beneficiaries to new medical interventions, especially if the costs are high and the efficacy has not been demonstrated. Depending on what type of insurance individuals have, they may or may not have access to new forms of surgery, transplants, or new drugs. Experimental procedures are excluded in virtually all plans, but the reclassification of an intervention from experimental to accepted practice is often a judgment call that will be made at different times by different plans. If Medicare moves along the spectrum toward more of a defined contribution model, and less of a defined benefit model, the possibilities for differential access to new technologies multiply.

Still a third general concern about technological progress in health care is our seeming inability to forecast and manage the large societal consequences that are associated with new technology. On one side of this debate are the technological imperialists, who believe that technological progress is a good in itself and that bureaucratic efforts to control progress are counterproductive and threaten our international leadership in science. On the other side is a group of modern day Luddites, who see extreme dangers in technological progress and who advocate much stronger planning, assessment, and regulation of technology.

This chapter considers the implications of one of the new technologies in the pipeline, the total artificial heart, and a related family of technologies, ventricular assist devices. The artificial heart is an excellent example of the generic problem of technology management for Medicare because (1) its ultimate clinical efficacy is uncertain and subject to a relatively long process of refinement and improvement; (2) the demand for such a technology among the Medicare population is potentially enormous—many persons with end-stage heart disease are theoretically potential candidates; (3) its adoption reflects economic, political, and ethical considerations; and (4) if successful, it belongs to a class of technologies that "create a clinical ability to treat previ-

ously untreatable terminal conditions by some long-term maintenance therapy, where unit cost, patient volume, and changing epidemiology drive costs.
The treatment of diabetes, end-stage renal disease, and acquired immuno-
deficiency syndrome (AIDS) are examples."[3] A successful total artificial heart
program would create a new class of Medicare survivors with subsequent
needs for medical and long-term care services.

The development of the artificial heart is important for the argument in
this book in that it represents a prototypical technology contracting problem
for Medicare: it illustrates the problems of dual interests in coverage, the need
for a new structure of agency at the congressional and individual levels, and
the need for a coherent approach to purchasing. Finally, the culmination of total artificial heart technology will represent an important Medicare resource
allocation and policy problem in its own right: it has been estimated that the
artificial heart will be eligible for full FDA approval in about the year 2005, precisely when the baby boom population will be crossing the threshold to eligibility for Medicare coverage.

A Primer for Technology Assessment

In order to understand the policy design issues in Medicare's adoption of new
technologies, it is necessary to build on some basic definitions, concepts, and
theory of technology diffusion. It is also important to understand Medicare's
current approaches for coverage and payment of new technologies, though in
many specific cases the policy and management approaches are idiosyncratic.

New technology in health services can take the form of new procedures,
new devices, or new drugs. Within these categories lies a heterogeneous collection of biotechnology, materials, medical appliances, administrative mechanisms (such as modern information systems), and clinical interventions. To
further complicate matters, many of the advances in medical technologies
emanate not from some linear and observable chain of events in medical research and development but, instead, grow out of applications of ideas, material, and approaches developed in some other arena of science or engineering.
Although discussion about technology growth in medicine has traditionally
been associated with new and sophisticated surgical approaches, such as endoscopy or laser surgery, innovation in procedures can be fostered by much
less dramatic changes in the ability to process information or other changes in
care management.

Technology is a flow, not a stock. At any moment in time, technological
improvements are in various stages of development from the seeds of an innovative idea in basic research, to halfway and three-quarter technologies already

in widespread use. Some technologies will be cost reducing, leading to lower cost and more effective health services. The standard theory of technology diffusion envisions new devices or procedures moving through a predictable cycle of early and often experimental high-cost/low-volume use followed by increasing clinical acceptance and decreasing unit costs. Because technologies have their own life cycles, it is often not useful to label a device, procedure, or drug as cost saving or cost increasing from a snapshot in time. Technologies that are cost-increasing substitutes for other approaches to care often become cost-saving approaches as they mature and increase their volume. The first electronic calculators were very expensive substitutes for slide rules; over time their unit cost decreased to the extent that sophisticated calculators are now given away as marketing promotions. Drug therapies often exhibit more complicated patterns of diffusion because of the routines of testing, approval (and nonapproved use), and patent protections.

Pipelines by which technologies come to be perfected and adopted for payment can be extremely long and idiosyncratic, not amenable to management and regulation. Richard Rettig's account of how hemodialysis and renal transplantation came to be candidates for Medicare coverage and payment begins in both cases at the turn of the century.[4] Dialysis became viable through incremental changes in surgical technique (e.g., subcutaneous shunts); drugs (e.g., heparin); materials (e.g., Teflon); and mechanics, spread over time, place, and industrial settings. Kidney transplantation became possible through parallel developments in surgery and improved immunosuppressants. The ability to deliver end-stage renal disease services evolved through largely separate funding and demonstration efforts in the National Institutes of Health (NIH), Public Health Service–funded centers under the Kidney Disease Control Program, the Regional Medical Programs of the late 1960s, and the Veteran's Administration. By 1972, all of the pieces could be assembled into a benefit: the technology existed to produce a clinically beneficial service that demonstrably saved lives, and an organized delivery system had been geared up.

The growth of medical technologies can, in theory, be controlled in three ways. If the market for medical care functioned competitively, the growth and demand for technologies would be driven principally by consumer demand and willingness to pay. Pharmaceutical and medical device companies would bet on the effectiveness of their future products and would allocate their research and development portfolio so as to maximize profits subject to the constraints of consumer (and physician) demand. Even in the face of insurance, consumers would contract with third-party payers who limit their expenditures on new devices and products.[5]

Because medical innovations often come out of basic research sponsored by the government, a pure market-driven solution to the growth of technology is neither feasible nor appropriate. As Kenneth Arrow demonstrated more than thirty years ago, the inherent uncertainty of research and development, the increasing returns to investment in research with scale, and the difficulties of limiting access to information will lead societies to underinvest in research without governmental intervention.[6] This centrality of government research and development support to the development of new technology means policy has a more strategic role in managing the sector than in most other markets. Traditionally, the management of health sector research and development, primarily through the NIH, has occurred at some distance from the management of the costs and priorities of the health sector. Since the values and long-term purposes of particularly basic research are primarily driven by knowledge development, good reasons have separated decisions about the NIH portfolio from the more strategic and relatively short-run concerns of health policy. As will be demonstrated later in this chapter, however, this separation can produce serious downstream consequences for the Medicare program.

The standard criteria for technology assessment include assessing risks, costs, benefits, and effectiveness. Depending on the application, these criteria will be combined into formal risk-benefit, cost-benefit, or cost-effectiveness analyses. Cost-effectiveness analysis allows a new technology to be weighed in a common metric, such as years of life saved, against other alternative uses of the same resources.

It is necessary to understand two somewhat technical refinements of basic cost-benefit and cost-effectiveness analysis for applications to Medicare-covered technologies. First, many interventions produce benefits beyond saving lives, and the ability to conceptualize and measure these effects will be crucial to the ultimate assessment. Even when the principal benefit will be a life saved, the quality of life associated with that intervention is a crucial dimension of the value of the service. A technology or procedure that saves a life but leaves the patient in a persistent vegetative state or in chronic pain with no ability to function socially has lower value than a procedure that restores the patient to perfect functioning. The necessity of calibrating cost-effectiveness measures for these quality-of-life differences has given rise to techniques that, for a cost-effectiveness analysis, adjust the value of the year of life saved for the quality of life associated with that intervention. The most common of these measures, the quality-adjusted life year (QALY), provides a weighting or adjustment for the life year saved.[7] If the resulting condition of the patient were a state of perfect functioning (without pain or limits in social or other function), the year of life saved would have a value of one. If the resulting condition left the patient in a condition that he or she judged to be equivalent to death, then the resulting year of life saved would have a value of zero.

Second, the technical ways in which future costs and benefits are treated and valued in a population of older persons will have a significant effect on the ultimate quantitative assessment of costs and benefits. The arithmetic reality of most interventions affecting Medicare beneficiaries is that they will generate a relatively short stream of future benefits because life expectancy in old age is by definition so low.[8] In addition, the accounting for all of the future costs of treatment, including those unrelated to the intervention itself, is the theoretically proper standard for cost-benefit assessment.[9] Thus, if an individual with end-stage heart disease is saved and subsequently demands expensive cancer treatment, then the total cost of care incurred is properly attributed to the original cardiac treatment itself. The somewhat macabre economic reality is that the subsequent cancer treatment would not have occurred if the patient had died from the original presenting heart disease.

These technical issues of using QALYs and cost-effectiveness assessment present themselves in the artificial heart case I discuss later in the chapter. A significant issue in evaluating the merits of artificial heart technology will be the quality of life associated with living with a mechanical device after the operation. These patients will inevitably experience subsequent morbidity, some of which is associated with the procedure and the device, some of which is the natural by-product of living longer and having future opportunities to get sick. To date, the Medicare program has developed no institutional resources that combine scientific, economic, and ethical dimensions to consider these questions.

The Governmental Context of Technology Assessment

The difference between the principles and the practice of technology assessment is large.[10] The United States has never been effective or aggressive in technology assessment or regulation. Susan Foote's analysis, for example, illustrates how efforts to control costs and expand the liability system run headlong into governmental values of safety, innovation, and access to new devices.[11] Indeed, the closing of the Congressional Office of Technology Assessment (OTA) in 1995 symbolized the ambivalence the Congress has had about prospective evaluation and control of technologies. A small bureaucratic cemetery could be created in memory of agencies created to conduct technology assessment and subsequently disbanded.[12] Organized public technology assessment has long gone on in the FDA under its authority to review drugs and, more recently, medical devices.[13] The National Center for Health Care Technology was established in 1978 and closed because of lack of funding in 1982. The Office of Health Technology Assessment, formerly housed in the National Center for Health Services Research and then in the Agency for Health Care Policy and Research (AHCPR), was also supposed to advise on Medicare technology policy. It was eliminated in the most recent AHCPR reorganization. The Congressional Office of Technology Assessment was disbanded in 1995 as a result of budget reductions. The Institute of Medicine (IOM) closed its Council on Health Care Technology in 1990. As a result, the United States has no formal mechanisms for national technology assessment; indeed, the United States and France are the only major industrialized countries without a major agency of technology assessment influencing national health policy making.[14]

Although occasional discussions and analyses of technology occur in the Congress's Medicare payment commissions, the General Accounting Office, and the Congressional Budget Office, these are largely ad hoc and descriptive. In the private sector, a variety of targeted technology assessment projects go on among the associations (such as the American Hospital Association [AHA]), in large insurance and managed care companies, and in specialized consulting firms. The growth of pharmacoeconomics within pharmaceutical firms and among a group of specialized consulting firms represents the demand for more sophisticated cost-effectiveness justification for FDA approval and for acceptance into drug formularies.

How Medicare Decides about New Technologies

Medicare's basic approach to paying for new technologies was established in the original law in 1965. In general, medical services reimbursed by Medicare must be "reasonable and necessary," further defined as "safe and effective, not experimental, and appropriate." The task of determining what services are safe and effective is carried out by the FDA. In reimbursement, technology growth is treated differently in hospital, outpatient, and physician payment systems. A recent analysis by Susan Foote demonstrates the overwhelming obstacles that Medicare has faced in trying (over twenty-five years) to implement a rule that operationalizes this congressional standard to pay for what is reasonable and necessary. She describes this situation as a case of "regula mortis," or a dead rule.[15]

Until the merger of the two Medicare commissions, the Prospective Payment Assessment Commission (ProPAC) was responsible for evaluating a group of technologies believed to be significant drivers of hospital costs and that have the potential to improve the quality of patient care. These selected technologies must also be midway in their process of diffusion, affecting be-tween 5 and 75 percent of the relevant class of Medicare patients. On the basis of judgments about the cost-increasing effects of these technologies and the number of beneficiaries that will use them, the commission made recommen-dations to the Congress about the percentage increase in Medicare hospital costs attributable to scientific and technological advance.[16] ProPAC also at-tempted to take into account a number of other considerations in its final rec-ommendation to Congress: the importance of small technology advances not covered in their formal analysis, the expected response of patients and doctors to change, the influence of external market conditions, and outcomes findings.

ProPAC reports that since 1996 it has adopted a more "qualitative" ap-proach to these assessments. Between 1987 and 1997, ProPAC recommended increases in operating payments to hospitals of 0.3–1.0 percentage points for scientific and technological advances. For fiscal year 1998, the commission recommended an update of 0.4 percent for scientific and technological ad-vance, based on a review of changes in cardiovascular drugs, devices, and procedures; radiology, imaging, and nuclear medicine; biotechnology; and management information systems.

For physician payment, the reforms that were begun in the Omnibus Reconciliation Act of 1989 (OBRA) required HCFA to take into account changes in technology when recommending annual updates for the volume performance standards. The PPRC and other bodies have attempted to ac-count for the influence of new technologies on individual physician practices, but the conceptual and measurement issues involved in these estimates have been daunting.[17] Although a general update was provided in physician pay-ment, it had about the same level of underlying justification and analysis as the hospital payment update. In neither case were technology payment poli-cies used strategically to alter Medicare's coverage and cost structure.

Changes in the 1999 Balanced Budget Refinement Act (BBRA) and the 2000 Benefits Improvement Act (BIPA) required HCFA to update its payment methods for both outpatient and inpatient services to better account for new technology.[18] As it stands now, Medicare payment takes account of new tech-nologies for payment purposes in a variety of ways: if large, new capital outlays characterize the organization and practice of medicine, increases may be re-flected in the base payments; if particular procedures associated with specific diagnoses involve expensive new technologies, increases may be reflected in changes in the relative weights given to payments in those categories; if a par-ticular new technology is associated with a narrowly defined procedure or di-agnosis, reclassification of the case or changes in coding may be undertaken. For example, in Medicare's outpatient payment system, certain ambulatory payment classification groups that are influenced by new, high-cost drugs, bi-ologicals, and medical devices are identified for specific pass-through pay-ments as supplements to the basic payment.[19] BIPA required HCFA to develop new methods for incorporating technology into hospital payments through classification and coding, to collect data on the costs of new technolo-gies with the goal of reassigning cases to payment groups, and to provide a form of pass-through payment to hospitals that takes account of new technol-ogy, but in a budget-neutral way.[20]

In 1994 HCFA proposed to formally require cost-effectiveness analysis in a limited way as part of decisions to expand coverage. HCFA (CMS) indi-cated it would be "flexible" in its definition of cost effectiveness and would not require such analyses in every coverage decision.[21] Under current policy, CMS makes coverage decisions subject to the Administrative Procedures Act, a cumbersome process involving numerous steps of due process and public comment. The effect of this process is to delay the uptake of new coverage even when it may be effective and cost saving and to prolong coverage of pro-cedures and devices even after they are obsolete.[22] In 1998 HCFA established the Medicare Coverage Advisory Committee to formally review in a public process the merits of covering new technologies in the areas of medical and surgical procedures; drugs, biologics, and therapeutics; laboratory and diag-nostic services; diagnostic imaging; durable medical equipment; and medical devices and prosthetics. The new process involves explicit criteria for decision making. The early experience of this process has been mixed, with concerns raised about the lack of standardization in the process, the quality of underly-ing evidence, and the lack of connection to coverage decisions and costs.[23]

Taken together, these mechanisms represent a largely passive and weak effort to incorporate technological advances into Medicare coverage, payment, and informational approaches. On the payment side, small percentage in-creases in payments are justified by broad assessments of technology, and some internal technical adjustments to coding practices and weights may also be justified. On the coverage side, the resources and institutional support pro-vided to the Medicare Coverage Advisory Committee are an appropriate but extremely modest beginning along the path toward evidence-based technol-ogy assessment, not to mention the broader consideration of cost, ethical, so-cial, and political implications of new technologies.

The Artificial Heart

No emerging technology more dramatically illustrates the policy dilemmas that underlie the growth in the intensity of health care in Medicare than the development of the artificial heart. This development illustrates the inherent role of politics, the potential societal and program consequences of a passive approach, and the weaknesses of congressional (and Medicare's) institutional supports for undertaking technology assessments.

The significance of the artificial heart also stems from the prevalence in the population of severe coronary disease, which is responsible for about 700,000 deaths annually. The quest for an implantable total artificial heart foreshadows the difficult ethical, clinical, and financial decisions that will arise in decision making about access to other innovative therapies for the aged. The artificial heart debate is also important for symbolic reasons, for its potential impact on the health of persons with severe cardiac disease, and for the statements it makes about the priorities we attach to different health care claims from basic prevention to dramatic end-stage interventions. The artificial heart is an extraordinary issue because it conjures up a set of literary and cultural images that give special significance to the human heart. It also represents (in the same way that space exploration does) the very frontier of technology in the public eye. Largely for these reasons, the media has covered and propelled the artificial heart in a way that it has done with few other technological developments.

The development of the artificial heart has progressed right to the cusp of a clinically effective, broadly usable device. Ventricular assist devices, designed to support the pumping of the heart, have been in widespread use since 1994, when the FDA approved the first device for use as a bridge to keep a patient alive until a human heart became available for transplant.[24] In the United States, three devices with different mechanical properties—the Heart-Mate, Thermo Cardiosystems, and Novacor assist pumps—have provided substantial opportunity for clinical investigation and testing en route to a permanent device, even though they were originally approved as temporary implants. Numerous patients have returned to work and other activities with the artificial heart devices, and there have been reports of some candidates actually being successfully weaned from the pumps after a period of respite for their damaged hearts. Still, significant clinical obstacles and quality-of-life issues remain.

History

The quest for a total artificial heart has been long and halting. Development began in the late 1950s at the Cleveland Clinic, with the first federal funding granted in 1964. Since then, federal support of the artificial heart program has been dispersed over projects targeting the development of emergency-assist devices, partial-assist devices (mechanisms to provide pumping support in either the left or right ventricles), and a permanent, implantable, total artificial heart. All told, the federal government has devoted more than a billion dollars in funding the development of mechanical-heart technology.

The recent era of total heart implants began in 1982 when Dr. William DeVries implanted a Jarvik-7 artificial heart in Dr. Barney Clark. The operations and subsequent experiences of Barney Clark and William Schroeder received enormous media exposure and professional reaction, much of it negative. Barney Clark's low quality of life was distressing and received widespread public attention, raising visible questions about the ethics of this experimentation.

While a moratorium on permanent artificial heart implants was in place, the use of artificial implants as a bridge to the transplant of a human heart was widespread and clinically successful. However, significant ethical questions have been raised about the number of these bridge procedures, their clinical management, and the priority that bridge patients receive in the allocation of scarce human hearts.

Bureaucratic and corporate interests also drove the evolution of the artificial heart. The actions and interests of large institutions, such as the National Heart, Lung, and Blood Institute (NHLBI), the arm of the NIH responsible for administering the federal program of research in this area; the Food and Drug Administration (FDA); large university programs; and a number of private corporations were driving forces behind both the underlying basic science and clinical applications. In the early days of experimentation with total hearts, the Humana Corporation invested enormous sums of its own private capital in a program with a goal of experimental implants for a hundred patients. The debate over the future of the total artificial heart quickened in the spring of 1988, when the NIH announced that it would suspend public funding of four major contracts for the development of the total artificial heart. This announcement drew immediate and forceful response from strange bedfellows, Senators Orrin Hatch and Edward Kennedy, both from states receiving substantial federal research dollars for development of the artificial heart.

Under threats that the NIH would lose considerable autonomy over their own research decisions, the leadership of the NIH capitulated and reinstated the contracts. The *New York Times,* in an unusually strong editorial, accused Kennedy and Hatch of "terrorizing the National Institutes of Health" and engaging in the manipulation of contracts "in a way that lards their own pork barrels."[25] The openly political debate over the federal funding of the artificial heart program reinforced a long-standing concern by many observers that the development of the total artificial heart was being conducted without sufficient public debate, scientific and ethical scrutiny, or oversight. A 1991 Institute of Medicine (IOM) study of the total artificial heart program, reported extensively below, came to the somewhat curious conclusion that although the technology would produce higher costs for lower benefits than any known procedure in use, its development should proceed.[26] The news account of the IOM report in *Science* carried the byline: "An Institute of Medicine panel says the device may be a bad social bargain but recommends further federal research anyway."[27]

After this report, the technical development of an artificial heart and related ventricular assist devices progressed rapidly. Substantial progress occurred in the miniaturization, reliability, and endurance of the mechanical components. Innovations in materials for membranes in the devices have been extraordinary. In addition, a great deal of clinical research and testing has been devoted to managing the problems of bleeding, clotting, and infection that plagued the early implants.

Development of artificial heart devices has been carried out by three consortia. Pennsylvania State University and 3M Corporation, the Texas Heart Institute and Abiomed, and the Cleveland Clinic Foundation and Nimbus are all testing and developing new devices. Each of these devices provides separate pumps for each ventricle, wireless transfer of signals and electrical power, pumps that are directly implantable into the chest, and power supply and electronic canisters that are implanted in the abdomen. Animal testing and refinement have been underway with testing in humans already receiving limited approval from the FDA. The Jarvik-7 evolved into the CardioWest Total Artificial Heart and is now the subject of an FDA Investigative Device Exemption that allows testing in six heart transplant centers. The original Jarvik-7 was implanted in 198 patients through 1992, and its successor, the CardioWest Heart, was implanted in 86 patients between 1993 and 1996.[28] In 2000, a more recent successor to the Jarvik-7, the Jarvik 2000, was implanted in a patient in Israel.

On July 3, 2001, the first of AbioMed's AbioCor artificial hearts approved for testing by the FDA was implanted at Jewish Hospital in Louisville, Kentucky. The titanium and plastic device, about the size of a grapefruit and weighing less than two pounds, is powered by an external battery pack. The stated expectation for the first round of experimental devices is for patients to live to sixty days, effectively doubling the life expectancy of these patients who have no other options.[29] Press reports indicated that the hospital was deluged with calls from individuals looking for information on how and where they could have the surgery performed. Depending on the success of the FDA approval process, AbioMed anticipates having their artificial heart ready for commercial distribution in 2004.

Despite this tremendous scientific progress, there continues to be little serious debate about the long-term consequences of this technology for potential recipients, public program costs, or public health more broadly. A Medline search for 1993–2000 did not uncover a single article addressing policy, economic implications, or social implications of artificial heart technology.

In political parlance, the artificial heart program has "big mo," big momentum, for the development of a viable implantable device. Large institutional, corporate, and political interests are now firmly aligned with the future development of this technology. The competition to develop a compact, reliable, and durable total artificial heart is now international and it is fierce.[30] Although the technical problems facing development of the artificial heart are formidable, they pale in comparison to the ethical, social, and economic dilemmas that the availability of this technology represents. With the current special interests behind the artificial heart program, it is hard to imagine how the development of this technology could be derailed. Despite formidable clinical obstacles, the pursuit of a total artificial heart will go ahead. Beyond the clinical development lies the hard work of shaping a social policy response—particularly a policy response for Medicare—to the availability of this technology.

Costs and Demands

Developing a reliable, compact, and clinically effective total artificial heart implant will continue to require significant public expenditures, first in research and development and then in reimbursement for health services. Candidates for ventricular assist devices and total artificial hearts include individuals with congestive heart failure (brought about by coronary artery disease and numerous other causes) and viral infections of the heart. Patients may have either failure of their left ventricle's ability to pump blood through the body's arteries, the right ventricle's ability to pump blood to the lungs to be oxygenated, or both. Heart transplantation has been an important and increasingly clinically successful treatment for a limited group of patients with end-stage heart disease. However, only about two thousand hearts become available for transplantation each year. Especially for older persons, the availability of appropriate hearts at the right moment is extremely limited, and some evidence suggests that the availability of organs for transplants varies considerably by sex, race, health insurance coverage, and other socioeconomic characteristics in addition to age.[31]

In addition to transplantation, significant progress is being made with new drugs, new surgical procedures, new devices for electrical stimulation, and more speculative research on xenotransplantation, cellular transplantation, and tissue engineering. The effect of all these innovations on reducing the ultimate pool of candidates for mechanical devices is unknown. Many of these interventions are likely to postpone, but not necessarily eliminate, the need for mechanical assistance.

The size of the potential population of heart recipients who would be candidates for mechanical circulatory support devices ranges from the IOM 1991 estimate of 35,000 to 70,000 cases annually, to a more recent National Heart, Lung, and Blood Institute (NHLBI) study group estimate of 35,000 to 105,0000, depending on coverage, financing, clinical criteria for transplantation, and the availability of the clinical services to perform the procedures. How many of these patients would be candidates for a total artificial heart is difficult to quantify, largely because the effectiveness of various forms of partial ventricular support is unknown. For example, some cardiac specialists believe that left ventricular assist devices, if implanted early enough, would preempt the failure of the right ventricle. The IOM committee estimated that by the year 2010 between 10,000 and 20,000 patients with end-stage heart disease would need total artificial hearts, with another 25,000 to 60,000 eligible for other forms of mechanical assist devices.[32] The NHLBI study group estimated a total pool of 100,000 patients for long-term, out-of-hospital mechanical assistance, with perhaps a population of 5,000 to 10,000 as candidates for a total artificial heart.[33]

The costs of artificial heart implants include the costs of the device itself; the costs of the medical procedures, personnel, and hospitalization; and the costs of subsequent care. The 1991 estimates of the costs of the device were $100,000 in the base case. Hospitalization for the period surrounding the operation costs $57,000, and other evaluation costs amounted to $45,600, assuming four patients evaluated for each successful candidate for surgery. Thus, the total initial costs of an artificial heart amount to about $200,000 per patient. Estimates of the initial cost of the AbioCor device (from the company itself) were $75,000 for the device, and $175,000 for the procedures.[34]

The IOM's assessment of the lifetime costs of an artificial heart, taking into account survival and subsequent health care costs, amounts to $327,600 per patient, discounted at 3 percent per year. The cost per quality-adjusted life year was estimated at $105,000 when compared with conventional medical therapy for patients with end-stage heart disease.[35] Given the available estimates of potential recipients and expected costs, this technology would impose on society new medical costs of $2.5 to $5 billion annually.

Obviously, the costs and social diffusion of the technology will be profoundly affected by the age and other clinical criteria that are ultimately chosen. In addition to age criteria, the availability and generosity of Medicare reimbursement will affect the diffusion of the total artificial heart. Gregory de Lissovoy has examined the impact of the availability of Medicare reimbursement for heart transplants and found that economic incentives have affected judgments about the suitability of patients at different ages. He observes that "prior to Medicare's coverage decision, financial realities reinforced the clinical rationale for selecting only younger patients. Now the federally insured sixty-five-year-old patient is on an equal footing with his or her privately insured juniors."[36]

The interpretation of cost estimates is a microcosm of the larger debate about the costs and trade-offs of spending on health services. Some observers see the artificial heart as a huge new extension of the health care industry, an engine of increased costs without justification. Others point out the obvious trade-offs with access to care for the indigent, public health, and primary care alternatives. Comparisons have been drawn between the cost of a single implant and the number of days of hospital care that could be purchased, the amount of preventative programming that could be offered, and the numbers of indigent people who could receive basic health insurance. The imagery on the other side is equally compelling: the costs of the artificial heart have been favorably compared to now accepted procedures such as liver transplants, the purchase of nuclear submarines, or relatively small fractions of other governmental undertakings with very questionable social benefit. These expenditures compete with other possible interventions both for heart disease and more broadly for improving the public health.

Daniel Callahan has argued that the pursuit of the artificial heart sends out the wrong signal to policy makers concerned about the cost implications of providing health insurance. "Fear of uncontrollable government expenditures has frightened legislators and others away from any national health insurance program. . . . The trouble is the [artificial heart] research may be a success, and the heart will become a required part of any health care program. Programs of this kind would scare off possible supporters of a good national health insurance program."[37]

Decisions about eligibility and access to this technology, particularly for older individuals with end-stage heart disease, will be a significant public policy contest played out over the next ten years. This issue will eventually be most sharply brought into focus when Medicare is forced to rule on coverage and reimbursement for total artificial heart technology. At that time policy makers may be staring at a technology that has the potential to extend the lives of thousands of older individuals. Although the critics of the end-stage renal disease (ESRD) program in Medicare will holler that a similar "mistake" is being made, the pressure to expand coverage will be politically very difficult to resist. In ESRD, the dilemmas were prototypical: a new technology, a claim made on public resources, a variable potentially eligible population, and an eager group of providers ready to capture the reimbursement made available by this new entitlement. As in the case of the artificial heart, lives were hanging in the balance.

Quality of Life

The highly publicized cases of Barney Clark and William Schroeder in the mid-1980s had a chilling effect on the early deployment of artificial heart technology and heightened concerns about the ultimate quality of life for recipients. In the subsequent use of ventricular assist devices and bridge hearts, significant complications have included bleeding, kidney failure, infections, respiratory failure, and clotting.

For the patient with an artificial heart, the reality of being dependent on machinery for basic organ functioning may bring on profound depression or emotional distress. Complex psychological issues, such as the patient's own body- and self-image, the patient's reaction to the reaction of others, and the potential stigmatization that go along with these devices may occur. Predicting how all of these many reactions will play out is especially difficult in light of the cultural and symbolic significance of the human heart. In early generations of artificial heart technology, the equipment will continue to be relatively bulky and cumbersome. Like many other devices that provide life support (e.g., mechanical ventilation), the possibility of failure and the uncertainty of the technology bring anxiety and emotional worry for the duration of the patient's life. Of course, all of these reactions will be conditioned by a host of factors, such as the spiritual values and social supports of the patient.

In the IOM study, a detailed assessment of quality-of-life considerations was also produced in order to evaluate the potential cost effectiveness of artificial hearts. The IOM committee examined the literature and experience of patients with organ transplantation, with other implanted devices, and with the initial artificial hearts.[38] The IOM study identified the need for consistent information about the health status, quality of life, and cost implications of the technology for the various parties involved: patients, clinicians, and payers. The committee believed that one of the more subtle determinants of the psychological effects of artificial hearts (and thus its effects on quality of life) will be its societal acceptability. Its societal acceptability, in turn, will be determined by the evidence and public sense of the cost worthiness of this intervention. This suggests a health policy version of a Catch 22: if early quality of life is perceived to be low, the social stigma and public perception of the artificial heart will subsequently undermine the quality of life of subsequent recipients.

The IOM study produced quantitative quality-adjusted life year (QALY) estimates as inputs into its broader cost-effectiveness analysis. The analysis took into account physical health states (e.g., vitality, physical activity, time in bed), mental health, social and role functioning, self-care responsibilities, and survival expectancy. The analysis also took into account the time that recipients would spend in hospital and intensive care unit settings. The estimated mean utility level for total artificial heart recipients was 0.66 in an average state, compared to 0.75 for a human heart transplant patient and 0.08 for a patient with conventional medical treatment. As discussed earlier, these estimates compare to QALY benchmarks of 1.00 for a state of perfect health and 0.00 for a state equivalent to death. Taken together, the cost and QALY estimates indicate that the artificial heart would cost $105,000 for each additional QALY gained over conventional therapy.

Already the artificial heart has had an underground life of development and application, with some impressive publicity leaking out. Although left ventricular assist devices have been used in trials and as bridges to transplants, stories exist of elderly patients who have successfully utilized artificial hearts, including patients who have subsequently been taken off the mechanical assist devices. Dr. Mehmet Oz of Columbia has reported on numerous patients who have returned to work, including a jazz musician who went out on a concert tour with his early implanted assist device.[39]

Medicare Policy Making for the Artificial Heart

The artificial heart story illustrates the weakness of our institutions and tools for technology assessment. Part of this problem is the usual situation of fragmentation of responsibility over unconnected domains of the federal government. The National Heart, Lung, and Blood Institute, the Congressional Office of Technology Assessment, the FDA, HCFA, the National Center for Health Services Research, and ProPAC, as well as extragovernmental bodies, such as the National Academy of Sciences, were all potential players in the game of technology assessment. As it has played out, not one of these agencies provided substantial leadership in assessing the large-scale ethical, social, and economic implications of this technology. Since the 1991 IOM study, the National Heart, Lung, and Blood Institute has provided the most significant analyses, but its mandate is primarily to assess the scientific merits of pneumatic research on cardiac assist devices. Rather than fault these agencies, however, perhaps a different lesson could be drawn from this experience: technology assessment is inherently indeterminate and politically vulnerable when mounted from a national, bureaucratic platform such as the Office of Technology Assessment or Agency for Health Care Policy and Research.

However, Medicare's ability to decide on coverage and payment for new technologies is a fundamental issue for its future costs, effectiveness, and political sustainability. Medicare's ability to make prospective decisions about coverage and payment for mechanical cardiac assist devices is a good test of its larger ability to manage the costs and ethical implications of the broader panoply of new technologies in the pipeline. Should Medicare pay for technologies whatever their cost? Should Medicare pay for new interventions and devices that have low initial quality of life, even if they are lifesaving? What thresholds of costs and quality of life, if any, should guide Medicare coverage and payment decisions? What freedom of choice should be extended to beneficiaries who are willing to pay for either experimental interventions or interventions that have extremely high cost-to-QALY ratios?

Gregory De Lissovoy's finding is extremely important for understanding Medicare's policy problem in allocating resources to new technologies. The artificial heart story potentially exhibits the classic pattern of technology diffusion and adoption: (1) technology is developed as a basic scientific hill to climb; (2) the technology is deployed and becomes clinically effective through trials; (3) a "vanguard" of patients gains access to the technology; (4) through political logrolling, Medicare beneficiaries become eligible for a clearly effective technology that saves lives, but at high cost; and (5) with reimbursement, access equalizes for Medicare versus other eligible candidates.

A useful place to start in thinking about Medicare's process and organizational resources for evaluating new and uncertain technologies such as the artificial heart is to reflect on the basic theory of Medicare's agency. Medicare decisions have two interested parties: the beneficiary and taxpayers. If beneficiaries were enrolled in a purely private insurance arrangement with no public principal, then carriers would cover new technologies in the short run that met the tests of accepted medical practice—not experimental—and did not represent a new category of covered services. In a world with rapidly changing technology, perfectly informed consumers might demand plans with significant option features, where new services would be covered with higher premiums or substantial copayments to control costs. Over the longer term, conventional policies would incorporate new technologies as they became medically accepted and demanded by doctors and enrollees.

In practice, though, beneficiaries are not confronted in advance with the prospect that they may have choices to make about therapies with different probabilities of success, cost, and quality-of-life consequences. By the time one has end-stage heart disease and the technology is available, the value that individuals (and society) will place on saving a named life is almost unlimited.[40] Simply put, an individual with end-stage heart disease will have no other lifesaving choice but a human transplant or mechanical assist device. As Robert Tools explained his decision to participate in the AbioCor trial and become the first recipient of a fully self-contained artificial heart, "I had no choice, I knew I was dying. My doctor told me." The alternative is palliative care and short-term therapies, often delivered in intensive care units.

From the theory I presented in chapter 3, disinterested taxpayers would support the inclusion of services and technologies that produced substantial externalities. Devices that increased social functioning, drugs that reduced infectious disease, therapies that improved mental health and quality of life would presumably be on society's short list of demanded new technologies.[41] Some technologies will simply produce widely different assessments of benefit for society and for individuals. Still other interventions may be highly valued by beneficiaries but not deemed deserving by the Congress and administrative decision makers.

Since public budgets are limited, then both taxpayers and beneficiaries may reasonably expect that cost-benefit and cost-effectiveness tests would apply to the adoption and payment for new technologies. New devices, interventions, and drugs with high costs that fail to produce externalities and maintenance or improvements in quality of life become much more difficult to justify. As Richard Rettig has demonstrated, however, Medicare currently has virtually no administrative or political machinery with which to weigh these considerations.[42]

Linking Technology Assessment to Policy, Payment, and Practice

Technology growth can theoretically be controlled "at the wellhead," where applied research and development occurs, or "at the pump," where administrative and clinical decisions are made about acquisition and use of new devices, procedures, and drugs. The advantage of controlling technology at the wellhead is that, with properly executed control, society would not waste resources on unproductive research and development, clinically ineffective services, or poor outcomes. Unfortunately, such control requires the administrative wisdom of Solomon, in which the development and application of science can be perfectly forecasted, its diffusion perfectly predicted, and its costs and benefits known far in advance.

Such control also presumes that technology assessment can be a fundamentally rational process, not undermined by the influence of economic actors with a commercial stake in the product, the self-interested decisions of politicians with pork-barrel interests in research funding and commercial development, or the scientific community's motives for advancement and credit. The history of technology assessment and even the narrow case study of the artificial heart recounted in this chapter demonstrate that such expectations for a rational and deterministic process of technology assessment are naive. Here again, politics and rational policy analysis meet head on. Lehoux and Blume's study of technology assessment in different countries and contexts reinforces this idea that assessment is an inherently political undertaking.[43] Their recommendations involve broadening the disciplinary bases for technology assessment (including the political environment), as well as creating new organizational homes for this form of policy guidance:

> HTA [health technology assessment] should be informed by perspectives that discern what is at stake when a technology is developed and promoted by engineers and manufacturers, used by health care providers, introduced into patients' lives, paid for by third-party payers, and preferred over other interventions. This entails (1) an effective broadening of the disciplinary perspectives upon which HTA is relying, (2) the renewal of research methods that are used, (3) the redesigning of the organizational structures in which HTA is produced, and not least of all, (4) a fundamental reconsidering of the nature of technology, which remains HTA's main object of inquiry.[44]

Control of technology "at or near the pump" means that new mechanisms of payment, risk bearing, and even rationing will need to be accepted as part of the Medicare contract. Instead of thinking of each new technology as an item to be added to the list of entitlements or eligible for increased reimbursement, a much more purposeful process of discovery, analysis, decision making, and administration will be necessary. No simple solution will be completely adequate to address this prospective problem of determining the merits of particular technologies, the boundaries of experimental versus warranted coverage, or the range of choices that should be afforded to individuals in the gray area of unproven technologies. But for sure, such a process of assessment will not occur unless organizational invention occurs: where there is no accountability for the costs of new technology entering the system, or where the accountability is diffuse, no agent will surface to make the hard choices that technology management at the pump necessarily entails. An agency approach can help in determining the respective roles that can be played by federal administration, Medicare purchasing, individual choice, and provider behavior.

Prudent purchasing of new technologies requires the following elements. First, careful selection of technologies needs to be undertaken in advance by Medicare administrative and policy-making arms. In other words, setting priorities is required. Charles Phelps and Stephen Parente's test for expected gain in technology assessment provides useful guidance for such selection: analysis will produce valuable information for those technologies that (1) affect large numbers of potential users, (2) will have high unit costs, (3) have high levels of uncertainty, and (4) have a marginal cost that is likely to decline as use expands.[45] My artificial heart example meets all of these tests for useful and valuable technology assessment.

Information about the relevant clinical indications, costs, risks, benefits, quality-of-life implications, and effectiveness of emerging technologies will be a necessary but not sufficient ingredient for technology management. Such assessment is technically difficult and needs to be closely linked organizationally to the decision making about coverage, payment policy, and information for beneficiaries. This is a version of Eisenhardt's closing the distance. Because this information has a substantial public good character, it needs to be publicly subsidized and managed. Indeed, the growth of pharmacoeconomics on the private side of the drug and device industry is an important signal of the necessity for relatively objective and disinterested analysis to be fed into the decision process for Medicare. A large industry of private health technology assessment has grown up with uneven methods, some significant conflicts of interest, and no necessary connection to public priorities.[46] The virtual hegemony of the industry over technical information as devices and interventions develop is an example of information asymmetry, which places consumers, payers, and administrators at a distinct disadvantage in ultimately making prudent coverage decisions.

Second, payment constraints need to be apparent to the agency responsible for administering Medicare, as well as to the providers and plans that will bear risk. One of the great insights of Burton Weisbrod's analysis of the linkage between insurance, payment mechanisms, and technology is that constraints that are imposed at the point of service delivery (through such mechanisms as managed care and prospective payment) have a way of signaling back to basic, private-sector decisions in research and development.[47] Although Weisbrod looked at the apparent chilling effect of managed care and reimbursement policy on research and development with great concern, the lesson of this story should also give policy makers interested in mediating the cost effects of technology growth some reason for optimism.

If Weisbrod is correct, there is a form of market intelligence built into the technology pipeline. Implementation of strict prospective payment and other utilization constraints means that plans and providers bear the risk of bringing on new equipment, devices, procedures, and drugs. A better solution for both developers and payers of health services would be an evidence-based system for technology assessment, not simply the blunt instruments of prospective payment. As Rettig has pointed out in his analysis of managed care arrangements, the existence of financial risk motivates both the utilization of health technology assessment and decision making about coverage and payment.[48] John Eisenberg has described many of the benefits of linking technology assessment to coverage and what he calls the "community of practice."[49]

The experience with diagnosis-related groups (DRGs) provides some preliminary evidence that, indeed, prospective payment policies will affect the rate of diffusion of new devices with desirable and undesirable consequences. Cochlear implants, a new and more expensive alternative treatment for counteracting hearing loss, was never fully deployed because it was assigned to a DRG that did not pay its average costs, at least for the early period of its use.[50] Scientific evidence had demonstrated its efficacy, FDA approval was granted in 1984, and large numbers of Medicare beneficiaries with the requisite hearing loss to make them candidates for the implant were available. After a protracted debate about the proper payment category and amount, cochlear implants were eventually assigned to a relatively low DRG in 1988. Medicare paid for only sixty-nine implants nationwide in 1987, leading 3M, the original manufacturer of the device, to discontinue marketing and further research. Three of the original five manufacturers that won FDA approval for the device left the market.

Eisenberg has also emphasized the importance of bringing together many of the disparate federal resources for technology assessment.[51] While Eisenberg was mostly interested in bringing together the disparate federal intellectual resources for technology assessment, there are also interesting strategic questions in technology assessment that cross agency boundaries. For example, under current arrangements, Medicare (as a payer) often bears the burden of decisions made much earlier in the determination of property rights and subsidies provided to a new technology. An interesting version of this problem of property rights and public subsidy occurs at the time that research is ready to bear fruit in commercial application. In the case of the artificial heart, the interesting question will be the terms under which the total artificial heart is brought to market, given that a substantial portion of the development costs have been borne by the National Heart, Lung, and Blood Institute (NHLBI), a public entity, and a substantial payer for the technology is likely to be the Medicare program, a public entity. The expert panel discussion has recognized the difficulty of this role for the NHLBI and has recommended that the subsidy for research and development for the total artificial heart be diminished as the device gets closer and closer to market. The broader question of how the public interest and, more specifically, Medicare's interest in issues of funding, patients, and pricing will need much more attention in technology assessment as science, commercial interests, and clinical practice are increasingly intertwined.

Technology and Beneficiary Agency

The introduction of new and dramatic technology, such as the total artificial heart, illustrates a more general shortcoming in beneficiary agency in Medicare. In the theory developed in chapter 3, decision making about high-cost, first-generation technology, such as a total artificial heart or ventricular assist device, falls into a category in which the beneficiary's interpretation of the merits of a particular technology may conflict with that of the Medicare principal as represented by the Congress. What is interesting, however, is that we do not know what decision fully informed beneficiaries would make about the use of a particular technology such as the total artificial heart after they have fully considered the costs, quality of life and social functioning, the uncertainty of outcomes, and so forth. It may be that with proper agency for beneficiaries, this category of health care decision would fall into quadrant II rather than into quadrant I (see table on page 73). With proper information and support for decision making, Medicare beneficiaries and the Medicare program may actually come to the same choices about the desirability of an artificial heart as the public sponsor or principal. Empirically, we know precious little about how decision making for high technology care would be affected by alternative forms of beneficiary agency.

Because decisions about new technologies, whether they be about emerging pharmaceuticals, devices, or procedures, involve a complex interplay of personal, family, and clinical considerations, new forms of organization for beneficiary agency will be needed to fully support beneficiary decision making and care. An example of sophisticated beneficiary agency in the current delivery system is the interdisciplinary teams that have been organized to work with patients and families in complex transplantation procedures, such as liver transplantation. Numerous issues arise in these cases—the suitability of the candidate for an organ transplantation in the first place; the patient's receptivity to the psychosocial, medical, and behavioral consequences of the transplantation; and the adequacy of the patient's support system. These cases can be even more complex where financial, cultural, or religious issues come into play. Seemingly small considerations, such as translation and medical literacy, can derail or complicate well-informed decisions.

The best transplantation services involve interdisciplinary teams of surgeons, primary care physicians, nurses, social workers, and, from time to time, other allied health professionals, such as ethicists or spiritual advisors working closely with the patient and his or her family. What is interesting about these services is how variable they are; provision of these services generally depends on the motivation and leadership of the clinical and administrative staff in a given health care system, not contractual requirements or incentives provided by the payers.

In order for Medicare beneficiaries who are facing care involving high technology to have these forms of agency available in a systematic way, versions of a process-oriented contract would be necessary. These contracts would look most like the "bundled" or package payment arrangements currently in existence that specify the preoperative, procedural, and postoperative services required in order for payments to be made. While this would require innovation in the contractual approach that Medicare brings to its purchase and payment for health services, it may be warranted in selected procedures such as the high technology cardiac procedures envisioned in this chapter. Even in strict cost-benefit terms—not to mention the powerful clinical and ethical arguments for grounded decision making in these cases—the benefits of proper agency and support for beneficiaries may be tremendous compared to the costs of devices, procedures, and follow-up care to implants that were ill-considered.

Conclusions

The artificial heart story represents a kind of parable for Medicare and technology. It illustrates the inherent political character of technology development (in this case involving the industry, academia, and legislators such as Hatch and Kennedy), the information asymmetry between public and private interests, the weakness of organizational agency for assessing technology, the weakness of beneficiary agency, and the potential downstream consequences for Medicare as the family of assist devices, including the total artificial heart, get ready for commercial introduction.

A 1994 workshop on the total artificial heart, organized by the National Heart, Lung, and Blood Institute, produced the following conclusions (among others), which remain valid for responding to the development of ventricular devices and the total artificial heart:

- Decisions for research support, development, and application of new and evolving technologies are political processes serving a wide variety of public and private interests. There is currently no systematic method of coordinating and integrating these various interests. It is appropriate that attempts be made to establish a mechanism of managing this complex array of interests.
- Analogous to the developing mechanisms of managing the delivery of medical care, there should be a mechanism for managing technological development and applications.
- There will, in the foreseeable future, be a sizeable population that could derive benefit from effective long-term mechanical circulatory support.
- The development of an effective total artificial heart (TAH) is technically feasible within five to ten years.
- Cost-effectiveness analysis is a useful method to guide decision making throughout the investment phases of innovative medical technology development.
- The funding of clinical trials should include long-term information on the quality-of-life and economic effects imposed upon patients and their families.[52]

Medicare needs to develop substantial capacity for prospectively assessing significant new technologies, such as the artificial heart, as they unfold. It is not sufficient for the Institute of Medicine (IOM) or any other distant actor to study these technologies as an abstract problem of science policy. The impressive 1991 IOM report devotes only three pages to Medicare-related issues in artificial heart technology, and even there the analysis is quite general. For example, the report simply asserts that "Medicare, in particular, can be expected to scrutinize [the artificial heart] closely because many of the potential candidates for TAHs and VADs will be Medicare beneficiaries; the Medicare program is likely to be required to pay for more MCSSs than any other third-party payer, if it decides to cover broad MCSS applications."[53] The report does not consider the mechanisms or criteria that Medicare might use to conduct this scrutiny or make hard decisions.

As this story demonstrates, the Medicare program has no significant institutional capacity to plan, evaluate, incorporate in benefits and payment, or ration significant new technologies in any systematic way. Moreover, the program has virtually no institutional capacity to collaborate with the other significant actors in technology development, such as the NIH, in assessment and technology policy.

The treatment of technology is in many ways a microcosm of the larger reform challenge for Medicare. A two-step process is necessary. First, legislative and executive leadership of the program must engage the public in a long-term and ongoing discussion of the risks, costs, benefits, ethics, and societal impacts of new technologies. The artificial heart illustrates the need for this discussion in a dramatic form. The closest recent example of such a public deliberation occurred in response to the president's decisions (and open engagement of the issues) about the use of stem cells in research.

An even stronger version of this public deliberation would take into account the trade-offs that will be necessitated by the adoption of many new high-cost interventions. New biologics, drugs, tests, and devices will be competitive with our financial and organizational capacity to provide "low-tech" approaches to personal care, chronic care, long-term care, and community supports for beneficiaries. Making these judgments is the practical work of deriving the modern Medicare social contract.

Second, significant development of organizational agency to perform technology assessment must be created for the Congress to carry out its role as a prudent principal over the Medicare program. Logically, the nexus of accountability for this process of assessing the artificial heart and other significant evolving technologies should be an arm of the Congress, such as a reconstituted MedPAC or its administrative sponsor, the GAO. Other experiences with technology assessment in the Congress, such as the Office of Technology Assessment (OTA), have always had the property of being at arm's length from economic or coverage decisions in Medicare. Thus, the specific audience for the assessment was never obvious. Moreover, interest group opposition and criticism of technology assessment findings (particularly findings critical of new technologies) never had a countervailing force, a pure public interest in the results of technology assessment. Finally, this case illustrates another weakness of agency at the level of individual beneficiaries in the Medicare program. With new technology, even when reimbursed, the capacity of beneficiaries to make "good decisions" becomes the paramount issue. New technology adds uncertainty, quality-of-life issues, and often high cost to the mix of already difficult clinical, family, and ethical considerations. Building new supports—including the involvement of new professionals and agency at the bedside—will be a critical reform in service delivery to accompany the organizational changes in the government's capacity for technology assessment. Only when capacity has been built all along the pipeline of technology diffusion can we expect more prudent resource allocation and use of new technologies such as the artificial heart.

Life is a play with a badly written third act.

—Molière

It's not that I am afraid to die. I just don't want to be there when it happens.

—Woody Allen

CHAPTER SIX

A Medicare Contract for End-of-Life Care

A "Good Death"

A good death occurs when we have control over the timing and means of our passage, when we are surrounded by our loved ones, and when we are relatively free of pain.[1] David Eddy's controversial account of the death of his own mother—expressed in her own words after numerous surgeries and treatments—eloquently illustrates this goal at the individual level: "I've lived a wonderful life, but it has to end sometime and this is the right time for me. My decision is not about whether I am going to die—we will all die sooner or later. My decision is about when and how. I don't want to spoil the wonder of my life by dragging it out in years of decay. I want to go now, while the good memories are fresh. Help me find a way."[2]

As will be demonstrated later in this chapter, this seemingly simple request for a good death is exceedingly difficult to honor in American health care. The forces of medical practice, reimbursement, and the organization of care often conspire to wrest control of this passage from patients (and their families), to escalate the level and invasiveness of care in the period leading up to and the moments near death, and to situate the experience in hospitals, often in intensive care units—56 percent of decedents age twenty-five and older die in the hospital,[3] and another 19 percent die in nursing homes. The limited data we have indicates that 40 to 70 percent of adults who die each year suffer unnecessary pain, and 10 to 30 percent have their wishes ignored by providers.[4]

End-of-Life Care and Medicare

Medicare and the larger public are not disinterested parties to these decisions: 12 percent of the national health care budget and 28 percent of Medicare expenditures are attributable to end-of-life care. Roughly 80 percent of all persons who die in the United States are covered by Medicare.[5] As in other forms of Medicare provision, the geographical variations in practice are tremendous, indicating that there is some potential gain in efficiency, appropriateness, and quality of care from closer scrutiny and better contracting for care at the end of life. Indeed, much of what we know about the epidemiology and medical costs of those who die comes from examination of Medicare data, yet we have converted little of this information into purposeful policy for improving the quality of end-of-life care.

Statistically, many beneficiaries will face end-of-life decisions in the near term, not as some distant abstraction. The life expectancy for an eighty-five-year-old white male is 5.1 years; for a white female, life expectancy is 6.4 years (for nonwhites life expectancy is slightly longer at older ages). Recent estimates from the Mortality Follow-Back Study indicate that about 216,000 older persons who died in 1990 experienced little or no decline in physical or mental functioning during the last year of life. However, about 169,000 decedents experienced both physical and mental impairments and were institutionalized for the majority of their last year of life. About 100,000 decedents ages eighty-five and older experienced serious physical impairments and required assistance through much of their last year of life.[6]

On their own, many of these beneficiaries will not prospectively take steps to manage the course of their end-of-life treatment. The only formal requirements that Medicare will place on them will be to question the existence of an advance directive at the time they enter the hospital or join an HMO. Some will not choose to create formal or informal advance directives because they are essentially comfortable with the expected treatment arrangements, because they are myopic, or because they exhibit more deep-seated denial. All of this suggests that the agency problems are central: to create the structure of information and incentives that will bring patients and providers together to do something they would not necessarily do of their own volition.

Second, improving the appropriateness and quality of care at the end of life will require detailed and technical work on payment policy, information, and the organization of care, albeit through a different lens than has characterized Medicare policy to date. This is why Joanne Lynn's work, reviewed at the end of this chapter, is so provocative. It raises questions about whether progress can be made in improving Medicare-sponsored end-of-life care without more general reform affecting the chronically ill, whether they be labeled terminal patients or not.

As it currently exists, the Medicare payment policy creates numerous obstacles to coordinated, palliative, home-based care in situations where the beneficiary and her or his loved ones would desire it.[7] Separate payment systems, none with particular incentives for encouraging the elements of palliative or supportive end-of-life care, operate in physician, hospital, home-care, and skilled nursing systems. Because none of these systems has particular risk adjustment that correlates with end-of-life care, powerful incentives operate against providers becoming known for, or emphasizing, end-of-life services or, more generally, chronic care. To do so would invite risk selection of potentially very sick and costly patients to the quality provider. Of course, the exception to this rule on the payment side is the Medicare hospice program, which provides specific prospective payment for palliative, spiritual, home-based care for terminal patients. While this benefit and its history is reviewed below, it is important here to recognize that it still reaches a relatively small portion of Medicare decedents, fewer than 20 percent.

Virtually all patients and their families will face difficult judgments about the appropriateness and boundaries of end-of-life care. With the coming growth and further aging of the old and disabled population, these issues of decision making, appropriate care, and cost will be increasingly at Medicare's doorstep. The tremendous advances occurring in the technology of acute medicine and intensive care will complicate these decisions still further.

This chapter asserts that policy for end-of-life care is best understood first as a public-policy problem of writing a "good contract" to achieve a "good death." The public interest in this contract is twofold: first, to empower Medicare beneficiaries (acting as principals) to exercise the requisite control over the decisions made by their agents so as to achieve the best chance of a good death; and second, to represent the interests of society in using resources prudently in these end-of-life decisions. The contract, however, involves broader elements of information and agency for vulnerable Medicare beneficiaries, the adoption of guidelines that embody accepted principles of chronic and palliative care, and the promotion of delivery systems that do not balkanize care among physician, home health, skilled nursing, and hospital settings.

To some, it may seem disrespectful to reduce the exquisitely compli-cated considerations that go into directing end-of-life care into the rhetoric and logic of a contract. To others, the incursion of Medicare into these deci-sions may seem overly paternalistic. Conceptually, however, the provision of end-of-life care is an appropriate contractual exercise: all patients would like this experience to go according to their wishes, yet often the critical behaviors and decisions are made by someone else, especially their physician-agents. Thinking of this episode of care as a contractual problem helps to articulate the interests involved; to evaluate the problems of information, risk, uncer-tainty, and agency involved; and to assess the properties of policy instruments that may be appropriate.

This chapter develops the logic of this contract in the following steps. First, I review evidence on the high cost of dying in Medicare. This story is im-portant because the perception of enormous sums going to futile care at the end of life is what fuels many policy makers' interest in this topic. Second, I briefly discuss the rationale and experience of the two major policy initiatives designed to alter Medicare end-of-life decision making. Increased use of hos-pice care and advance directives are considered to be the major possibilities for influencing Medicare's high cost of dying. Third, I review the major piece of scientific evidence about both the problem of end-of-life decision making as well as its potential solution. This study, the so-called SUPPORT initiative (Study to Understand Prognoses and Preferences for Outcomes and Risks of Treatments), presents a number of implications, positive and negative, of how to think about the design and prospects of an end-of-life contract. Then, I consider the challenges in reframing end-of-life care for policy and medicine. Finally, I develop the outline of Medicare policy design in this area: the ele-ments of a Medicare contract that would enhance the opportunity of benefi-ciaries and their families to experience a good death.

Medicare and the High Cost of Dying

Historically, the issue of death and dying in Medicare has been framed in Medicare as the problem of "the high cost of dying." One of the most quoted statistics about Medicare is that about 28 percent of Medicare expenditures go to 5 percent of the beneficiaries who die in a given year.[8] Expenditures for care during the last sixty days account for half of all resources consumed during the last year of life. James Lubitz and Gerald Riley, two of the major students of Medicare payments in the last year of life, have uncovered little change in the magnitude and pattern of this spending since 1976.[9]

The literature on the costs of death and dying illustrates a straightforward but not especially instructive result: individuals who die consume substantial health care resources, whether it be in the acute care or long-term care setting. Since almost by definition most of these individuals will be very sick, it is not surprising that they will consume a large proportion of any insurer's resources. Medicare's coverage of an old and disabled population means that not only are the vast majority of annual deaths occurring under the coverage of the program, but considerable comorbidity and coincident illness will complicate both the decision making at the end of life and the interpretation of data.

Careful longitudinal analysis of Medicare spending suggests that the high-cost-of-dying argument may be overstated because estimates are drawn from a cross-sectional and retrospective perspective. In other words, we infer that decedents cost a great deal because we look at those who die and, counting backward, add up the amounts that were spent on their care. Alternatively, M. Gornick and others' prospective study of those enrolled in Medicare compared the long-term expenditures on those who died over the next sixteen years with the costs for those who survived. Three insights emerge from this longitudinal perspective: (1) The sixteen-year pattern of spending for decedents looks much more similar to the spending on survivors than one would expect, given the high-cost-of-dying argument. Roughly half of the Medicare beneficiaries who began the study at age 65 died within the next sixteen years. Their lifetime spending by Medicare was $29,950 (in 1989 dollars). The survivors in this group accounted for expenditures of $20,897, but they had yet to incur end-of-life expenses. (2) For older cohorts followed over a sixteen-year period (cohorts age 75 and older, 85 and older), the difference between spending on survivors and decedents switches. The adjusted spending on survivors actually exceeds spending on decedents in these cohorts. (3) The average annual spending for decedents decreases with age. This suggests that resources may be more carefully rationed, intensity of end-of-life care decreased, or selection of different, lower-cost, end-of-life care occurs at older ages.[10]

Anne Scitovsky's extensive review of the literature on the costs of dying provides the basis for several general conclusions about the relationship among costs, age, and treatment patterns for survivors and decedents. First, Medicare spending is indeed high for decedents, roughly seven times greater than for survivors, in the immediate window before death. This differential shrinks, however, the longer the period viewed before death. Second, the extent of Medicare spending on acute services immediately before death appears to decline with age. However, nursing home spending for decedents appears to increase with age, perhaps completely offsetting the reductions in end-of-life intensive care observed on the acute care side. Scitovsky concludes that high-cost, aggressive care appears to be confined to a relatively small group of Medicare beneficiaries, perhaps less than 5 percent of all persons who die.[11]

A small body of literature (often based on small samples) has attempted to estimate cost savings that would occur from greater use of hospice or advanced directives.[12] Despite the evidence provided by SUPPORT and the National Hospice Study, the notion persists that substitution of lower cost interventions would be associated with referral to hospice or advance directives. The literature shows varying effects of substitution: patients with advance directives generate inpatient Medicare charges 68 percent lower than patients without documented directives;[13] patients enrolled in hospice generated a 63 percent reduction in expenditures in the last month of life compared to nonhospice patients;[14] and patients generated similar expenditures for both interventions.[15] Two major methodological problems limit the inferences that can be made from this class of studies. First, selection effects present an overwhelming challenge to any study that claims savings from advance directives and hospice. The act of executing an advance directive signals that this beneficiary is different, in important unmeasured characteristics, from a beneficiary who chooses not to sign a directive. Similarly enrollment in hospice is a significant indication that this beneficiary (and his or her doctor) has come to terms with the inevitability of dying: the characteristics that go along with this realization may have led to lower costs of care even in the absence of a hospice benefit. Studies that do not control for these effects either statistically or through randomization need to be viewed with suspicion. Indeed, the one randomized trial of hospice and the two randomized studies of advance directives found no statistically significant savings from these interventions.

The second important threat to such studies is the period effect. Virtually all of these studies, and especially the studies with strong research designs, were done in a different era, the early to late 1980s. For many phenomena, the passage of a decade represents a significant change in either the intervention or the context. David Kidder, for example, notes that changes in payment rates and policy toward the length of the benefit period for hospice may threaten the small estimated savings detected in their study.[16] Major changes that have occurred in the knowledge base about patient decision making, the introduction of managed care, and the larger societal changes that have occurred in attitudes about death and dying mean that the research base for policy in this area is profoundly out of date.

Ezekiel and Linda Emanuel stimulated an interesting discussion of the economics of dying in a study published in the *New England Journal of Medicine*.[17] In a heuristic designed to illustrate the limits of savings on the care of terminally ill patients, the Emanuels conclude that "best case" savings through hospice, advance directives, and reductions in so-called futile care would reduce national health care spending by close to $30 billion, 3.3 percent of all health care spending. Interestingly, this exercise produced very different reactions. Many observers have looked at the costs of care for beneficiaries who die and concluded that even if we were to save all of the resources that are allocated to decedents, the costs of Medicare as a whole would not be substantially affected. Others see the glass half full, arguing that the magnitudes implied by the Emanuels' analysis are sufficient to cover the uninsured or contribute to other worthy social purposes.

Hospice as the Medicare "Solution"

The enactment of the Medicare hospice benefit in 1982 as part of the Tax Equity and Fiscal Responsibility Act (TEFRA) was a radical step at the time it was enacted toward institutionalizing end-of-life care. Legislation to provide coverage for hospice care in the Medicare program was first introduced by Representative Leon Panetta in 1980, but neither the concept nor its political support had matured sufficiently to gain serious consideration. Between 1980 and 1982, a number of hospice activists and the nascent National Hospice Association lobbied extensively and garnered committed sponsors in both the House and the Senate. Hearings on a Medicare hospice benefit in March 1982 launched a serious drive in the Congress, with influential sponsors, to include hospice under the Medicare umbrella.

A number of objections were raised at the time: Because national experience with hospice had been so limited and hospice providers were so diverse, many observers wondered about the cost implications, the quality and service implications of different provider types, and the relative merits of alternative reimbursement systems. Since the National Hospice Study was in progress at the time, the administration urged a delay until the cost implications could be more adequately understood. In the midst of this debate, however, the Congressional Budget Office issued a report concluding that significant cost savings would result from a hospice benefit.

Despite the administration's objections, the investment of several key congressional leaders in a Medicare hospice benefit was too great. In the chaos that surrounded the Senate debate over TEFRA, the hospice benefit was introduced as an amendment close to midnight on July 22. The bill's chief sponsor was Senator Robert Dole, and some of the Senate's leading spokespersons— Senators Chiles of Florida, Glenn of Ohio, and Heinz of Pennsylvania—spoke eloquently about the rights of the terminally ill. With some parliamentary maneuvering, the bill was passed on a voice vote and later reconciled with the House version in conference.

With Medicare reimbursement, the hospice movement in the United States took a dramatic turn. What began as a grassroots, counterculture movement in health care became a licensed, certified, reimbursed, regulated, and formalized service. Although the growth in hospice organizations was precipitous, the number of Medicare-certified organizations grew slowly, numbering only 633 by 1991.[18] The benefit itself paid for physician services; nursing care; home health aide and homemaker services; medical social services and counseling (including nutrition and bereavement support for family members); physical, occupational, and speech therapy; short-term inpatient care for pain control or respite care; and medical supplies and equipment (including drugs for pain control).

Eligibility for the hospice benefit rests on a physician's determination that the patient is terminal, meaning that the physician expects the patient to die within a six-month period. Payment for hospice is prospective but determined by the days of care rendered. Hospices are provided a flat payment per patient day, but the actual payment amounts depend on whether the patient is provided routine home care, general inpatient care, or continuous home care. Since these payments cover all of the supplies and services provided under the hospice benefit, hospice providers are at risk if patients require more expensive treatments, are admitted for expensive hospitalizations, or require extensive therapy. On the other hand, hospices that are able to maintain strictly palliative care with a substantial volunteer base, or minimize their costs in other ways, can retain considerable financial returns under the Medicare benefit. This realization has spurred interest in hospice from large health systems and has stimulated the growth of a for-profit hospice industry

In theory, hospice care can be efficient because low-cost interventions, such as social support, are substituted for high-cost, high-tech, end-of-life interventions. The imagery of this cost saving is avoidance of an episode in an intensive care unit, with associated expensive monitoring and diagnostic work that ultimately yields no benefit for the patient. In practice, whether this substitution of hospice for acute-care interventions actually generates savings depends on the timing of the decision to enter a hospice program. Depending on the time path of a patient's medical expenses under a regimen of conventional care and the time path of hospice expenses, the use of a hospice alternative can be less expensive, more expensive, or a wash.

The available data on the trajectories of care for potential hospice patients suggest that the greatest medical costs are often closely clustered at the very end of life. At the same time, the longer before death a hospice approach is initiated, the greater the benefits of hospice treatment. It is less effective if implemented in the days immediately before death than if begun when more time is available.[19] Neither the patient nor the family can make the adjustments and preparations that hospice engenders unless there is adequate time.

Thus, in the decision about the timing of enrollment in hospice, there is an underlying trade-off between cost savings (versus conventional acute care) and capturing some of the benefits of hospice services. Enrollment in hospice very close to the time of death will, on average, produce large relative cost savings, but it will undermine some of the inherent benefits of the hospice approach. Enrollment relatively early in the course of a patient's terminal illness will allow the hospice approach to produce its greatest benefits for patients and families. However, it will not necessarily save resources for Medicare over conventional alternatives.

An analysis of the distribution of hospice costs versus the costs of conventional care under Medicare reveals that the expected cost savings would be small in any case, but also that under certain assumptions hospice can actually be a more costly form of care than conventional acute care approaches.[20] Under one set of assumptions, hospice care is the more expensive alternative for all intervals except for the final one to five days before death, during which time there is no difference in reimbursement. Under a more conservative set of assumptions that captures changes in hospitalization (before the actual period of cost savings), hospice savings are substantial during the period close to a beneficiary's death but diminish sharply as the period of time moves further back from the time of death. These data also indicate that the potential cost savings appears to vary widely depending on the type of hospice organization. Freestanding and home-health-agency-based hospices show the greatest potential for cost savings over conventional care, while, not surprisingly, hospital- and skilled-nursing-facility-based hospices indicate the least potential.

Until now, hospice has operated as something of an enigma in Medicare. The benefit was mounted with a wealth of good intentions, a paucity of good data about its effects, and under the influence of a number of politically astute interest groups with divergent intentions about the concept itself. The pessimistic view of this enterprise is that it is simply providing some health care providers with the opportunity to capture surpluses—allowing for the cost of terminal care to be shifted in new ways, especially to families, and providing outcomes that are not discernibly different from conventional care. The optimistic view is that a great deal of good is being done by the hospice movement even if there are few hard scientific or economic data to prove it. The goodwill, competence, and caring that are provided by many hospice organizations are, at face value, extraordinary, and it would be exceedingly difficult to account for these benefits in the metrics of health services research and evaluation.[21]

Hospice, then, provides the first leg of any Medicare contract for end-of-life care, though the incentives are still not completely aligned for physicians to make optimal decisions from either a patient care or societal economic standpoint. For the typical fee-for-service oncologist, for example, a referral to hospice means the end of his or her own supervision of and reimbursement for treatment. In agency terms, the incentives for this oncologist are not neutral with respect to the referral of the patient. For the hospital, referral to hospice means the end of inpatient acute care, although under prospective payment and increasingly under managed care contracts, early discharge is advantageous. For hospitals that own hospice organizations, the incentive is to discharge patients to their own units. Unfortunately, for doctors and hospitals, this set of incentives encourages the use of hospice simply as a discharge strategy, leading to later, rather than earlier, decisions about referral. Current evidence suggests that hospice care is used relatively infrequently and late in the course of most terminal illnesses.[22]

Timing is everything in both the economics and the effectiveness of a hospice approach, and in many cases palliative care is ordered too late to generate significant savings or to improve patients' quality of life. Spiritual counseling, relationships with family, pain management, social support, and other aspects of effective hospice care require considerable "lead time," yet most hospice orders occur in the last weeks, if not the last days, of care. All of this suggests that hospice care needs to be more carefully and fully integrated into the design of incentives and, ultimately, into the organization of delivery systems. Many new integrated delivery systems have strong hospice components and protocols. For patients, the hospice option needs to be placed on the radar screen much earlier in the course of doctor-patient discussions about advance directives for end-of-life care if there is to be increased uptake. The experience of the Patient Self-Determination Act in simply mandating the implementation of these advance directives, however, is sobering.

The Patient Self-Determination Act

Passage of the Patient Self-Determination Act (PSDA), part of the 1990 Omnibus Reconciliation Act, brought the federal government explicitly into the business of defining the requirements of health providers and educating beneficiaries about advance directives. PSDA required all health facilities participating in Medicare and Medicaid—including hospitals, nursing homes, home health agencies, hospices, and health maintenance organizations—to inform patients about their rights with respect to refusal of treatment and the opportunity to execute an advance directive.

The requirements of the act were to be implemented at the time the patient was either admitted to the facility or, in the case of an HMO, enrolled in the plan. Providers were required to document in the patient's record whether or not the advance directive had been executed. The PSDA was implemented in various forms among medical facilities and plans. Many providers took the act as a perfunctory regulatory requirement and either simply passed along written material to patients or communicated the opportunity to execute an advance directive as part of a hurried admissions process.

In the legislative debate and in the requirements of the law, the goals of PSDA were vague and ill defined. Advance directives were considered to be a "good" thing in their own right, and little consideration was given to the costs, benefits, or potential efficacy of such a law.[23] It was presumed that the costs of the law would be borne by the providers (and their payers); no earmarked financing accompanied this new mandate. Indeed, because the requirements of the act were so divorced from either financing or organizational reality in hospitals, some ethicists worried in the early implementation of the law that it might be targeted at disadvantaged patients with poor insurance coverage.[24] The rules published by HCFA to implement the act left considerable discretion to providers and plans about the exact nature of the communications involved, how the advance directive was to be documented in the medical record, the content of "community education" required by the law, and even which patients were actually covered by the requirements of the law.[25] Not surprisingly, early accounts of the implementation of PSDA in hospitals showed enormous variations in response, ranging from hospitals that took the most perfunctory attitude and could not document the incidence of advance directives to hospitals that demonstrated significant increases in the execution of do-not-resuscitate (DNR) orders.[26]

As a piece of the Medicare contract for end-of-life care, the PSDA was probably not a bad idea; but as a piece of policy, it was terribly designed and executed. PSDA was an unfunded mandate for hospitals and plans. It was directed at a moment in patient care—the admissions process—that could not be more inopportune for a deliberative consideration of advance directives. It was directed not at physicians or other caregivers proximate to the patient, but rather it concerned faceless procedures that leveraged no relationship or personal attachment to the patient. Indeed, in many facilities, the act was implemented with paperwork, audiotapes, or closed-circuit television. The mandate was issued in vague rules that allowed providers to avoid any accountability for the quality or even the quantity of advance directives. It is possible that PSDA was even counterproductive, instilling further cynicism among providers about the seriousness of the advance-directives agenda. PSDA left physicians out of the loop in terms of eliciting and structuring the discussion of patient preferences for end-of-life care. PSDA brought no sophistication or fore-thought to the subtle issues of cultural sensitivity and accommodation to the "message" implied by the solicitation of an advance directive.[27] Finally, the PSDA did impose costs, not the least of which may have been on patients who were taken through an often ineffectual and burdensome exercise.

The SUPPORT Study

Despite the advances of this literature in recent years, policy making for death and dying in old age inevitably confronts enormous ignorance about the nar-rower questions of the clinical appropriateness and cost implications of care for the very ill. Most current research provides only the most indirect evidence that inappropriate care is, or is not, being provided. Anne Scitovsky, for ex-ample, infers that inappropriate care is probably not being provided, because Medicare spending for acute hospital services goes down with age.[28]

The best evidence about the characteristics of end-of-life care, as well as the difficulties in changing decision making, comes from the Study to Under-stand Prognoses and Preferences for Outcomes and Risks of Treatments (SUPPORT).[29] This study selected over 9,000 patients with advanced disease to assess the management of end-of-life care and to document the nature and quantity of physician-patient communication over a four-year period. The cri-teria for selection into SUPPORT generalizes to about 400,000 admissions per year, with another 925,000 individuals estimated to have similar levels of ill-ness out in the community. The authors of the SUPPORT study estimate that patients falling under the study selection criteria account for 40 percent of all deaths.

The first phase of the study attempted to document patterns of end-of-life communications between doctors and patients, the incidence of ag-gressive treatments, and characteristics of treatment experiences—such as the presence of significant pain—at the end of life. This phase revealed significant problems in communication, planning, and management of end-of-life care. Less than half of all physicians knew whether their patients pre-ferred not to have CPR performed. Almost half of the do-not-resuscitate orders were written within a two-day period before death, indicating little ad-vance consideration. Data on the settings and management of pain at the end of life indicated substantial use of intensive care: 38 percent of patients spent ten days or more in intensive care units before death. Family members reported that about half of the patients suffered moderate to severe pain before they died in the hospital.

The second phase of the study tested an intervention designed to improve communication and decision making: physicians were given daily forecasts of the functional status of patients, estimates of the survival probabilities out to six months, and assessments of patient quality-of-life preferences for different forms of end-of-life care. Trained nurses were involved in the care team in order to better elicit preferences, explain options, and facilitate planning of care. The SUPPORT study expected that the intervention would produce earlier and "better" treatment decisions, improve the quality of life immediately before death, and reduce resource use.

Despite a carefully designed protocol and an extensive investment in the intervention, the SUPPORT study produced no statistically significant improvements in the indicators of improved management of end-of-life care. No improvement occurred in the number or timing of do-not-resuscitate orders; physicians' knowledge of patient preferences; ICU utilization, incidence of coma, or use of mechanical ventilation before death; or the reported level of pain before death. The intervention did not produce any significant reduction in hospital resource use.

What is so stunning about these results is that, in many ways, this study represented a best-case opportunity to change behavior and decision making. The Robert Wood Johnson Foundation invested $28 million in this analysis and intervention. Physicians at the participating institutions had expressed willingness to participate and had suggested elements of the intervention itself. Nurses were given discretion to customize the intervention to the particular circumstances of the case, and the entire study presumably operated under a very strong Hawthorne effect. In fact, the intervention should have been reinforced by external events: the PSDA, the intensive discussion and intervention of medical ethics in these decisions, and increased use of guidelines and attention to pain management and palliative care. Data were provided to physicians in a timely manner. Nurses were judged to be "committed, energetic, and highly trained." The results of SUPPORT were regarded by the investigators themselves as "troubling" and have stimulated intense discussion among clinicians, researchers, and ethicists. Some reviewers of the data are simply uncertain of its implications: for example, the seemingly high incidence of reported pain at the end of life may represent a trade-off between pain and sedation, not necessarily a failure of clinical sensitivity.[30] Some observers believe that the SUPPORT findings may actually reflect the triumph of patient preferences, not the unwarranted intrusion of medical technology. By this interpretation, patients with bad but not "really bad" prognoses may wish for advanced and intensive care, often eschew do-not-resuscitate orders until the last minute, and often experience extended stays in ICUs.[31] Patricia Marshall argues that the intervention itself—especially lodging the responsibility for communication with the nurse—merely reproduced the failure of communication that characterizes the doctor-patient relationship in modern hospital care.[32] Some have read the SUPPORT findings as incontrovertible evidence that hospitals are simply the wrong place for most patients to die. George Annas concludes that "if dying patients want to retain some control over their dying process, they must get out of the hospital if they are in, and stay out of the hospital if they are out."[33]

Franklin Miller and Joseph Fins have concluded that hospitals must be reformed both structurally and philosophically to change "practice routines, clinical education, and physical spaces."[34] They make the analogy of the reform of hospital practices for childbirth, which they argue has been transformed within hospital practice in the last two decades to accommodate an alternative "nonmedical" model of delivery, to give mothers substantially more control, and to include family members in the process. They propose the creation of new hospice-like alternative care units within hospitals, physically adjacent to ICUs, where patients could move seamlessly from intensive to palliative care at the appropriate moment. These units would be staffed by teams who are expert in negotiating end-of-life decisions and providing palliative care. Like much of the literature in this field, however, they do not articulate the financing, regulatory, and market arrangements that are necessary, perhaps as preconditions, for these changes to occur.

End-of-Life Care as a Policy Problem

One could argue that the circumstances of dying are largely the province of individuals, their families, and physicians. One could also argue that the fundamental questions of caring are more proximate to the patient, involving the specific doctor and team providing care; the policies and management of the hospital, nursing home, or hospice; and the families and loved ones surrounding the patient. Many would argue that the high stakes, emotions, and nuances that go along with life-and-death decisions cannot be reconciled with the general and blunt instruments that are often the tools of public policy. Clearly, all of the parties close to the decision making at the end of life are critical, and as research findings in this chapter illustrate, their behaviors will be extremely difficult to change. The role of doctors in these decisions is complex, ever more so with the recent controversies over physician-assisted suicide and euthanasia.

However, end-of-life care also belongs at least partially in the domain of policy, regulation, organization, and finance.[35] Such care almost by definition does not fit into the traditions or ethos of medical practice, suggesting that public policy has an important role in either fostering or regulating changes in end-of-life care. Medical practice that expands its purview beyond purely curative goals has a more ambiguous mission, and its ability to self-regulate is more suspect. As Franklin Miller and colleagues have argued, "any treatment whose purpose is to cause death lies outside of medical practice, which is defined here as medically indicated interventions aimed at promoting health and healing and alleviating the suffering of patients. Currently accepted standards of comfort care allow for the use of aggressive palliative treatment and may indirectly or unintentionally contribute to a patient's death."[36] Indeed, expanding the goals and agenda for end-of-life care beyond the traditional medical model invites other professional and cultural perspectives into the debate, including nursing, social work, and communities of faith.

The possibilities opened up by more direct and proactive management of the dying process also open up the possibilities for abuse, especially the maltreatment of vulnerable populations.[37] Indeed, the visibility of physician-assisted suicide cases, the recent spate of state legislation, and the resort to ballot initiatives for physician-assisted suicide in states suggest that these questions are becoming increasingly public and increasingly policy oriented. In the absence of an explicit policy discussion about end-of-life care, society is confronted with questions of end-of-life care on the basis of extreme cases—such as the Jack Kevorkian cases—instead of a more measured and deliberate approach that would occur in the context of policy making.

The inability of policy to confront and ameliorate some of the questions of end-of-life care is resulting in increased polarization of the issues, diversion of policy questions into the courts and into public referenda, and the increased fracturing of the medical profession. Public opinion polling has shown a dramatic increase in the percentage of the population that would support the legalization of euthanasia in situations where a disease cannot be cured.[38] Increasingly, mainstream medical practice is accepting or at least acknowledging palliative care, withholding of treatment, and even physician-assisted suicide. For example, in a recent study of physicians in Washington State, 53 percent of responding physicians thought that physician-assisted suicide should be legal, and 40 percent indicated that they would personally be willing to assist a patient with suicide.[39]

With a broadening of the boundaries in both medical practice and medical ethics, issues of death and dying will increasingly become the province of public policy. Questions of reimbursement, regulation, and monitoring will impinge on what was formerly a virtually private sphere. However, the linkage between policy and decision making about death is delicate.

At the same time, the recent upsurge in interest in care for seriously ill, older persons reflects a sense that a "win-win" situation exists for public policy. The 1997 Institute of Medicine (IOM) report on end-of-life care, *Approaching Death*, established a set of consensus principles for such care, as well as an agenda for research and policy for the Congress.[40] The IOM process suggested that fixing the circumstances in which older persons die could potentially improve patient care, help resolve a set of ethical problems in medicine, and ultimately help deploy societal resources fairly and efficiently. Subsequent to the IOM report, active programs of research, policy analysis, and advocacy have emerged, such as the Last Acts program sponsored by the Robert Wood Johnson Foundation, the Soros Foundation's Project on Death in America, and the Center to Improve Care of the Dying's MediCaring demonstration projects.

Policy can intercede at several levels to influence the care of the dying. At high levels of reimbursement and regulatory policy, broad incentives for the venue, content, and intensity of care are established. There is widespread belief that these incentives distort the choices available to patients and their families. For example, it is not surprising that only 21 percent of deaths occur outside of institutional settings when one considers the difficulty of receiving payment and accessing professional services at home.

The role of public policy down at the level of doctor-patient decision making is more delicate. Physicians have their own views about the boundaries of appropriate care, pain, suffering, and resource use. Family members and proxy decision makers bring their own interests and values into these decisions. Questions of patient competence further complicate this decision making. Nonetheless, even here Medicare policy may have a role. Through specific payment incentives, program requirements in exchange for financing graduate medical education, and the development of practice guidelines, Medicare already plays a large implicit role at the bedside. Through all of these vehicles, it could play a more explicit role in influencing the communications and decisions that occur between doctors and patients. More generally, through research, information policy, and the promotion of broader approaches to policy and practice, Medicare policy could play a leadership role in influencing quality of care.

In actual medical practice, the models of care that are available to many Medicare beneficiaries at the ends of their lives can be traced back through a long and complicated story in the history of medicine: (1) the attributes of doctors and other care providers who select into medicine, (2) the aggressive and

curative nature of medical education and practice, (3) the management and organization of hospitals (and nursing homes), (4) the regulatory context of
medicine (including malpractice), (5) the information and communication
that traditionally extend to families and patients, and, (6) not least, the preferences and attitudes that patients themselves bring to these decisions.[41] Physicians outside of oncology, critical care, and some other select subspecialties
deal relatively infrequently with dying patients and have little background and
expertise to deal with the psychosocial aspects of preparing for death.[42] The division of labor in modern medicine, especially in hospitals and now increasingly in managed care, means that interactions with patients are broken up
into small, discrete increments, among a host of clinical specialists.[43] However, the emerging roles of primary care practitioners and the reorganization
of delivery systems provides new opportunity—at least in theory—to elicit advance directives and improve ongoing doctor-patient communications about
end-of-life care.[44]

The problem of making appropriate decisions about end-of-life treatment would be relatively straightforward if "terminal illness" had a clear-cut
definition. If patients could be sorted in a binary way into those who are "dying" and those likely to survive, then most elements of policy design and management of care could be organized around these designations. This concept
was implicit in the movement during the early 1990s to create a diagnosis-
related group (DRG) for end-of-life care, which ultimately resulted in a (non-
reimbursable) code being created for palliative care. In many respects, the
hospice benefit in Medicare fits this model of clear *ex ante* definition of terminal care: physicians determine that a patient is expected to die in the next six
months, eligibility is determined, the patient is enrolled with separate specialized providers, a distinct program of palliative care is initiated, and a separate
prospective payment system for care is engaged.

However, many diagnoses and patients do not predictably sort into this
dichotomy of dying or surviving. Daniel Callahan argues that this problem is
getting harder with medical progress and the increased incidence of chronic
conditions in old age: "Predictions of death, unless virtually imminent, become increasingly problematic. Who among us does not know of someone,
stricken by a supposedly fatal cancer who is still alive months or years after a
predicted death? The slow, but variable course of most chronic diseases alone
makes it difficult to say when death is on its way. When to that uncertainty is
added the further impact of life-extending therapy, whose purpose is to stretch
the borderline and the practice of brinkmanship, whose purpose is to resist
the idea of a fixed limit, the location of the gate between life and death becomes more indeterminate."[45]

Nicholas Christakis's extensive analysis of prognostication in medicine provides an important further complication to this model of conditioning treatment (and payment) on a forecast that a patient is terminal.[46] Christakis reveals how deeply embedded the problem of prognosis is in the concept of modern medicine. Little training or reinforcement of prognosis is provided in medical education or subsequent practice; little professional encouragement exists in medicine to face the difficult moral and ethical responsibilities that come with predicting a patient's demise; and few institutional supports exist to promote the kinds of communication that would follow from more forthright efforts to define and "foretell" patients' prospects. Christakis traces this dilemma of prognosis in the literature, textbooks, and training of physicians. Other research shows that the treatment of end-of-life care in medical texts and education is limited.[47]

Most analysts now understand that "the dying" are not an easily discernible or identifiable population group, especially when viewed prospectively. Epidemiologists tell us that the vast majority of deaths in old age are attributable to a small number of broad diagnoses: heart disease and its close cousins (atherosclerosis, hypertension, congestive heart failure), diabetes, cancer, complications from Alzheimer's and other dementias, and infections, often resulting from inpatient treatment. But death often results from combinations of many of these causes. Beyond these "official" causes of death usually lie other sources of serious illness or disability waiting in the wings to present themselves, if only the primary cause of death did not occur first. Sherwin Nuland's summary of autopsy studies paints a picture of the aging process in which physiological vulnerabilities are cropping up in virtually all organ systems with advanced age, but only the order of deterioration is uncertain. This underlying physiological reality leads to an important insight for the clinical (and resource) decision making that should occur:

> When an elderly man is offered the possibility of cancer palliation or even cure, provided he is willing to endure debilitating surgery or radical surgery, what should be his response? Will he suffer through the treatment, only to die of his ongoing cerebrovascular atherosclerosis the following year? After all the cerebrovascular disease is likely the result of the same process that so decreased his immunity to malignant growth that he developed the cancer that is trying to kill him. But then again, different manifestations of the aging process proceed at different rates, so it may be much longer than he anticipates before his stroke exerts its claim. Such possible eventualities can be estimated only by evaluating the present state of his nonmalignant process, such as the degree of his hypertension and the status of his heart disease. These are the kinds of considerations that

should go into every clinical decision involving older people, and wise physicians have always made careful use of them. Wise patients should do the same.[48]

To entertain such eventualities in decision making without inviting ethical abuses and discrimination against the very old and vulnerable requires both a commitment to agency for the patient on the behalf of doctors and providers and a commitment of resources for doctors, nurses, and social workers to attend to a broader clinical array than the immediate diagnosis and treatment. It would also require a commitment to deal with a set of psychosocial issues that attend such difficult clinical decisions. Part of the explanation for our current inability to face up to these decisions ahead of time is that our payment and delivery systems have such powerful reasons to focus on immediate treatment, cure, and discharge.

A Medicare End-of-Life Contract

An astonishing number of possible solutions to the problem of improving end-of-life decision making have already been offered, some unusual: for example, more public interest law specializing in the rights of dying patients or the revocation of medical licenses for those physicians who do not properly respect and treat the pain of dying patients. Missing in almost all of these interventions, however, has been a systematic policy construction that incorporates powerful incentives and financing arrangements to improve agency as physicians, families, and patients manage the process of end-of-life care.

Consider the incentives under Medicare reimbursement. For inpatient care, a patient with congestive heart failure falls under a DRG that in turn is based on an average (one time) expected length of stay. Once in the hospital, both conventional treatment and the incentives of prospective payment are to restore or at least stabilize the patient's functioning, adjust medications and determine the needs for respiratory or other ongoing therapy, and prepare the patient for discharge. The hospital may be a Medicare-supported teaching center in which payments are made for residents to hone their diagnostic and therapeutic skills, with a strong emphasis on applying state-of-the-art medicine and curing disease. Incentives for clinical research and advancing new therapies reinforce an ethos of aggressive treatment in the hospital setting. The hospital clearly has an incentive to organize home health, hospice, or other resources for a smooth and timely discharge of the patient, but there are no inherent incentives for the hospital to deal with the more difficult and longitudinal issues, such as managing this condition from the moment of discharge to death, particularly as a process of managing often multiple chronic conditions until death.

Overcoming these powerful incentives will ultimately require a Medicare contractual approach that addresses training (and retraining), workforce issues, physician payment incentives for evaluation and management in primary care, information, and hospital regulation and payment. The goal for this contract is on the one hand simple, but on the other hand extremely difficult to implement. The Institute of Medicine report *Approaching Death* nicely articulates this goal in its first recommendation: "People with advanced, potentially fatal illnesses and those close to them should be able to expect and receive reliable, skillful, and supportive care."[49]

A policy process that would lead to a transformed Medicare program for end-of-life care—a new contract—must involve the following steps: (1) The Medicare sponsor establishes coherent coverage, payment, practice guidelines, and quality-of-life outcome measures for end-of-life care. This policy design maps to an approach to purchasing high-quality health care, to be implemented in the contracts written with hospice providers, managed care organizations, and individual providers (including hospitals, physicians, nurses, and social workers). (2) The Medicare program develops the proper resources—measurement instruments, educational interventions, trained professionals—to implement a regime of high-quality care at the end of life. (3) Providers and plans are monitored for the quality of palliative and end-of-life care, quality-of-life outcomes, and family satisfaction with care.

In establishing this contract, it is useful to reflect on the theory of Medicare provision developed in chapter 2. Even in decisions about end-of-life care, there are at minimum two distinct interests in the decision: Medicare (which represents society's financial and social interest in the care of older persons and the disabled) and the patient (including the wishes of family and loved ones). Medicare will obviously have a more general and limited interest in these decisions than the beneficiary. Medicare itself has no tradition or standing for inserting itself into the individual decisions of doctors and patients, but it does have an interest in seeing that resources are used prudently and the societal interest in care is upheld. Since expensive intensive care has an opportunity cost, Medicare has an interest in seeing that the societal contribution to that care at least serves the interests of patients. A stronger version of the Medicare contract, one that sees Medicare as a prudent purchaser of care, would also demand that end-of-life care be cost worthy, that the benefits in terms of quality of life and quantity of life roughly justify the pain, risks, and economic resources consumed.

The Beneficiary as Principal

Much of the pain and risk of decision making near the end of life is obviously borne by the severely ill patient. The psychosocial risks of poor contracting include a painful and undignified process of dying. Interestingly,
the specter of this outcome, like that of residing in a nursing home, is one
that troubles many older persons long before they are in the position of making decisions about end-of-life care.[50] In other words, the "disutility" that
comes from the uncertainty and lack of control over end-of-life care occurs
earlier in life for many people. If individuals felt greater confidence that they
would experience a dignified and relatively pain-free experience at the end of
life, they would benefit from this peace of mind for many months and years
in advance. In part, the aversion that many feel to end-of-life care and decision making is a by-product of poor public and private advance contracting
mechanisms.[51]

Even in cases of undeniable patient competence to make decisions,
important cognitive problems in carrying out this contract arise for end-of-
life care. First, clinical depression, prevalent in old age anyway, is often a by-
product of the knowledge and circumstances that go along with serious or
terminal illness.[52] Depression interferes with the beneficiary's willingness to
engage in discussion and decision making about end-of-life care and clouds
the ethical basis on which such decisions (particularly to withhold or forgo
treatment) can be made. Even in the absence of clinical or diagnosable depression, manifest denial of the reality or implications of serious illness prevents
many beneficiaries from engaging in meaningful discussions or confronting
difficult decisions.

The literature on cognitive bias alerts us to another class of cognitive
problems, often more subtle but still quite consequential for end-of-life decision making. Well-known cognitive biases are likely to exert an influence on
beneficiaries' willingness to entertain the idea of making end-of-life arrangements, much less participate in the process in a wholly "rational" way. Using
Kahneman and Tversky's heuristics, for example, we would expect beneficiaries to distort the likelihood of the risks of death depending on their exposure
to other end-of-life experiences. Beneficiaries may misperceive the risks associated with their diagnosis or condition. Beneficiaries may misperceive the
consequences of treatment, even when they have been carefully and accurately described. Beneficiaries may misunderstand the quality-of-life implications of a course of treatment. For example, some evidence exists that patients
are predisposed to be overly optimistic about their prognoses, despite the information they are given.

Even if doctor-patient communication could assure that patients accurately understand risk, consequence, benefit, and other attributes of the decision at a point in time, there would still remain the problem of the inherent instability of the patient's condition, circumstances, and preferences over time. Patient preferences about what to do in a life-threatening situation are often unstable. Transforming experiences, such as conversations with loved ones, the direct experience of pain and suffering, or exposure to other patients in similar circumstances, may fundamentally change a person's attitude or preferences about life-sustaining care, even from day to day. Finally, the underlying competence of the patient to make decisions may vary over the course of treatment and may be difficult to assess at a moment in time.

All of this illustrates the cognitive difficulties of eliciting valid and useful advance directives from older persons. The lesson for Medicare is that the advance directive agenda cannot be tackled casually at the level of individual cognition and decision making. The idea, implicit in the PSDA, that beneficiaries can simply provide this form of subtle (and consequential) guidance in the course of filling out hospital admissions forms is flawed. Part of an effective Medicare contract, then, must be a more systematic and scientific approach to eliciting patient preferences for end-of-life care.[53]

From both a clinical and a policy perspective, developing effective supports for end-of-life care planning and management will take time and considerable public investment. In the meantime, considerable progress can be made in structuring information resources and communications that help patients better understand options. The evidence about how few patients understand their options for end-of-life care is extremely troubling and represents an obvious area for policy improvement.[54] Providing these supports is an appropriate role for beneficiary agents. The role and necessity for general improvements in beneficiary agency will be revisited in chapter 7. This case study of end-of-life care illustrates its importance in a particularly meaningful clinical context—when beneficiaries are navigating the exigencies near the time of death.

The Role of Families

Family and other loved ones also bear the consequences of a poorly managed process: often these individuals are robbed of the opportunity to spend the last days and hours with the patient on issues that matter and instead are forced to advocate for certain clinical decisions to be made or particular services to be provided. The involvement and "standing" of the family in end-of-life decision making is a problem that has occupied medical ethicists, and examples from particular clinical contexts, such as the administration of cardiopulmonary resuscitation, have illustrated the significant financial and psychosocial consequences of end-of-life decisions for families.[55] Because the dominant value in mainstream ethics is that of individual patient autonomy, it is difficult to go beyond almost rhetorical statements that the interests of family members should be taken into account. Weaker versions of a patient autonomy model "balance" the interests of family members, especially when the patient's treatment decision has the effect of imposing significant costs or hardships on others. Even here, the issues are complex. Numerous studies have documented the disparities between family (or other proxy) treatment decisions and the stated preferences of the patient.[56] Especially when families have conflicts of interests—support and care responsibilities or bequest motives, for example—the reliance on family preferences, absent strong guidance from the patient, is problematic. But in most cases, it is likely again that the interests and values of families can be reconciled with the interests and values of the patient with effective planning and care management.[57]

A public policy perspective on this question is slightly different. Here, the question is how Medicare should take into account family interests in shaping the incentives, practice requirements, and accountability of end-of-life care financed by Medicare. Interestingly, CMS has abandoned efforts to make children financially accountable for the care of parents. In 1983, the Reagan administration proposed that states look to patients' families for contributions to long-term care expenses whenever Medicaid resources were required. The idea was that if taxpayers were to be charged for these expenses, then next of kin had a responsibility to contribute. In the resulting controversy, the issue of family responsibility was widely discussed, and ultimately the administration rescinded its initiative to garner family contributions. In effect, this experience defined for policy purposes the limits of family financial accountability for older persons' medical expenses. In finance and in agency relationships, Medicare recognizes the beneficiary as the only party of interest.

As a political and policy matter, Medicare may choose to encourage communication with family and others in end-of-life decisions. For example, in Linda Emanuel's protocol of structured deliberation, family members and others have a role in end-of-life planning but only as they are identified and brought into the process by the patient.[58] In any case, as Medicare is currently configured, children or other family members do not have standing in payment or clinical decision making; they are simply not principals in the end-of-life contract. A process approach to redefining end-of-life care could require that family involvement at least be considered a component of care management. To do this well would potentially require the involvement of social workers and other professionals in the process.

The Professional Context for Agency in End-of-Life Decisions

Most discussions of clinical practice and policy design for end-of-life care presume that physicians are appropriate agents in the decision making that must occur.[59] The physician's ability to elicit and implement the patient's wishes with respect to end-of-life care is limited by a host of factors—inherent in medicine more broadly—that have nothing in particular to do with issues of terminal or futile care.[60] Physicians bring considerable concerns themselves to the perceived involvement of patients in decision making and to the perceived levels of inappropriate or burdensome care being provided.[61] Physicians bring individual assessments of prognosis and the probabilities of treatment outcomes and consequences to each case.[62] Physicians bring individual preferences for certain therapies, such as a distinctive preference for withdrawal of one form of life support versus another.[63] Studies on physician decision making with respect to end-of-life care have demonstrated the influence of variables such as specialty, religion, or region.

In other words, depending on the "draw" of the attending physician (given the same facts of the case), the patient will receive varying forecasts of the likelihood of different outcomes and varying advice. The selection, training, and reward system of physicians, however, strongly conditions their ability to perform as effective agents for patients at the end-of-life. As has been widely discussed in the medical literature, individuals who select into the medical profession tend to be achievement and goal oriented, problem driven, and competitive. Almost everything about medical school training reinforces the propensity to aggressively pursue curative care, to eschew limits, and to emphasize medical over psychosocial approaches.

No consensus exists over the proper standards of agency for physicians in managing end-of-life care. In theory, a pure agent fulfills the wishes of the principal as if that person were present and had access to all of the information available to the agent. In other words, pure agency approaches a form of pure surrogacy where the judgment is purely consistent with the preferences of the principal. In a situation of pure agency, the physician merely implements the preferences of the patient, given the asymmetric nature of the information available to doctor and patient. Alternatively, proxies or agents could employ a "best-interest" standard, where broader considerations and a looser fit with the patient's prior expressed wishes is expected. In further departures from a pure agency approach, the physician's own assessments of quality of life, distributive justice, and other extrinsic considerations take on greater weight. Rarely does the agent or the agents of the patient exhibit the kind of disinterest and detachment in the decision that might be desired in principle. Conflicts of interest and deep-seated emotional investments abound in these decisions.

Formally, the contracting problem between doctors and patients is a forward exercise in which principals and agents are agreeing to some protocol of care out into the future, potentially so far ahead that preferences and circumstances may change. This means that advance directives do indeed have to be advanced. Documented, structured conversations, probably beginning at the time of eligibility for Medicare, would establish a deeper record of guidance and communication than characterizes current practice. This also means that either some process for updating or some other form of validation of preferences is necessary. As mentioned above, "transforming experiences" (time with a loved one, experiencing pain and suffering, etc.) may fundamentally change a person's attitude or preferences about life-sustaining care. Stronger versions of a planning process for end-of-life care envision the involvement of interdisciplinary teams, including nursing, social work, clergy, and other relevant professionals.

Medicare's Role

Because Medicare is also a principal in this contract, how can the interests of the public in end-of-life care be defined and executed? Joanne Lynn has proposed that a new program be created to fit in between traditional Medicare and hospice alternatives for the care of the dying:

> A care delivery system could be designed around the important priorities: relief of pain and other symptoms, maintenance of function and control, support of family and personal relationships, avoidance of impoverishment, trustworthiness and continuity, attentiveness to meaningful activities, and spiritual issues. Such a program could be called "MediCaring" to emphasize its link to the commitment that society once made to the elderly with the establishment of the Medicare program. . . . The incentives and barriers that now make hospital services readily available and impede access to supportive services could be rearranged. Coronary artery bypass surgery for those with serious, eventually fatal conditions could become as hard to get as the daily services of home health aides are now. Having a separate, identifiable low-technology MediCaring program would permit the incentives, barriers, financing, and supply of services to be tailored to the clinical needs of this target population.[64]

Although the sentiments and logic for a separate new Medicare program to service this population is understandable, from a contracting point of view, it would compound Medicare's existing problems of policy and contract design. Eligibility and payment could be further balkanized; the incentives for providers to exploit reimbursement substitutions could increase; and the complexities facing beneficiaries could escalate.

Even though a full articulation of Medicare's solution for end-of-life care will require an extensive political vetting of the issues over a period of time, both a process and a potential conclusion can be defined. It is perhaps most important to state what such a process and outcome should not attempt: Congress, CMS, and other parties to the Medicare contract should not attempt to prescribe the exact circumstances in which care should be allowed (in the tradition of an "allowable expense" or, conversely, the particular end-of-life care that should be denied). While politically appealing, these forms of microregulation of practice cannot possibly address the varieties of clinical complexity, uncertainty, and patient preferences that will attend individual end-of-life decisions.

Alternatively, Medicare can feasibly promote a requirement for providers who participate in the program to have guidelines and practices for determining appropriate end-of-life care, including limiting treatment for Medicare beneficiaries. Such a requirement would have two effects: (1) at a national level, the political and policy process of scripting such a requirement would inevitably stimulate a broad and hopefully constructive debate about social responsibility, ethics, and the economics of intensive care; and (2) at an institutional and plan level, such a requirement would force physicians, hospitals, and other providers to actively develop mechanisms for communicating, deciding, and justifying end-of-life treatment decisions.

End-of-Life Care in Medicare Managed Care

Managed care organizations provide the opportunity for providing organizational agency for both beneficiaries and the public interest in end-of-life care. In theory, managed care organizations could provide the basis for integrated care—including palliative and hospice care—that segues from hospital and acute care for very ill patients.[65] Until now, very little of this integration and sequencing of care has occurred in Medicare managed care, in part because hospice is "carved out" from the managed care benefit. In other words, when a beneficiary is diagnosed as terminal, the payment and oversight of care moves away from the managed care organization and into the hospice. In a few cases, managed care organizations have started or acquired hospices, but they still are often discrete entities for the purposes of payment and clinical decision making.[66]

In managed care, placing hospitals and physicians at risk fundamentally shifts the traditional incentives to do more at the end of life. Although in the popular press there are significant worries about the exploitation of the elderly and some anecdotes about managed care plans introducing "managed death" practices and guidelines, there are few examples of these practices occurring in a systematic way. Nonetheless, because the incentives to undertreat are so powerful, especially for patients whose prognosis is poor, the contract in a Medicare managed care environment should look very different from the alternative contract in fee-for-service. Here, Medicare's role can be defined in terms of risk bearing, information, purchasing, and oversight.

Complete financial risk, as occurs in Medicare risk contracts, encourages the plan to be accurate in prognosis, to establish a plan of managed care, and to limit the costs of this care. Medically, the plan faces little incentive to either take medical risks or necessarily assure the quality of well-being for the enrollee. In extreme terms, the incentives in full-risk managed care are to disenroll the beneficiary, to limit potentially beneficial but costly care, or otherwise to underserve the patient. A more modest incentive response would involve limits on ineffective care and some substitution of social supports for acute medical care. The little evidence that exists about the treatment patterns of Medicare HMO patients at the end of life is consistent with these incentives, with HMO patients receiving less "potentially ineffective care" when compared to fee-for-service patients.[67]

In sum, in managed care environments, where plans are bearing financial risk, Medicare's primary role is to convey information to beneficiaries, monitor closely end-of-life practices by plans, and assure the accountability of providers for end-of-life care. Since the plan already faces incentives to limit care, especially intensive care at the end of life, the accountability concerns actually run in the opposite direction to much of the "high cost of dying" literature. Medicare has the power as a purchaser to encourage more information sharing with the patient and a greater use of information tools in end-of-life care at the plan level. Some plans have incorporated advance directives and other advance planning in their systems of care.[68] In its payment systems, Medicare could establish a weaker form of risk bearing but still retain prospective payment for patients who are terminal. This system, analogous to the current payment system for the Medicare hospice benefit, would require both physician and patient to agree to a terminal diagnosis. The Medicare program could also influence the uptake and consistency of quality end-of-life care practices by requiring performance reporting on these aspects of care. These measures have not been a feature of the National Committee for Quality Assurance (NCQA) approach to reporting and accreditation of health plans (HEDIS), but work by the Foundation for Accountability and the Institute of Medicine provides an initial basis for these measures.[69] Finally, for Medicare to require guidelines for end-of-life care would be especially reasonable for Medicare risk plans.

The Design of Guidelines

Since it is very difficult to structure outcome-based contracts for terminal care anyway, managed care arrangements lend themselves to *process-based* monitoring of end-of-life care in much more routinized ways than the virtually unobservable practices in the fee-for-service sector. In a managed care Medicare purchasing model, Medicare can demand guidelines and protocols for delivery, perhaps established on a plan-by-plan basis, for end-of-life care.

Guidelines for hospice enrollment for patients with noncancer diagnoses, initially developed by the National Hospice and Palliative Care Organization, have been in use since 1996.[70] These original guidelines have been modified by Medicare intermediaries, and further modified and interpreted for use by individual hospices.[71]

At the patient level, Linda Emanuel's framework of structured deliberation, for example, lends itself to guideline implementation in a managed care environment and is entirely consistent with the ideal of contracting for a "good death."[72] Emanuel argues that this process of structured deliberation can be highly routinized, in the same way that medical histories or informed consent can be elicited and can be incorporated into standard medical practice using valid and appropriate instruments. Her framework would include a process of eliciting permissions and orienting patients, involving proxy decision makers in the advance discussions, and discussing scenarios of care that are relevant to patients' circumstances. This process would produce a written record as well as a set of purposeful conversations that would in principle carry over to actual decisions, whether or not the patient was competent at the time of critical end-of-life choices.

In addition to requiring guidelines and practices for advance care planning, Medicare can insist that its resources for end-of-life care be used prudently, that they not be spent on futile care. Much of the ethics literature on medical futility is based on a standard in which there is no benefit to further treatment. Even by this standard, considerable debate rages among ethicists about responsibilities to the patient, the obligations to provide treatment, obligations or responsibilities to withhold treatment, and so on. In the midst of this debate, the concept of futility is evolving from a clinical concept into a broader social, legal, and policy construct that has implications for the design of Medicare policy.[73]

In order to understand both the limits and power of futility as a policy concept, it is important to distinguish several classes of potential treatment.[74] Treatments are strictly medically futile if no amount of resources could produce benefit to the patient. A more difficult set of cases involve treatments that have some very small probability of producing benefit (either some increment in life expectancy or some temporary maintenance or restoration of functioning). To make matters both more complicated and more realistic, imagine that these treatments sort out by cost: some interventions will produce marginal benefit at very low cost and some at very high cost. For some diagnoses and treatments, it may be more realistic and useful to think of the medical care choices in terms of both their probability of success and their cost. Some expensive care has a very high likelihood of contributing to survival, and other care has a low, but nonzero probability of contributing to survival. Obviously, the health care system can alter the relative costs of dying by moving along this spectrum. At the very end of this spectrum, where the likelihood of survival is very low, the costs potentially high, and quality of life unacceptable, advance directives and hospice care are relatively accepted and uncontroversial.

The evaluation of end-of-life care choices must go beyond the simple implications suggested in the "high costs of dying" literature. Implicit in much of the current literature is a notion that if only the "forecasting" could be improved in our low probability/high cost cell, then perhaps large savings could be captured with no discernible impact on mortality rates and quality of life. The problem with this view is that the clinical experience leading up to death is more dynamic than it is static, making it very difficult to preview for patients the array of potential clinical, quality-of-life, and survival choices.

Although some clinicians and ethicists question whether definitions of futile care can be operationalized and used in practice,[75] such definitions have been in place in many institutions and plans since the early 1990s. The Santa Monica Hospital Center, a pioneer in this movement, defines futile care as "any clinical circumstance in which the doctor and his consultants, consistent with the available medical literature, conclude that further treatment (except comfort care) cannot, within a reasonable possibility, cure, ameliorate, improve, or restore a quality of life that would be satisfactory to the patient." Santa Monica Hospital gives as examples an irreversible coma or persistent vegetative state, a terminally ill patient where care only serves to "artificially" delay the moment of death, or patients who face the prospect of permanent ICU care. Santa Monica Hospital and other institutions have implemented guidelines that systematically deal with cases where either the patient or the patient's family would challenge the propriety of limiting treatment.[76] Interestingly, the guidelines provide two fallbacks for patients or families who object to the physician's determination: patients can either find another provider (doctor and/or hospital), or they can resort to private payment for care even if it is deemed futile after this process of review. In principal-agent terms, the patients and their families still have the right to exercise their authority over the terms of care they expect, albeit with different physicians and hospitals as agents.

In a situation with two principals, such as characterizes end-of-life care provided for Medicare beneficiaries, different judgments can be rendered about the appropriateness of care by each of the principals. Guidelines provide a vehicle for Medicare to define its interests and boundaries in paying for end-of-life care, while still preserving the role of patients and their families in defining their own expectations and preferences for care. As described in chapter 3, the initial expectation is that in the vast majority of cases the interests of *Medicare-as-principal* and *beneficiary-as-principal* will be the same for end-of-life care.

Finally, Medicare has an interest in assuring that end-of-life care for high cost/low benefit/high uncertainty diagnoses and conditions is informed by the best evidence and prognostic acumen available. The challenge here is not to implement futile care or end-of-life guidelines but rather more general interventions that attend to both the clinical and social aspects of care in cases that involve dementias, congestive heart failure, or other prevalent chronic conditions.[77] Pain management and cancer represent the areas in which guidelines, palliative care, and end-of-life decision making have come most closely together.[78]

Conclusions

What do we know about the policy problem of end-of-life care in Medicare? First, it is well established that many Medicare beneficiaries have aggressive end-of-life care and die in hospitals, often with substantial pain that could be alleviated with better palliative care. Second, the preferences of these patients are often not known to their physicians, and twenty-five years of advocacy for advance directives has not fundamentally changed the instruments, information, and communication that accompany decision making at the end of life. Significant obstacles lie in the way of getting patients to "announce" their preferences for end-of-life care in clinically meaningful ways, especially before the fact. Third, physicians bring many predispositions to these decisions: the problems of prognostication, physician values, incentives, and communication from doctor to patient are formidable. Fourth, although the costs of end-of-life care are high, it will be difficult to achieve substantial savings. Fifth, efforts to change the mix of physician, hospital, and patient dynamics, such as the SUPPORT initiative, have been largely unsuccessful. With the exception of Medicare hospice policy and the Patient Self-Determination Act, few incentives or systematic policy reinforcements exist that shift the propensity of physicians and hospitals to treat patients with all possible intensity and vigor until the very end.

Given this mix of facts and experience, is there any reason to expect a sudden and dramatic change in Medicare-financed end-of-life care? The answer most certainly has to be no. The inertia in medical training and practice is so great that no mix of tinkering with the Patient Self-Determination Act or altering the information available at the bedside can be expected to change decision making in fundamental ways. No amount of nuanced discussion of the issues among ethicists in the medical literature will shift these practices in the short to middle term. Since the current world of research does not definitively characterize the magnitude of this problem, much less provide evidence about effective strategies in this complex world of doctor-patient decision making, it is clear that we are a long way from designing effective interventions. The lack of evidence that the Patient Self-Determination Act has either changed decision making or altered use of resources is further reason to proceed carefully, purposefully, and in a targeted way in the quest to achieve the elusive "win-win" solution that so many believe would accompany changes in the care of the dying. Daniel Callahan, who has looked at this mix of practices and traditions in great detail, has concluded that even modest changes in end-of-life care will require shifts at a societal level in broad attitudes toward death and dying, in the culture of medical-decision making, and in the actual techniques of decision making and communication at the end of life.[79] Perhaps the most necessary innovation would involve changes in the conversations that occur between doctors and patients, and between patients and other caregivers. For these conversations to have the nuance and effect that will lead to changes in care planning and management, an array of changes in professional skills, systems of care, and related policy and management supports will be required.[80]

Clearly this is a problem that is subtle and complex, and expectations about the power of policy and practice interventions need to be modestly calibrated. But both Medicare and beneficiaries have extraordinary interests in seeing better decision making and practice at the end of life. The key issue for

Medicare policy design lies not in specifying the particulars of an end-of-life care intervention at this point, but rather in the acceptance that improved decision making for end-of-life care constitutes a worthy contractual problem in its own right for Medicare reform. Indeed, if the experience with advance directives, hospice, SUPPORT, and other interventions demonstrates anything, it is that improvements in end-of-life communication, decision making, and care will require experimentation, multiple interventions, and considerable research and development. To develop and implement instruments for assessing patient preferences for treatment at the end of life will require a program of decision research of the scale that usually characterizes cancer trials, drug testing, or genetic therapies.

Ezekiel Emanuel estimates that increased use of advance directives and hospice has the potential to reduce end-of-life expenditures by 25 to 40 percent during the last month of life, 10 to 17 percent over the last six months of life, and 0 to 10 percent over the last year of life.[81] The relatively weak evaluation literature on cost savings from advance directives and hospice implies that the savings could be zero but certainly not negative. Thus, a major end-of-life initiative for Medicare might be based on a "bet" of a very small percentage of forecasted end-of-life expenditures, with the goal of reducing inappropriate care by at least that amount. More important is that this initiative would bet that systematic attention to research and development, instrumentation for doctor-patient communications and advance directives, practice guidelines, payment policy, and regulation would improve quality of life and the prospects of a "good death" for beneficiaries.

As part of the process for developing a better end-of-life contract, Medicare could invest in research and development that develops viable instruments, payment incentives, and accountability standards for end-of-life care. To be successful, Medicare will need to implement and evaluate end-of-life care not in the style of the Patient Self-Determination Act but rather in a more realistic mode: with payment, incentives, information, and oversight. Although the SUPPORT program generated mostly negative publicity, its aftermath created a great deal of policy learning about the requirements and subtleties of these end-of-life interventions. In effect, the debate and deliberation that followed SUPPORT was a good result, even if the investigators were disappointed that their particular intervention was unsuccessful. Broaching policy in this area necessarily requires a foundation of significant research and development that produces a scientific and clinical basis for communicating end-of-life decisions between doctors and patients.

A second ingredient of this contract is reimbursement that finances the ongoing generation of end-of-life care plans between doctors and patients or, in the case of managed care, between plans and Medicare enrollees. In order for physicians, patients, hospitals, hospice, and other providers to make significant progress in designing new approaches to end-of-life care, Medicare must pay for the time and administrative overhead for developing and documenting a plan for end-of-life care.[82] In reimbursement terms, the conversations and decisions that are required to create an advance directive must be treated as analogous to procedures. Plans could be audited and beneficiaries interviewed to determine the costs and efficacy of this approach. The prevalence of advance care plans and the utilization of alternative end-of-life treatments (e.g., hospice versus ICU days) would be a reportable measure of provider performance.

As a condition of Medicare participation, providers could be required to implement guidelines for limiting futile care that is paid for by Medicare. As in the Santa Monica Hospital case, the exact details of these guidelines can be left to the individual providers and regional purchasers. Although clinicians may challenge some of the nuances of these guidelines, such as what constitutes "adequate time" or when treatment is "medically indicated," these bands of discretion are entirely appropriate when defined at a policy level. Medicare can require that providers have guidelines and procedures for limiting futile treatment but not specify at a micro-level the clinical requirements for making this determination. The incentive arrangements of the Santa Monica Hospital Guidelines are also roughly right: hospitals bear some responsibility (and costs) for identifying alternative providers in the event that patients or families disagree with the determination that care is futile; patients and families bear the cost of further treatment if, after this clinical due process (complete with ethics review), the patient's care is still regarded as futile. In other words, the guidelines do not ultimately prohibit care that is futile, they merely limit the economic responsibility of taxpayers or other payers for care that "cannot, within a reasonable possibility, cure, ameliorate, improve, or restore a quality-of-life that would be satisfactory to the patient."

For care that is not strictly futile, but where costs are high, the probability of benefit is low, and the uncertainty of prognosis is high, Medicare has a more limited but still significant role. Here the agenda involves strategic development and implementation of practice guidelines for selected diagnoses such as congestive heart failure. In these more ethically and clinically ambiguous cases, the issue is less about structuring so-called terminal care and more about encouraging appropriate and cost-effective chronic and palliative care.

In the regional purchasing arrangements that are discussed in chapter 7 as a reform strategy, Medicare could capture many of the innovations that are occurring in palliative, hospice, and chronic care in selected markets in the country but are not possible in a one-size-fits-all nationally administered program. In Oregon, for example, the prevalence of advance directives for nursing home residents is reported to exceed 80 percent as a result of extensive education and outreach.[83] Regional purchasing agencies could contract, monitor, and advocate for better end-of-life care arrangements than are possible under current national Medicare administrative arrangements. It is an example of shrinking the distance between Medicare-as-principal and providers who exhibit different practice patterns in different regions. Such a regional approach to reform exploits the geographic variation that characterizes Medicare end-of-life care, as it does other aspects of Medicare delivery.[84] Such a regional approach could exploit what is already known about the local market influences on an end-of-life care.[85]

Even with strong inducements for advance planning and directives, beneficiaries may still make an informed and rational choice not to execute an advance directive. Nonetheless, this solution recognizes the role of the beneficiary as a principal in the contract and Medicare's role as a supplier of a public good—the information and wherewithal for beneficiaries to execute an advance directive if they choose.

The sophistication of the debate over policy for the dying has evolved considerably since the original observations in the early 1970s about the "high cost of dying" in Medicare. The current state of the art provides little empirical basis for expecting significant savings from the promotion of advance directives or the further marketing of hospice benefits. Many very sick patients utilize substantial medical resources but recover, while others use substantial resources and die. However, the broader Medicare challenge involves structuring an array of incentives and practices such that decisions carry out patients' wishes and so that society's health care resources are more appropriately allocated. Medicare pays for heart transplantation, but the program does not directly reimburse doctors, nurses, and social workers for simply and directly engaging patients in advance planning for their experience of dying. Through its activities with carriers and intermediaries, quality assurance activities, and regulation of fraud and abuse, Medicare makes a substantial effort to guarantee certain standards of access, facility standards, and financial integrity. Yet the program has little capacity to assure that patients do not experience pain and can exercise control over the "pathway" of their death.

As the major programmatic initiative in Medicare to provide appropriate care for terminal illness, the Medicare hospice benefit is probably under-utilized and substantially misused because it is not embedded in a larger concept of decision making for care at the end of life. For many beneficiaries, this benefit is not utilized at all or used too late in the course of illness to make much of a difference. All of this suggests symptoms of poor contracting and inadequate agency for beneficiaries.

CHAPTER SEVEN

Principals and Agents, Realities, and Medicare Reform

Introduction and Summary

Instead of entering into the Medicare reform labyrinth with a particular fix for financing or coverage—such as a premium-support model for financing or the Federal Employees Health Benefit Plan (FEHBP) model for administration—consider the problem of Medicare reform as an exercise of tackling and solving a series of principal-agent problems. This approach to Medicare reform is less about the search for a global fix—a magic bullet—than it is about the systematic building up of institutions, incentives, and information resources to be legislated and implemented.

This final chapter pairs a set of reform ideas with each of the Medicare realities introduced in chapter 1. In each case, the reform ideas are considered through the lens of the principal-agent framework developed throughout the book. Conceptually, these reform ideas grow out of a purchasing model for Medicare reform (described below), a model that imagines the administrative sponsor of the program acting in a stronger role as a principal in contracts with plans and providers—seeking the kinds of information, quality, and outcomes-orientation that would follow a formal contractual approach to management of the program.

Chapter 1 described five realities for Medicare reform that provide the context for any reform of Medicare's governance, institutions, and policy design: (1) Medicare is big and complicated, (2) beneficiaries are vulnerable, (3) everything varies by geography, (4) government administration is halting, and (5) providers are nimble. These realities provide important touchstones for discussions of the reform ideas in this concluding chapter. For other approaches to Medicare reform, these realities can serve as a filter for considering the feasibility of stylized approaches to policy and management. For example, the current interest in moving coverage and benefits to a "consumer-driven" paradigm, where beneficiaries are given a defined contribution and sent out to shop and choose health coverage, needs to be assessed in light of the financial, social, and even cognitive vulnerability exhibited by many of Medicare's beneficiaries.

Chapter 2 argued that Medicare's political origins and its subsequent history have created a pathway, a set of promises, symbols, institutions, constituencies, and expectations that cannot easily be eschewed in the name of some highly stylized and ideologically pure version of health care coverage and delivery. The situation for Medicare is analogous to John Chubb and Terry Moe's analysis of the problem of school reform, where the productive ground lies in considering institutional reforms as part and parcel of the larger reform project: "the last decade's 'revolution' in School reform has been restricted to the domain of policy, leaving the institutions of educational governance unchanged. In our view, these institutions are more than simply the democratic means by which policy solutions are formulated and administered. They are also fundamental causes of the very problems they are supposed to be solving."[1]

So, too, the challenge for moving Medicare reform ahead is to think simultaneously about institutions, politics, and policy. It is necessary to wrap an environment of institutions around the policy ideas in order to assure effective policy deliberation, as well as the possibility of implementation. The policy game described in this book focuses on identifying a set of reform approaches that are respectful of Medicare's path and politics, yet represent significant opportunities for improving the quality and economic performance of the program. Although many possible reforms can be analyzed and evaluated using a principal-agent perspective, this chapter will examine one such model: a regional/purchasing approach to Medicare.

Chapter 3 outlined an alternative toolkit, using the concepts, literature, and analytic approaches from agency theory, for understanding issues of

Medicare service delivery. This framework identifies a number of structural issues that lead to difficulties in Medicare policy making and management. Most fundamental, Medicare is a program that operates under the auspices of two principals—the public, who pay for the majority of Medicare services through taxes, and individual beneficiaries, who pay through premiums, deductibles, copayments, and out-of-pocket payments. A preoccupation with the agency problems involved in Medicare delivery leads to an analytic emphasis on the *contracts* that guide plan and provider behavior, *information* sources in the system (and their behavioral effects), *incentives,* and the administrative and *organizational oversight* of the program.

Chapter 4 investigated how agency for Medicare managed care might be redefined in legal, organizational, and financial terms. The chapter first recast Medicare's structure and history with managed care in agency terms. Interestingly, the legal history of Medicare managed care suggests that the organizational accountability of plans—their organizational *agency*—has never been definitively established. The chapter asked how the goals of managed care could be respecified in contracts written with plans and providers: for example, what forms and modalities of health prevention and promotion should be actively encouraged (through incentives and information) in managed care? How should incentives and information, such as risk adjustment and reporting on quality of plan performance, be conceptualized? In particular, how should the interface between social, chronic, and long-term care and the traditional forms of acute services for managed care models be encouraged and reimbursed? Should versions of S/HMOs and Program of All-inclusive Care for the Elderly (PACE) or other forms of managed care delivery be further developed and tested? What forms of care management and integration of services should be promoted for beneficiaries?

Chapter 5, the first of two case-study chapters, demonstrated the significance of technology assessment in the long-run costs and coverage of Medicare, using the artificial heart as an example. That chapter illustrated the important role that the march of technology plays in increasing costs and intensity of care. Decisions about coverage of new procedures, drugs, and devices are inherently difficult and will require the best thinking about quality-of-life consequences, resource use, and ethical implications. The capacity to conduct ongoing, substantial, and rigorous technology assessment is an important capacity for congressional policy making for Medicare. It is part of the agency that the Congress should play for the public in defining benefits, coverage, and payments to be provided by the Medicare program. Technology assessment has a large public good component and is appropriately performed in close proximity to purchasing and payment decisions. Bringing technology assessment more formally into the evolution of Medicare coverage, benefit design, and payment policy will require organizational invention as well as structural reform in congressional oversight of the program. In order to promote prudent use of technology at the beneficiary level, new approaches to supporting clinical decision making for beneficiaries will be necessary. Again, this will require the invention of new forms of beneficiary agency, a topic discussed in more detail later in this chapter.

More broadly, redesign of the structure of congressional deliberation, oversight, and analysis of Medicare policy would make it possible to consider priorities for resource allocation in Medicare. Priority setting, much less priority setting over time, is an exercise almost nonexistent in the current policy machinery for Medicare. Conceptually, if we asked what care and services would yield the greatest improvements in quality of life for Medicare beneficiaries (or even more conservatively, quality-adjusted life years—QALYs), we would undoubtedly produce an allocation of resources dramatically different from current Medicare. No one is asking this question in a systematic way.

Chapter 6, the second case-study chapter, looked at Medicare's treatment of end-of-life care from an agency perspective. It asked how one would design a contract that serves the interests of beneficiaries and the public and supports care that leads toward a "good death." What elements of quality palliative and end-of-life care should be made available to beneficiaries? Can processes of care, communication, the involvement of interdisciplinary professionals, and provision of information be achieved so that this most important moment of Medicare service delivery better serves its principals? Tackling these questions by using the tools of contracts and agency, as opposed to debating abstractions and slogans, is the fundamental approach of this book.

With this background, the book concludes with a look ahead, considering a set of reform ideas that recognize both Medicare's realities as well as its agency dilemmas. This discussion begins with a brief overview of a purchasing approach to reform. While other approaches lend themselves equally well to an agency toolkit, the ideas presented here serve both to introduce some new thinking about Medicare reform as well as to illustrate how an emphasis on agency concepts helps motivate and analyze alternative reform approaches.

A Purchasing Orientation for Medicare

With the exception of a series of reports by the General Accounting Office (GAO), relatively little translation of the experience of managing health benefits and promoting health care quality from the private side has made its way into Medicare policy and practice. Although the private record is itself arguably spotty, numerous innovations and systematic approaches to private benefits management deserve more analysis for the purposes of conceptualizing Medicare reform.[2] In their particulars, many of these plans have tackled health promotion and wellness, analyzed data on provider practice patterns, and engaged in selective contracting in a serious way to address both cost issues and quality of care.[3]

What would administration of a purchasing paradigm for Medicare look like? Two sources of ideas, evidence, and analysis exist for understanding the potential design of a purchasing approach to Medicare reform: (1) the private sector experience with purchasing coalitions and approaches; and (2) the public sector consideration of health alliances and purchasing cooperatives during the debate over the proposed Clinton Health Security Act. Indeed, perhaps one of the only positive legacies of the Clinton health proposal is that it provided a foundation of some provocative thinking on administrative redesign of national health systems.

Employer Approaches and Coalition

Experiments in employer coalition and purchasing models emerged during the early 1990s and received a great deal of attention during the Clinton reform debate. The basic philosophy behind these models was that *value* in health care could be enhanced by bringing to bear tools of quality improvement, information about and data analysis of provider performance, the use of incentives to reward quality and outcomes, and the purposeful use of contracting arrangements to structure relations with plans and providers. The more innovative coalitions engaged in education and communications programs; quality forums around particular areas of clinical practice, such as cardiac surgery and caesarian section rates; and identification of best practices among contracting providers.[4]

The Midwest Business Group on Health went one step further, initiating a set of discussions on public-private purchasing coalitions, including representatives from HCFA, state Medicaid programs, private employers, and business coalitions. Examples of these partnerships—the MEI partnership with Racine government and schools in Racine, Wisconsin; the Greater Detroit Area Health Council; the Buyer's Health Care Action Group partnership with the State Department of Employee Relations in Minneapolis; the Massachusetts Health Care Purchasing Group; the Business Health Partnership and Utah Health Care Purchasing Alliance in Salt Lake City; and the Foundation for Health Care Quality and State Department of Health partnership in

Seattle—illustrated many of the problems and prospects of achieving scale and cooperating on the purchasing side of health care.

An important insight from this experience was the potential power of tackling quality and information issues at a regional level. Pragmatic interventions for improving features of health care delivery—such as accessibility of service, dealing with the politics and intransigence of local hospitals, and consideration of the meanings of data and evidence at a local or regional level—were facilitated in some limited ways by these partnerships. These partnerships also showed some beginning capacity for dealing with the political and administrative dimensions of achieving quality improvement from plans and providers—building relationships and trust, building shared understandings of the problems to be addressed, and providing a "table" or venue for greater communication and work on regional health care delivery issues.[5]

At the peak of the debate about managed competition as the framework for health system development and health reform, there was some limited analysis of the potential of purchasing models and their potential for Medicare and Medicaid. The Progressive Policy Institute, for example, put forward a sketch of a proposal based largely on privatizing the insurance coverage for Medicare beneficiaries, but it had elements of an information and purchasing infrastructure at its core.[6] However, the overall record of purchasing cooperatives, especially cooperatives for small employers, has not been encouraging.[7] Cooperatives did not reach significant scale, did not show evidence of reducing prices, and elicited overt and covert opposition from insurers and insurance agents. Arguably, what is missing from this record is a fair test, one that involves supportive policy and participation by government purchasers, such as Medicare or Medicaid, that would bring these cooperatives up to a critical mass in regional markets. The Clinton reform plan stimulated widespread analysis and debate over the concepts of purchasing cooperatives and health alliances.

Health Alliances

The proposed health alliances in the Clinton reform plan represented an effort at a large-scale organizational fix to problems of insurance coverage, pricing, marketing, and regulation. Although the concept of the Clinton health alliances had a political shelf life of less than eighteen months, vestiges of these organizations live on in so-called private health purchasing cooperatives and several state reform initiatives. Critics of the alliance concept argued that the workings of the market, coupled with limited small-market insurance reform, would solve the key problems of insurance coverage and pricing without the need for organizational invention. Proponents of alliances argued that they were "market makers," the necessary administrative foundation for fair and productive competition among managed care plans to happen, especially in the face of risk selection and strategic behavior by plans.

The proposed Clinton health alliances were remarkable in their scale, complexity, and potential command of resources; indeed a good case can be made that health alliances represented one of the most complex and consequential organizational inventions in modern political history. They combined elements of a benefits office (recruiting and processing enrollment and transfers); the defense department (procurement of large quantities of complex products under conditions of accountability); a regulatory agency (overseeing insurance marketing practices); a consumer union (collecting and disseminating quality information); an administrative law agency (hearing grievances); and a negotiating body.

Health alliances in the Health Security Act differed substantially from other health insurance purchasing cooperatives that have been proposed and discussed in the literature.[8] In the administration's proposal, health alliances were regional organizations, either government or nonprofit, that recruited and enrolled beneficiaries, negotiated premiums and contracted with accountable health plans, administered risk adjustment of payments to plans, and monitored and disseminated information (e.g., report cards) about the performance of these plans. The alliances would establish and enforce rules for fair competition among health plans. In the details of the alliance proposal were strategies for preventing medical redlining and other strategic behavior by plans. Alliances were geographically bounded, typically mapping over large metropolitan areas or states but under no circumstances spilling over state boundaries. Alliances were to be governed by a board of directors drawn from participating employers and employees but not individuals who, by occupation or relationships, represented conflicts of interest. Most presentations of the alliance concept emphasized their nonpolitical nature; advocates of health alliances saw them, like the national health board, as quasi-public bodies that would be dominated by consumers of health care, not providers or experts.[9]

Throughout the literature on health insurance purchasing cooperatives (HIPCs) and health alliances, the notion of an HIPC functioning as an agent of consumers and employers was stressed. Paul Starr, for example, argued that the role of HIPCs in health planning should be limited because "it will jeopardize their special role as agents of the purchasers. A purchasing cooperative should be recognized, first and foremost, as the arm of the purchasers—that is consumers and employers." This is a classic agency formulation, where the organization is designed to carry out the interests of the payers in strict terms.

Knee-jerk reactions of two types greeted the Clinton administration's health alliances proposals. One reaction was simply ideological, that alliances symbolized more government over less, the triumph of collective solutions over individual interests and choice. A second, and perhaps more damaging, reaction was that these organizations represented new "bureaucracy"—as it turned out, perhaps the most negative label that could be put on a policy proposal in the early 1990s. Alliances became a virtual poster child of what was wrong with the Clinton plan. A television advertisement between "Louise" and her friend "Libby" complained that these "mandatory government health alliances" would restrict the choices of health plans and doctors available to consumers.

For Medicare's paradigm to shift from a concept of financing or reimbursing services to a concept of actively purchasing services that respond to the health priorities for population health (as well as the preferences of individual beneficiaries), changes in the respective roles of individuals, the public administrative sponsors, and private plans and providers will be necessary. For individual choice and management of health services, beneficiaries will need to be empowered and supported in making health care decisions. To carry out the public interest in Medicare services, greater emphases would be placed on specifying desired outcomes in advance, contracting for particular forms and processes of care. An active purchasing approach would emphasize strong incentives for provider and plan performance, producing accessible and influential quality assessment, and tailoring Medicare's services to the geographical realities of the market.

In theory, a purchasing approach for Medicare has the potential to marry a progressive health agenda for aged and disabled persons with the use of contracting, market arrangements, and competition. While there is no inherent reason why reform that serves the interests of Medicare's most vulnerable beneficiaries cannot go hand-in-hand with achieving efficiencies in cost and quality, strong ideological currents have prevented these two agendas from coming together. However, Medicare's contractual arrangements must make it worthwhile for plans and providers to serve disadvantaged, sick, and socially isolated beneficiaries. In effect, the program, in its design, needs to reverse the incentives for risk selection and reward excellence in providing certain forms of care management for vulnerable patients. Medicare has a precedent for tailoring policy to vulnerable populations in its coverage and reimbursement for end-stage renal disease and hospice care. With careful design and implementation, a purchasing approach, coupled with a regional orientation and improved contracting (see below), could provide the basis for purposeful programming and payment for disadvantaged classes of patients.

The best outcome would be systems of care and provider competition that actually reward providers who affirmatively step forward to take care of vulnerable and sick patients.

Medicare Is Big and Complicated: Roles and Supports
for Congressional Policy Making

At the highest level of Medicare policy making, one can ask whether the Congress effectively acts as the agent of the public in designing and implementing Medicare policy. (Remember in chapter 3, the basic theory imagined that Medicare service delivery operates under two principals—its policy design intermingles an articulated public interest with the private interests of beneficiaries in seeking and managing care.) If the Congress, for structural and other reasons, is unable to articulate and represent the public interest as the ultimate principal in Medicare, then the program will be unable to manage the fiscal and economic realities posed by demographics and the federal budget, the changing needs of beneficiaries, and the pace of adjustment in the health care market.

Although a full treatment of the shortcomings of congressional policy making for Medicare is beyond the scope of this book, it is worth pausing on this problem to consider the principal-agent dimensions of congressional oversight of Medicare and to look toward some possible alternatives. Clearly, the Congress has demonstrated limited capacity for oversight, limited willingness or ability to respond to market change, and little appetite to counter the special interest capture of Medicare policy. In the spirit of the analysis of this book, are there ways to make congressional policy making for Medicare less "halting" and more responsive to the needs of beneficiaries and vendors through improved agency? Are there ways to assure that the Congress's guidance represents the public interest in services for beneficiaries?

Several political and structural problems can be identified in the congressional relationship to Medicare policy making and administration. First, Medicare's history has been characterized by divided government, meaning that in twenty-eight of the thirty-six years of the program's existence, the executive branch, Senate, and House have been held by different parties.[10] Within the Congress, oversight and policy authority is divided between the House Ways and Means Committee, and the House Committee on Commerce, the House Judiciary Committee (e.g., fraud and abuse), the Senate Finance Committee, and, to a much lesser extent, the Senate Labor and Human Resources Committee.[11] As a structural matter, the oversight of the long financial health of the program is outsourced to the trustees of the Hospital Insurance fund and the Supplemental Insurance Program. Year-to-year recommendations are now made by the Medicare Payment Advisory Commission (MedPAC) but, again, at some distance from the committee structure and with uneven coverage of Medicare issues: heavy on payment policy, relatively light on beneficiary and administrative concerns.

The incentives and rewards for Medicare policy making in the Congress are also out of phase with both the long-run financial concerns of the program and the short-run and often urgent needs for changes in payment, coverage, and management. The short-run influence of the two-year cycle in the House, the volatile, age-based politics of Social Security, and the geographically loaded politics of the budget process mean that few members have political reasons to tackle the inevitably controversial long-run issues necessary for changing the Medicare status quo. Because so little administrative discretion has been delegated by the Congress to the bureaucracy, the Medicare providers and beneficiaries are often held hostage for long periods of time until congressional attention returns to the specifics of their issues. Even then, Congress usually considers Medicare issues in the context of budget reconciliation rather than dedicating attention to Medicare policy.

The budget reconciliation context for Medicare policy making creates a seesaw of generosity and constraint in program benefits, coverage, and reimbursement, depending on the larger fiscal climate. A budget-cutting regime is applied to provider reimbursement policy when the Congress is facing deficits or fiscal constraints; expansion of the program occurs in the short-term environments of surplus. As a matter of public finance, this cyclical approach to reform and payment policy often has the perverse effect of putting plans and providers through reimbursement stringency at precisely the time when their finances tend to be most stressed. The budget surplus and the Medicare "lockbox" were the immediate context for considering the Medicare prescription drug benefit in 2001. With the sudden changes in the economy and fiscal policy that followed the September 11 terrorist events, a whole new budget and political context suddenly surrounded Medicare. Beneficiaries, providers, and Medicare's administration are all buffeted by these exogenous changes in budget-driven policy.

While on the one hand this congressional environment means that political checks and balances effectively prevent any large ideological or philosophical shifts in the program, it also means that significant and sustained attention has been difficult or impossible to achieve. Congressional attention to Medicare has always been balkanized, presidential leadership tepid, and interest group pressure divided and diffuse. Given this structure, issues of principle or structure of the program become suppressed in the politics of budget reconciliation, and attempts to frame larger reforms get token or episodic expression in bipartisan commissions such as the Pepper Commission, the Bowen Commission, and the National Bipartisan Commission on the Future of Medicare.

In the background, the Congress lacks the data, analytic, and intellectual resources to give sustained and expert attention to the project of Medicare reform. Congress currently receives input from a disparate set of institutions—the trustees of the funds, MedPAC, the Congressional Budget Office (CBO), the GAO, CMS, Health and Human Services' Assistant Secretary for Planning and Evaluation, committee staff—but ultimately relies on no closely held or substantial policy analytic infrastructure. For example, the Congress has no significant, ongoing resources to monitor and evaluate the implications of new technology for Medicare and the health system more broadly. The ability of the Congress to engage and provide sustained attention to the long-term reform issues facing Medicare (and health policy more generally) is in part a function of its analytic and support capacity. While both the intramural and extramural congressional capacity for policy analysis and formulation has grown in the past two decades, it has grown in a diffuse way. The relatively successful experience of the Physician Payment Review Commission (PPRC) in formulating physician payment policy has been eclipsed, and the future status, capability, and influence of MedPAC is uncertain.

Thomas Oliver's study of the establishment and behavior of PPRC for the Congress demonstrates how a well-functioning commission exerted control over the relevant information and dominated the agenda for physician payment in Medicare. When it was created, the PPRC defined its role as providing "independent" advice to the Congress and the Secretary of Health and Human Services. Although Oliver's account credits the PPRC and its role with achieving one of the major Medicare policy successes in its entire history, the structural lesson is actually more troubling for the larger agenda of Medicare reform. According to Oliver, who quotes David Smith:

> The creation of a body such as the PPRC is a testament to the protracted partisan conflict that exists between the legislative and executive branches of the federal government, and represents an attempt by legislators to break the characteristic "deadlock and drift" in policy under those conditions. This is extraordinarily difficult, however. The decentralized structure of the Congress and its patterns of behavior generally allow it to follow or respond to the president, but not take the lead. . . . Indeed the Congress devised the PPRC only after the executive branch did not come forth with proposals for a Part B counterpart to the new Medicare hospital payment system. . . . Under the circumstances, the development of

physician payment policy represented "an extreme example of what Congress can do, with little help and some active opposition from the executive branch."[12]

By tailoring the policy analytic support narrowly around physician payment (and its counterpart, the Prospective Payment Commission for Hospitals), the Congress neither created a strong and sustainable institutional policy engine for Medicare reform, nor did it connect the information and analytic capacity demonstrated by the PPRC (in the lead up to the Omnibus Reconciliation Act [OBRA] of 1989) to the later implementation and administration of the physician payment by HCFA. Meanwhile, the GAO, the CBO, the staffs of the several House and Senate committees have grown significantly, though (perhaps with the exception of CBO) without a well-defined institutional responsibility and mandate for particular policy analysis of Medicare reform.

It is also interesting that much of the intellectual capital surrounding the Medicare program has been developed and supported through the efforts of nongovernmental sponsors. In particular, a set of interested foundations— the Robert Wood Johnson Foundation, the Kaiser Family Foundation, the Commonwealth Foundation—have taken on an external role of monitoring and analyzing Medicare, especially the experience of the program under Medicare+Choice. It is not clear how influential or well integrated this work has been with either the priorities of congressional deliberation or even the technical input that is flowing up through staffs. Rather, the foundations and the broader health services research community appear to be playing the role of honest broker of information, with a particular emphasis on evaluation. However, all of this decentralized body of research and evaluation lacks an overall policy quarterback.

Respecifying and restricting the domain of Medicare policy will be as important as restructuring committee and analytic support for Medicare reform in the Congress. Chapter 2 illustrated the proliferation of transfers and what Guzmano and Schlesinger have called the "collateral" programs of Medicare.[13] As the discussion of budgetary politics in that chapter demonstrated, the number and complexity of Medicare's other agendas, such as the financing of graduate medical education or the granting of disproportionate share payments to hospitals serving indigent patients, means that Medicare policy deliberation can be captured by the special interests of providers, insurers, and other beneficiaries of federal spending. The politics of these issues are entangled in the structure of committee work and interest groups that surround them. It is difficult to imagine the Congress adopting an uncompromised role as principal for the Medicare program as long as the individual members and relevant committees are so encumbered with these collateral interests.

This discussion of the agency role of the Congress and the related commissions and executive agencies considers only the structural features of Medicare's politics in the Congress; it does not address the motives and involvements of interests groups, the paucity of recent presidential leadership over Medicare, or the nature of public opinion and voting that surrounds the legislative and administrative politics of Medicare. However, isolating and improving the performance of the Congress as an agent of Medicare policy, at least making it more streamlined and visible in its responsibilities for representing the public interest, would be a significant step in the larger project to make the program more responsive to public, beneficiary, and market concerns. The politics of reforming congressional structure and supports with respect to Medicare are daunting in their own right. However, this analysis should give reason to believe that reform of Congress-as-agent in Medicare policy itself is an important project. Some would argue that all else is secondary.

Government Is Halting: Creating a New Medicare Agency

Beneath this high-level agency problem of the Congress as the public's agent, a series of grittier agency problems—incentives, organization, information—specific to the Medicare program's relationship with plans, providers, and beneficiaries requires policy attention. The dysfunction of the former Health Care Financing Administration (HCFA), now the Centers for Medicare and Medicaid Services (CMS), as the administrative sponsor for Medicare means that a serious rethinking and organizational restructuring of the administration of the program is required. (This is not to diminish the necessity of also addressing the underlying structure of Medicare payment policies, benefits, intermediaries, information, and interface with beneficiaries in a unified way.)

Medicare was born with an idea that the central administrative function of the state was to pay claims for acute medical care with a minimum of control, oversight, and management. This idea was a product of the politics of the times. It emphasized avoiding "any supervision or control over the practice of medicine or the manner in which medical services are provided"[14] or, in particular, any affront to the AMA and organized medicine. The implicit contract was intergenerational, with younger workers paying for "necessary" medical services, and deferential to the judgment of medical professionals and providers. This was nowhere more evident than in the philosophy and practice of "cost-plus" reimbursement. For medical providers, these are now considered the good old days.

Over time, particularly as cost containment became a priority for Medicare payment policy, a partial shift in the governmental role and objective for program administration occurred. However, despite some significant forays in hospital and physician payment policy, the goals of promoting cost-effectiveness, facilitating beneficiary choice of health plans, rewarding quality, and encouraging innovative approaches to care have never been fully institutionalized in Medicare's policy design, organization, and administration. The overarching social contract has not been significantly updated or rearticulated, nor have new instruments for carrying out a revised social contract been seriously developed. Now, Medicare exhibits a form of path dependence, under which its philosophy of social insurance, the institutions that grew up around its payment policies, and its minor forays into competitive and market solutions to delivery have created a legacy that conditions all future reform options.

Chapter 3 asserted that public institutions (political and administrative) and private beneficiaries bear joint responsibility for purchasing and orchestrating health services under Medicare. These two parties serve as dual principals in the Medicare contract. The conceptual model for reform of the program developed in this chapter envisions that the Congress and the public administrative sponsor for Medicare, CMS, undertake a much more proactive and comprehensive role in defining the content and emphases of the benefit package in Medicare to more explicitly carry out the role of principal. In this model, the stance of the administration of Medicare would shift to that of a more active purchaser of health services, carrying out the public interest in health care for aged and disabled beneficiaries. For their part, beneficiaries would be given both better tools and more responsibility for choices of coverage and plans, as well as managing their own health care with their providers.

The limitations of HCFA, and now CMS, in administering Medicare's scale and scope of activities have been well documented and discussed.[15] HCFA has led an organizational life in which it has not been granted the administrative authority and resources to actively participate in the marketplace as a purchaser of health care for its beneficiaries, yet at the same time it has often been criticized for not behaving in this mode. The Congress has demonstrated profound ambivalence about the degree to which it would like to see Medicare use the tools of incentives, information, regulation, quality assessment, to change provider behavior. Timothy Jost characterizes the congressional involvement in the governance of Medicare as "frenetically active, intrusively micromanaging the program, but primarily for budgetary and ideological reasons."[16] Congress has been reluctant to delegate this responsibility to HCFA and especially reluctant to convey administrative discretion. I presented an extreme example of this phenomenon in chapter 2, where HCFA has been thwarted by individual members of Congress from implementing competitive pricing demonstrations, even though the Congress itself has mandated that this demonstration project be performed.

Hammond and Knott's analysis of control over bureaucracy helps frame the political problem of designing the Medicare bureaucracy in principal-agent terms.[17] Paraphrasing (and simplifying) Hammond and Knott, bureaucracies can be either autonomous (i.e., independent of presidential or congressional direction) or controlled by either the Congress or the president. In a situation where there are two principals, the Congress and the president, an agency such as HCFA can be either controlled or autonomous. In theory, HCFA could have been autonomous (1) if the president or Congress had been indifferent to its behavior, (2) if the principals had engaged in substantial conflict over the behavior of the agency, or (3) if significant information asymmetries had existed such that the agency controlled important sources of information. In the agency politics discussion of chapter 2, none of these conditions for autonomy appeared to exist. Both the president and the Congress have taken a significant interest in the agency and its decisions, and the information asymmetry that HCFA might naturally have enjoyed has never developed; it has been offset by the creation of numerous other resources for both congressional and executive control over information.

Perhaps no other function of the federal government provides a better opportunity for institutional invention and administrative reform than the development of a national health purchasing capability for Medicare.[18] The generic administrative problem involves creating effective contracting mechanisms, producing modern information and reporting tools, and establishing effective outreach and support for a vulnerable population interacting with a complicated service-delivery system. Whether a strong congressional function in Medicare policy making and a strong administrative function in Medicare purchasing could coexist is an interesting question of political and organizational design.

Under a strong version of administrative autonomy and authority, a newly constituted Medicare agency would be responsible for a set of functions that are national in scope and scale. This is consistent with the idea of the Medicare national board proposed in the original Breaux-Thomas proposal. As an executive agency, it would engage in the ongoing translation of the congressional will into standards of benefits and coverage that would extend to all Medicare beneficiaries. This translation involves complex questions that should be influenced by an ongoing process of analysis and inquiry coordinated across a broad spectrum of public and private organizations, including the federal resources of the Agency for Health Care Research and Quality, the National Institute on Aging, and the many other health-related agencies in the Department of Health and Human Services. The Medicare Agency would be responsible and accountable only for the design and oversight of the Medicare program *qua* delivery of health and social services for its covered aged and disabled beneficiaries. Under this model of administrative autonomy, the functions of the Medicare Agency would be strictly consolidated and streamlined, and collateral functions of Medicare, such as paying disproportionate-share hospitals and graduate medical education, would be jettisoned.

Contrast this model with CMS's current diffusion and fragmentation of administrative oversight of Medicare, as described by the GAO:

> CMS' management focus is divided across multiple programs and responsibilities. Despite Medicare's estimated $240 billion price tag and far-reaching public policy significance, there is no official whose sole responsibility is to run the Medicare program. In addition to Medicare, the CMS administrator and senior management are responsible for oversight of Medicaid and the State Children's Health Insurance Program. They also are responsible for individual and group insurance plans' compliance with the Health Insurance Portability and Accountability Act of 1996 in states that have not adopted conforming legislation. Finally, they must oversee compliance with federal quality standards for hospitals, nursing homes, home health agencies, and managed care plans that participate in Medicare and Medicaid, as well as all of the nation's clinical laboratories. The Administrator is involved in the major decisions relating to all these activities; therefore, time and attention that would otherwise be spent meeting the demands of the Medicare program are diverted.[19]

In principal-agent terms, narrowing and defining the process and outcome accountability for the Agency would provide the foundation for overseeing the Medicare contract as well as minimize the opportunities for organizational shirking, strategic behavior, and drift.

Obviously, to be effective, the agency needs to be given a mandate and the resources necessary to administer these national functions. Staff shortages and turnover, lack of computing and administrative infrastructure, and limited management and policy have all constrained CMS's ability to effectively manage the program. For example, the GAO has noted that CMS operates with only "49 senior executives to manage the two biggest insurance programs in the country and activities accounting for hundreds of billions of dollars in annual spending."[20] In administrative terms, this amounts to penny-wise and pound-foolish on a massive scale.

The administrative resource question can best be considered in cost-benefit terms. A 1 percent tax on Medicare payments would provide over $2.4 billion for national administration, research, guideline development, quality improvement, information and communications tools development, and evaluation. Instead of bragging that all of Medicare administration (including claims processing) takes only slightly over one percent of total expenditures, it is worth asking whether additional support (say in increments of one percent of expenditures) for the Medicare policy and purchasing function should be authorized up to the point where the benefits of increased administrative infrastructure (e.g., in efficiency and quality improvement) equal its costs.

Everything Varies by Geography: Regional Administration for Medicare

If Medicare is to solve a set of agency problems that arise at the level of plans, providers, and beneficiaries, then a new administrative structure tied to geography will ultimately be necessary.[21] The implication of much of the geographical variation documented in this book is that a modern administrative structure for Medicare can and should be built around regional purchasing organizations, Medicare regional sponsors.[22] The intellectual justification for regional administration and finance is based on the need to manage and reduce the regional variations in Medicare practice that have been extensively documented here and elsewhere. Taken together, Jonathan Skinner, Elliot Fisher, and John Wennberg estimate that these regional variations alone demonstrate inefficiency (i.e., expenditures with no observable incremental benefit) on the order of 20 percent of all Medicare outlays.[23]

The argument for regional administration is more subtle than the argument that Medicare utilization and service should be standardized. Observation of variation in Medicare services does not by itself reveal inefficiency; rather it provides a *signal* for management of the program that some deviation in practice is occurring, and an opportunity for further analysis, management, and perhaps improvement in quality and efficiency. Without regional administration, it is unlikely that the information resources, collaborative work with providers, and changes in contracting will be marshaled to address this variation. At the end of the day, it is theoretically possible that active regional administration would generate incentives and contracting for more, less, or the same service as currently provided, but the utilization would be directed and informed by more sophisticated understandings of the underlying Medicare epidemiology, provider service delivery, and trade-offs in resource allocation for that region.

In this model, regional sponsors would function as the direct contractors, payers, and beneficiary representatives with plans and providers in a defined geographical area. The organizations combine some of the features of old Blue Cross/Blue Shield plans (especially their community-rated character); modern purchasing cooperatives such as the California Public Employees' Retirement System (CalPERS), especially its contracting and information capabilities; and health alliances (especially some of the governance and regulatory functions). As a heuristic, think of these organizations as representing roughly 1 million beneficiaries (like CalPERS), though the exact configuration of the sponsor's catchment area would vary for rural areas and other geographical considerations.

If structured by state jurisdictions, the sponsors would often be smaller in terms of coverage, but could conceivably represent rural and other political dimensions of administration more effectively (see the discussion of regional budgeting below). The sponsors would likely be private nonprofit organizations, but they could also be quasi-governmental bodies. Likely candidates for this role include purchasing pools and organizations, respected insurers such as some Blue Cross/Blue Shield organizations, or intermediaries and carriers. Regional sponsors would be selected through a process of franchise bidding and contracting, consistent with what we have learned about the properties of successful franchise bidding arrangements.[24]

It would be important for the sponsors to either provide themselves or contract for an ambitious program of beneficiary agency, including services for plan and provider choice, coordination of retiree and Medicare coverage, coordination with Medicaid coverage, dispute resolution and grievance response with plans and providers, and counseling and decision support for medical and long-term care decisions. In these respects, the sponsor would incorporate many of the functions of a well-conceived benefits office for private firms, but with specialized capacity for dealing with aged and disabled beneficiaries.

The most important argument for creating the regional sponsor is that it would work collaboratively with other payers, plans, and providers to improve the quality of service, to implement guidelines, gather information, and manage observed variation in a region. Programmatic funds would be part of the regional budgets, allowing for partnerships and collaboration with other payers, as well as more intensive and constructive work to improve quality with plans and providers in the region. This kind of on-the-ground, developmental work on quality of care is virtually absent in the current Medicare program.

One of the major technical stumbling blocks in the organizational design of the Clinton health alliance proposals was the mechanism for determining premiums for plans and budgets for alliances. Because there was tremendous uncertainty about enrollment in plans, bidding by accountable health plans, risk adjustment and selection, and other important parameters, the proposed system of rate setting involved a complex negotiated back-and-forth among plans, alliances, and the national health board. The exercise of setting up regional administration and budgets for Medicare finesses many of these issues. Because the enrolled population is known in advance and a long history of payment policy exists as a baseline, the budgets for regional sponsors can in principle be established prospectively without resorting to many of the machinations debated in the Clinton plan. Over time, the process of regional budgeting should come together with a process for regional competitive bidding with plans and providers.

The concept of regional budgeting for Medicare has been around for some time. For example, a working group on Medicare reform that convened at the Harvard Medical School in the mid-1980s developed a bold proposal for reform based largely on a regional administrative structure.[25] Their proposal lodged responsibility for hospital care of Medicare recipients under a prospectively determined budget, shifting the risks of hospital costs (and the dilemma of hospital cost containment) to state governments. This change had the effect of changing the "distance" involved in Medicare transactions and devolving the administration of programs in much the same way that other social programs have been moved to state administration.

Although little analysis or justification of this radical shift in intergovernmental responsibility is offered in the various presentations of the Harvard proposal, some insight into its rationale can be gained from Rashi Fein's analysis of the relative merits of state versus federal control of the machinery of health care administration. Fein believed that states faced profoundly different problems of health care utilization and service delivery from state to state as well as variable capacity to manage: "The individual patterns found across the land are best understood and best addressed at a locus of control that is closer to those delivery systems and to the people they serve. California is not the same as West Virginia, and the systems and incentives that would best suit one are not necessarily appropriate for the other. . . . It is difficult to imagine that such a task can be performed from Washington or that if it were it would be found acceptable."[26] Fein acknowledged that there would be variability in the responses and capabilities of state government. In the principal-agent terms of this book, he saw the strategy of devolving the responsibility for administration as consistent with the behavior of a risk-averting principal: "If . . . we recognize that there is no guarantee that a government will always act wisely and appropriately, we may want to act as risk-averters. Multiple state programs are like a diversified portfolio: we will not do as well as we might have if we had bet on a single winning program, but neither will we do as badly if we were to commit a blunder."[27]

The Harvard proposal and other plans that advocate a regional approach to budgeting and administration address several of the critical agency problems in Medicare. Regional budgets help address the agency problem for Medicare by designating regional jurisdictions and organizations as the agents for resource allocation in health. The creation of regional budgets limits the risk to the public principal (the public fisc), presumably provides some efficiencies of scale in information gathering and monitoring, allows for regional variation in practice patterns to be managed, and potentially limits the opportunities for the agent to engage in selection practices. Although there has been little analysis of the informational costs, accountabilities, and advantages of higher and lower levels of regional aggregation in Medicare, it is clearly an important design issue that bears on the selection of states, or other bodies, as the geographical unit for designating intermediaries.

The concept of "administrative geography" has grown up in policy analysis of the devolution of social welfare programs to states, counties, and municipalities.[28] A social welfare definition of administrative geography as the "territorial boundaries that organize the eligibility, allocation, and delivery of program services" would be an appropriate conceptual starting point for drawing the boundaries of Medicare regional administration.[29] In social welfare policy, the relevant trade-offs include the difference between the scale and scope of labor markets versus the political and administrative boundaries mapped to cities and suburbs. In health care, the trade-offs will include the distinction between the boundaries of markets for plans and providers, and useful political and administrative jurisdictions for policy. For Medicare specifically, the challenge will be to design regional areas that have sufficient numbers of beneficiary lives (say, covered populations of one million) or markets of hospital services versus jurisdictions that are marked by insurance regulations, Medicaid programs, and constellations of retiree health plans.

Of course, a regional approach to Medicare resource allocation and administration will introduce a whole new set of political dynamics into the program. Here again, it is useful to think ahead about what principal-agent structures are desirable from a political perspective. If the Medicare regions map to health care markets, they will not correlate perfectly with either state political representation or necessarily congressional representation. This means the tendency to treat Medicare payments and resources as "pork" to be protected or captured by political representatives will be diminished. As the congressional history of protecting payments for hospitals in New York or establishing payment floors for managed care plans in Wyoming has illustrated, this kind of patronage Medicare policy can be economically inefficient, though politically understandable. On the other hand, mapping Medicare payment and administration to state jurisdictional boundaries could institutionalize a strong form of political checks and balances, where governors and other state political resources will care and advocate to the federal government for maintaining and enhancing Medicare payments and services in their states. It would also create more logical integration with the Medicaid program.

Providers Are Nimble: Improving Medicare Contracting

Managed care is about to pass Medicare by. Now, the Bush administration's goal to increase the proportion of Medicare beneficiaries enrolled in Medicare+Choice plans to 30 percent by 2005 seems extremely ambitious. The highly publicized withdrawals, the erosion of prescription drug benefits (and other supplementary benefits of participating in managed care), and the generalized backlash against managed care that has attended the patients' rights movement means that the early hopes for large-scale conversion of Medicare coverage to managed care have been dashed. It now appears that the future of Medicare managed care must lie in distinctive and attractive alternatives for beneficiaries, not perceived restrictions on their choice, denials of coverage, hassles, or other constraint.

The Congress never established a clear and coherent agenda for contracting with Medicare+Choice plans. Several broad agendas are possible for managed care: Medicare can use managed care approaches to achieve discounts in payments and overall expenditures; Medicare can use managed care approaches to coax innovations and restructuring of the delivery system; or Medicare can use managed care approaches to change the scope and quality of health care delivery to a defined population of enrollees. To date, the agenda has seemed to be mostly the first of these possibilities, to achieve some savings in overall expenditures, yet without the proper mechanisms to assure that these savings are not simply risk selection or other strategic behavior by plans.

The most promising direction for Medicare managed care is to emphasize the second two agendas: to promote innovations and restructuring of the delivery system and to change the scope and quality of services for beneficiaries. This harkens back to the original interests in HMOs as national policy, where it was believed that the incentives for prepaid health care would produce an emphasis on health prevention and promotion, and innovations in delivery. Now, an emphasis on integration of acute and long-term service and an emphasis on modern care management for chronic conditions can be added to these original goals. The payoffs of integrated delivery systems—organizations of care that combine and coordinate acute, postacute, subacute, chronic, and long-term care; social services; and hospice—while not yet demonstrated in the empirical literature, can potentially be significant for beneficiaries, many of whom will need care that moves them rapidly through these now largely discrete systems. The incentives provided by prepayment in managed care and a contractual framework that emphasizes these aspects of care and delivery are necessary to accomplish the hard organizational work needed to better integrate services. A framework of quality information and performance assessment of the plan is necessary to promote a philosophy of caring for the health of the whole covered beneficiary population. Designation of plans as the legally accountable agent for resource allocation and care management will be a necessary step, as illustrated in the legal and regulatory discussion of chapter 4.

On the payer side, an analogous need exists for coordinating and combining coverage to promote an intelligent allocation of resources. The PACE models, for example, have brought together Medicaid and Medicare resources to promote more coordinated community-based approaches to long-term care. Similar thinking and experimentation should occur at the interfaces of retiree health coverage and Medicare, and of Medigap coverage and Medicare.

The challenge from a design, incentive, and accountability perspective is to promote high-quality care for the sickest and most vulnerable beneficiaries by contracting with plans exactly for this response and rewarding them accordingly. The irony of the Medicare managed care experience is that the largest potential benefits of this model could in theory accrue to beneficiaries with cancer or chronic conditions, such as diabetes and congestive heart failure, and to those who face challenges to access. Unfortunately, much of the evidence gives reason to believe that the performance of managed care plans has been most suspect in these very areas. Little in the incentives and contracting for Medicare managed care has promoted systematic disease and care management for these vulnerable groups. On the contrary, the absence of appropriate risk adjustment for plans provided powerful reasons for the plans to avoid these patients and certainly not develop reputations for these particular modes of care.

The last part of the reform agenda for Medicare managed care does not involve financial change as much as organizational and administrative change. Medicare needs to establish a capable, stable, and respected business partner for plans. For quality plans to be induced back into Medicare managed care, the administration and contract must be perceived as fair, stable, and re-munerative. This will require a fundamentally different organizational spon-sor and contracting perspective. The sponsor will need to be more flexible and less bound by regulation and rule making. The sponsor will need to be geo-graphically closer and more substantively knowledgeable about the market and provider issues confronted by individual plans. Finally, the sponsor will need to engage in contracting with a longer-term horizon with an eye toward encouraging the participation of high-quality plans over a sustained period of time.

One of the most difficult problems of Medicare agency over the next decade will be its relationship with and management of individual providers in a fee-for-service world. Under even the most optimistic forecasts, managed care enrollment will continue to be a substantial minority of all Medicare beneficiaries. As a result of the 1997 Balanced Budget Act (BBA) changes, Medicare is at a crossroads in its relationship with individual providers in terms of the resources of CMS, intermediaries, and carriers. Medicare has not had great success in building either quality or information programs at the in-dividual level with participating providers. While some analysts see informa-tion systems and the Internet as a potential vehicle for creating stronger agency with individual physicians, hospitals, and other providers, substantial changes in behavior and systems would be necessary to make this direct-to-provider payment and management approach work effectively.

The key problem is not traditional utilization management, as histori-cally provided by intermediaries and carriers, which emphasizes the denial of payment for miscoded, unauthorized, or uncovered services. Rather, the chal-lenge is to assure that individual providers are providing the highest quality and appropriate services for individual beneficiaries. The most intriguing structural possibility here, made possible by changes in the 1997 BBA, is the use of commercial carriers to manage fee-for-service care. Here again, the concept of writing contracts to shape and provide accountability in fee-for-service care has significant potential. In effect, this would represent an exten-sion of Havighurst's concept of a contractual paradigm for consumers in health care.[30] For a Medicare beneficiary population, however, considerable agency would be required to make coverage, provider choice, and medical decisions accessible.

Private fee-for-service options made possible in Medicare+Choice pro-vide one such vehicle for creating agency in fee-for-service Medicare, though with some significant risks. As discussed in chapter 4, the private fee-for-service plan receives a capitated payment from Medicare and, in turn, admin-isters and pays claims for its enrolled beneficiaries. In return for taking on the administration and risk of these health care expenditures, the private fee-for-service plan is able to keep any surpluses that may result from claims less than capitated amounts. Thus, these plans replace public agency with private agency in Medicare delivery. If fee-for-service is going to be the modal approach to Medicare delivery, as it appears it will be, then new focus needs to be placed on structuring agency arrangements with individual providers (or intermediaries) that provide standards of quality, efficiency, and accountability that serve the interests of Medicare's two principals.

Beneficiaries Are Vulnerable: Improving Beneficiary Agency

The requirements for decision making around health plan choice have been well described and considered in the literature.[31] One of the takeaways from this literature is that the gap between information tools and cognitive wherewithal for consumers of health insurance and health services is great. This gap is arguably greatest for Medicare beneficiaries among all users of the health care system. Nonetheless, scattered throughout this literature is the finding that Medicare beneficiaries want information about their coverage, options, and health care itself, but they want it in a form that speaks to them and is not embedded in complex and irrelevant information. (The example given by Shoshanna Sofaer and Margo-Lea Hurwicz is that beneficiaries do not want information on pediatric immunizations.[32]) The implication of this literature is that substantial tailoring and customizing of this information needs to occur for a Medicare population. The longer-term implication is that plan, provider, and health care information will need to be fit to individual circumstances, which will require new forms of individual agency for beneficiaries.

Thus, cognitive and informational problems loom large in the agenda to convert Medicare beneficiaries to rational consumers exercising the form of plan choice envisioned in Medicare+Choice, much less engage in more active management of their own care. Despite some analysts' (and CMS's) enthusiasm about the potential role of information tools and the Internet in solving this problem, new organizational and interpersonal structures of agency and support will inevitably need to come into existence for beneficiaries to play this role of an active consumer and manager of their own care.

Distinct problems of agency confront beneficiaries when they need to make choices about health plans and coverage, when they make decisions about providers, when they are confronted with illness and hospitalization, when they lose a spouse or otherwise experience changes in their social supports, or need to make housing or long-term care decisions. It is easy to underestimate the psychosocial complexities of these decisions; cultural factors, religion and spirituality, life experiences and values, as well as trust in providers and organizations can all play a role.

The agency problem for beneficiaries is also confounded by the interests of family members and others in health care decision making. Often, family members, partners, and other caregivers have views about these decisions and will bear many of the consequences of them. Even decisions about coverage, plans, and providers can have significant downstream consequences for significant others; the choice of coverage can ultimately determine what options are available for such services as respite care, adult day care, and support services.

Where do beneficiaries go now for such agency? There are examples and resources throughout the health care and social services system, but for the most part they are small and unsystematic in their coverage and capabilities. Employers and human resource departments play some of this role for beneficiaries in retiree health plans. Hospital social work departments, agencies on aging, volunteer Medicare assistance programs, and now some specialized firms provide information and counseling on selected aspects of plan choice and health care decisions, usually at about the time home care or other long-term care needs are identified. Most recently, CMS has launched a national 1-800-MEDICARE information service, complete with an advertising campaign featuring actor Leslie Neilsen. Many states have developed information and assistance services for long-term care decisions, though these services are highly variable and are often unknown to residents at the moment they need assistance, such as when a hip fracture or serious illness has occurred.[33] It is interesting that no substantial market response has emerged to fill this need, but this is probably explained by the absence of any formal source of payment and the idiosyncratic nature of the perceived need for service.

The practical possibilities for institutionalizing agency for beneficiaries and their families are numerous, including existing health care providers, social service agencies, agencies on aging, volunteer and consumer-oriented groups, human resources departments, and community organizations. In most situations, physicians lack the inclination, the training, the time, as well as the expertise in counseling and other services to carry on the conversations and provide the care management that many beneficiaries require. At the same time, it makes sense for much of this agency to occur in close proximity to care delivery, ideally in the context of interdisciplinary teams that work with beneficiaries over time. It is only in the context of such arrangements that the kinds of nuanced conversations about such issues as planning end-of-life care can be envisioned.

In the framework developed in this book, strong beneficiary agency should be structured as either an integral part of the regional sponsor's activities or as a significant subcontract with the sponsor. These organizations should be available to beneficiaries and their families to assist in making plan and provider choices, to respond to questions about coverage and service, to explain quality and performance information about plans and providers, to help identify long-term care options and providers, and to serve an ombudsman role for grievances and claims problems. These organizations should have the character of "one-stop" social service provision and "plain talk" insurance provision. The organizations should bring social work, benefits management, and health administration capabilities to beneficiaries in an accessible form. In financial terms, this function should command a significant portion of the premium dollar for beneficiaries, perhaps as much as 1 to 5 percent of expenditures in order to carry out this complex and labor-intensive program of communications with beneficiaries.

Concluding Comments

Where has this exercise in conceptualizing Medicare reform through the lens of principal-agent relationships taken us? It has elevated the challenge of articulating the social contract for Medicare to the first order of business for Medicare reform. Before we can logically produce the instruments of payment and organization for Medicare, we need to be able to better articulate—as a political and policy matter—the broad purposes and objectives of the program. An agency approach suggests that these purposes be defined in outcome and process terms in order for efficient contracts to be written. It is ultimately the responsibility of our political institutions to articulate and implement this social contract in real legislation, regulation, and rules. However, instead of the usual discussion of defining the Medicare social contract in some broad rhetorical sense, it will be much more useful for actual policy formulation to gather some consensus around some selected and narrower high-priority domains of coverage and service delivery. In this book, I have tackled Medicare's challenge in the domains of end-of-life care, the uptake of new technology (e.g., the artificial heart), and the design of managed care arrangements. Not only do these represent some of the most significant policy problems facing Medicare broadly, they represent useful case studies for applying a principal-agent framework.

In its focus on theory, the analysis has identified a number of principles and goals for optimal contracting in Medicare. The program should strive to approximate the properties of outcomes-based contracts, or costless process-based contracts. In cases where the Medicare program and it beneficiaries have common preferences for the quantity and quality of health services, the primary challenge is to create forms of agency using incentives and information sources that encourage and discipline providers to provide that care. A significant amount of end-of-life care fits this case. In situations where the public interest and beneficiaries' preference may diverge, a more difficult problem of structuring agency ensues. Establishing policy for newly emerging technologies that are life saving, but extremely costly and with uncertain quality of life—such as the early artificial heart technology—represents an example of this problem. In this case, the first order of business is to create stronger organizational and informational supports for technology assessment and priority setting in Medicare. Many tools for creating improved agency for beneficiaries can be named, but it will also be important to preserve some instruments of agency, such as the integrity of the doctor-patient relationship, as markets and market regulation evolve.

Several of the most significant reform problems facing Medicare have been analyzed to produce a set of recommendations that are rooted in an agency approach. In response to the Congress's inability to delegate important administrative discretion to the Medicare bureaucracy, I propose a new scope of work and a new framework for congressional analytic support. For a Medicare managed care program in disarray, I propose a new contractual framing of care, with an emphasis on quality purchasing and integrated services, especially for the most vulnerable beneficiaries. For the inattention to technology policy—a crucial blind spot in updating care and gaining long-term control over costs—I propose a structure for analysis and input into congressional decision making and regional discipline over provider contracting. For end-of-life care, as well as other key areas of care management, I propose multiple levels of policy intervention, including a return to the development of and contracting for practice guidelines. All of these steps are framed by the idea of Medicare as a contractual undertaking.

For this contractual approach to be operational in Medicare, a new administrative structure, built around clarified agency and designating functions, is also proposed. This structure envisions that Congress will attend to longer-term policy issues and delegate administration of the program to an executive body. In principle, this means that the congressional committee(s) responsible for Medicare *qua* Medicare would restrict their attention to policy over payment, coverage and benefits, technology, and quality. The analytic resources of the Medicare actuaries, the committee staff, MedPAC, perhaps the GAO, and the Congressional Research Service would be consolidated into a close and responsive analytic capability for the Congress. The Secretary of Health and Human Services would create an elevated responsibility for the national administration of the program—its costs, quality, accessibility, and out-comes—in a new organization, named simply and appropriately enough, the Medicare Agency. The agency itself would have a limited role, establishing annual requirements for coverage and benefits, writing the contracts with regional sponsors that allocate the Medicare regional budget, overseeing national quality improvement of the program, and brokering a broad program of data collection and research (including the development and implementa-tion of Medicare guidelines).

At the regional level, new Medicare regional sponsors, operating under regional budgets, would take on responsibility for provider contracting, pay-ment (eventually in response to competitive bidding), promoting quality im-provement, communicating information to beneficiaries, and assuring strong forms of agency for beneficiaries. The regional sponsors would bring Medi-care's administration into closer proximity with the geographic variation that is endemic in Medicare, allowing for that variation to become a tool of effective management and quality improvement. Regional sponsors can be either quasi-governmental or nonprofit organizations and would be selected under a model of franchise bidding and renewal. The creation of regional budgets would allow for both flexibility and discipline in the system, forcing decisions about the adoption of new benefits and programs down to organizations that must live within a budget constraint. Restricting the size of the sponsor's catchment area would encourage pursuit of meaningful quality and access projects that are appropriate for that particular geographical area. The most exciting possibility of this model is the possibility of both public and private payers working together on quality improvement and information, as well as the possibility for payers to work collaboratively with plans and providers.

The regional sponsors would also assume the role of contracting with Medicare managed care plans, eventually under a regime of competitive bid-ding. (Because of the checkered history of the competitive bidding demon-strations, no significant testing of the feasibility and outcomes of these models has yet occurred.) For Medicare managed care to have a future, however, the plans will need to develop care management capabilities that transcend what is possible under simple, disorganized individual provider arrangements. This means that plans need to operate under specific contracts that develop excellence in particular modes of care that respond to the com-plex and often chronic health care needs of beneficiaries. The trick, then, for Medicare managed care is to flip the behavior of plans from positive risk se-lection and provider discounting to developing integrated systems of care that will take care of beneficiaries with diabetes, cancer, and other complex condi-tions at the highest level of care. This transformation will require innovation in payment and contracting (combining Medicare and Medicaid sources), a change in the modus operandi of plans, and ultimately a shift in the reputation and trust attributed to Medicare managed care plans.

A critical part of making choice work, beneficiary selection of providers work, and appropriate use of the health care system work, once providers are selected, will be the introduction of new forms of agency to be available to individual beneficiaries and their families. In this proposal, the loci of these organizations would vary depending on the resources and needs of particular communities. They would be funded, contracted, and overseen by the regional Medicare sponsor. They would not be token elements of reform, but rather a significant new feature of health care information and use.

I can now return to the problem posed at the beginning of this book and ask how this reform approach helps answer the question of whether new forms of rehabilitation therapy should be covered and paid for by Medicare. First, I recognize that the public has a joint interest in this decision and should develop the organization and techniques of technology assessment, especially with a quality-of-life orientation, to evaluate the merits of these new therapies. Second, (armed with this technology assessment) the Congress and Medicare Agency would transmit recommendations for coverage and payment to the regional sponsors for decisions about inclusion and guidelines at the level of plans and providers. Decisions about inclusion of these therapies would be operationalized in the contracts written with plans and providers. Finally, information and support for beneficiaries in making coverage, plan, and provider decisions would be built into the capabilities of beneficiary agents. Indeed, beneficiaries and families who have experienced the sudden complexities in making coverage and care decisions after a brain or spinal injury are paradigmatic candidates for improved Medicare agency.

In many cases, the ideas explored in this book either predate the original Medicare enactment or are products of the national struggle to achieve health care reform over the past three decades. Regionalization, emphases on quality, development of guidelines and outcomes, modernizing the administrative arrangements for Medicare, implementing risk adjustment, competitive bidding, market reform, purchasing, and producing accessible and valid information about plan and provider performance are all projects that have captured the agenda and sometimes the imagination of the health policy community in the recent history of reform. In each case, however, the problems are technically hard, demand sustained political attention, and ultimately require new political and administrative institutions. It is this latter agenda—building effective and sustainable institutions to support reform—that has been the poor stepchild of health politics and policy analysis.

Instead, our politics and policies have suffered from a form of attention deficit disorder. In recent history we have lurched from one preoccupation to another: from outcomes research and practice guidelines, choice, fraud and abuse, and now patient safety and medical errors, to name just four of the recent transitions. Our politics and policy formation seem incapable of maintaining the kinds of serious and sustained attention, as well as allocating the resources, that are required to make progress on these reform elements. Did we ever achieve the research and practice foundation for implementing guidelines in medicine? Did we ever achieve useful and valid report cards for beneficiaries? No, but still we have moved on to the next policy preoccupation. Progress on many of these fronts is not necessarily ideologically controversial; instead there is an absence of incentives, rewards, and accountability for our political and administrative organizations to see these changes though to completion.

It is instructive to look back on the history of Institute of Medicine (IOM) reports, to take just one illustration, as a benchmark of the translation of policy analysis and ideas into policy and practice. The IOM has produced significant reports on virtually every topic covered in this book: Medicare quality assurance, Medicare market reform, the total artificial heart, and end-of-life care. These book-length reports involve great expertise as well as a process for achieving consensus among those holding some diverse viewpoints. More than a dozen major reports have advocated the creation of a national organization and administration for health technology assessment.[34] Nonetheless, it is remarkable how little uptake has occurred in the wake of these well-conceived, reasoned recommendations. At least one of the explanations is the absence of institutional and informational mechanisms for translating these findings into policy attention over time.

If I use Harrison White's metaphor of agency relationship as a kind of social plumbing, then we appear to have some significant blockage in the flow of ideas and analysis into policy. Removing this blockage will require the creation of better institutional arrangements for both accountability for the program and its services and translating Medicare analysis and evidence into the world of politics and action. With institutional reform, we may have the possibility of incorporating social and policy learning into the long-term reform of the program. For Medicare reform to follow, politics and institutions must lead. Searching out opportunities for improved agency and writing "good contracts" are elements of an important toolkit for making the connection of politics and institutional change to the larger agenda of Medicare reform.

Chapter One

1. Sandra Blakeslee, "Therapies Push Injured Brains and Spinal Cords into New Paths," *New York Times,* August 5, 2001, sec. D, 6.

2. The resolution of dual agency problems in managed care arrangements is discussed extensively in Mark Schlesinger, "Countervailing Agency: A Strategy of Principaled Regulation under Managed Competition," *Milbank Quarterly* 7, no. 1 (1997): 35–87.

3. A short bibliography of book-length treatments in the Medicare reform literature includes Karen Davis and Diane Rowland, *Medicare Policy: New Directions for Health and Long-Term Care* (Baltimore: Johns Hopkins University Press, 1986); David Blumenthal, Mark Schlesinger, and Pamela Brown Drumheller, eds., *Renewing the Promise: Medicare and Its Reform* (New York: Oxford University Press, 1988); Mark Pauly and William Kissick, eds., *Lessons from the First Twenty Years of Medicare* (Philadelphia: University of Pennsylvania Press, 1988); Marilyn Moon, *Medicare Now and in the Future,* 2d ed. (Washington, D.C.: Urban Institute, 1996); Theodore R. Marmor, *The Politics of Medicare,* 2d ed. (New York: Aldine de Gruyter, 2000); Robert D. Reischauer, Stuart Butler, and Judith R. Lave, eds., *Medicare: Preparing for the Challenges of the Twenty-first Century* (Washington, D.C.: National Academy of Social Insurance, 1998); Andrew Rettenmaier and Thomas R. Saving, eds., *Medicare Reform: Issues and Answers* (Chicago: University of Chicago Press, 1999); Ronald J. Vogel, *Medicare: Issues in Political Economy* (Ann Arbor: University of Michigan Press, 1999); and Joseph White, *False Alarm* (Baltimore: Johns Hopkins University Press, 2001).

4. David Cutler, Kenneth G. Manton, and James W. Vaupel, "Survival after the Age of 80 in the United States, Sweden, France, England, and Japan," *New England Journal of Medicine* 333, no. 18 (November 2, 1995): 1232–35.

5. See, for example, Patricia Neuman, Diane Rowland, and Elaine Puleo, "Understanding the Diverse Needs of the Medicare Population: Implications for Medicare Reform," *Journal of Aging and Social Policy* 10, no. 4 (1999): 25–50.

6. Health Care Financing Administration, Office of Strategic Planning, Medicare Current Beneficiary Survey. Available in digital format from CMS.

7. Cathy Schoen, *Medicare Beneficiaries: A Population at Risk* (Menlo Park, Calif.: Henry J. Kaiser Family Foundation, December 1998).

8. Schoen, *Medicare Beneficiaries*.

9. Medicare Payment Advisory Commission (MedPAC), *Report to Congress: Medicare Payment Policy* (Washington, D.C.: MedPAC, March 2001), 21–47.

10. MedPAC, *Report to Congress: Medicare in Rural America* (Washington, D.C.: MedPAC, June 2001), 24–38.

11. Steven M. Asch et al., "Measuring Underuse of Necessary Care among Elderly Medicare Beneficiaries Using Inpatient and Outpatient Claims," *JAMA* 284, no. 18 (November 8, 2000): 2325–33.

12. Lauren McCormack et al., "Health Insurance Knowledge among Medicare Beneficiaries," October 20, 1999, draft.

13. Geraldine Dallek, *Consumer Protections in Medicare + Choice* (Menlo Park, Calif.: Kaiser Family Foundation, December 1998).

14. For a review, see John Wennberg, "Understanding Geographic Variation in Health Care Delivery," *New England Journal of Medicine* 340, no. 1 (January 7, 1999): 32–39; and Henry Krakauer et al., "The Systematic Assessment of Medical Practice Variations and Their Outcomes," *Public Health Reports* 110, no. 1 (January/February 1995): 2–12.

15. Elliot S. Fisher et al., "Associations among Hospital Capacity, Utilization, and Mortality of Medicare Beneficiaries, Controlling for Demographic Factors," *Health Services Research* 34, no. 6 (February 2000): 1351–62.

16. See, for example, Barry P. Katz et al., "Demographic Variation in the Rate of Knee Replacement: A Multi-Year Analysis," *Health Services Research* 31, no. 2 (June 1996): 125–40; Patricia A. Cowper et al., "Geographic Variation in Resource Use for Coronary Artery Bypass Surgery," *Medical Care* 35, no. 4 (April 1997): 320–33; and Gregory S. Cooper et al., "Geographic and Patient Variation among Medicare Beneficiaries in the Use of Follow-Up Testing after Surgery for Nonmetastatic Colorectal Carcinoma," *Cancer* 85, no. 10 (May 15, 1999): 2124–31.

17. Jack Hadley, Jean M. Mitchell, and Jeanne Mandelblatt, "Medicare Fees and Small Area Variations in Breast-Conserving Surgery among Elderly Women," *Medical Care Research and Review* 58, no. 3 (September 2001): 334–60.

18. Elliot S. Fisher et al., "The Implications of Regional Variations in Medicare Spending: Part 1, The Content, Quality, and Accessibility of Care," *Annals of Internal Medicine* 138, no. 4 (February 18, 2003): 273–87; Elliot S. Fisher et al., "The Implications of Regional Variations in Medicare Spending: Part 2, Health Outcomes and Satisfaction with Care," *Annals of Internal Medicine* 138, no. 4 (February 18, 2003): 288–98.

19. Robert Brook et al. "Appropriateness of Acute Medical Care for the Elderly: An Analysis of the Literature," *Health Policy* 14, no. 3 (May 1990): 225–42; Brook et al., "Predicting the Appropriate Use of Carotid Endarterectomy, Upper Gastrointestinal Endoscopy, and Coronary Angiography," *New England Journal of Medicine* 323, no. 17 (October 25, 1990): 1173–77; and Steven M. Asch et al., "Measuring the Underuse of Necessary Care among Elderly Medicare Beneficiaries."

20. Dartmouth Medical School, Center for the Evaluative Clinical Sciences, *Dartmouth Atlas of Health Care* (Chicago: American Hospital Publishing, 1998).

21. Edward F. Lawlor and Kristiana Raube, "Social Interventions and Outcomes in Medical Effectiveness Research," *Social Service Review* 69, no. 3 (September 1995): 383–404.

22. Lisa Green, *Medicare State Profiles: State and Regional Data on Medicare and the Population It Serves* (Menlo Park, Calif.: Henry J. Kaiser Family Foundation, September 1999); Barbara Gage, Marilyn Moon, and Sang Chi, "State-Level Variation in Medicare Spending," *Health Care Financing Review* 21, no. 2 (winter 1999): 85–98.

23. F. L. Lucas, D. E. Wennberg, and D. J. Malenka, "Variation in the Use of Echocardiography," *Effective Clinical Practice* 2, no. 2 (March/April 1999): 71–75.

24. H. Gilbert Welch, David Wennberg, and W. Pete Welch, "The Use of Medicare Home Health Services," *New England Journal of Medicine* 335, no. 5 (August 1, 1996): 324–29.

25. General Accounting Office (GAO), *Medicare Home Health Care: Prospective Payment System Could Reverse Recent Declines in Spending* (Washington, D.C.: GAO, September 2000), 20–22.

26. Stephen Jencks et al., "Quality of Medical Care Delivered to Medicare Beneficiaries: A Profile at State and National Levels," *JAMA* 284, no. 13 (October 4, 2000): 1670–76.

27. Jonathan Skinner and John E. Wennberg, *How Much Is Enough? Efficiency and Medicare Spending in the Last Six Months of Life*, NBER (National Bureau of Economic Research) Working Paper 6513 (Cambridge, Mass.: NBER, April 1998).

28. Herbert Simon, *Models of Bounded Rationality*, vol. 2 (Cambridge, Mass.: MIT Press, 1983).

29. This history is recounted in considerable detail in Bryan Dowd, Roger Feldman, and Jon Christianson, *Competitive Pricing for Medicare* (Washington, D.C.: AEI Press, 1996); and Bryan Dowd, Robert Coulam, and Roger Feldman, "A Tale of Four Cities: Medicare Reform and Competitive Pricing," *Health Affairs* 19, no. 5 (September/October 2000): 9–29.

30. The formal contracting issues are described in David Epstein and Sharyn O'Halloran, "Administrative Procedures, Information, and Agency Discretion," *American Journal of Political Science* 38, no. 3 (August 1994): 697–722; and Randall L. Calvert, Matthew D. McCubbins, and Barry R. Weingast, "A Theory of Political Control and Agency Discretion," *American Journal of Political Science* 33, no. 3 (August 1989): 588–611.

31. Vogel, *Medicare: Issues in Political Economy*, 64.

32. GAO, *Medicare Home Health Agencies: Closures Continue, but Little Evidence Beneficiary Access Is Impaired* (Washington, D.C.: GAO, May 1999).

33. An extensive description of these changes and their implications is provided in GAO, *Medicare: Home Health Care Utilization Expands While Controls Deteriorate* (Washington, D.C.: GAO, March 1996).

34. For a description of the 1997 Balanced Budget Act's Home Health changes, see Joint Economic Committee, *1999 Greenbook* (Washington, D.C.: U.S. Congress JEC, 2000), 131–41.

35. Robert Pear, "Medicare Spending for Care at Home Plunges by 45 Percent," *New York Times*, April 21, 2000, 1.

36. Bruce Vladeck and Barbara Cooper, *Making Medicare Work Better* (New York: Mt. Sinai Institute for Medicare Practice, March 2001), 3.

37. Health Care Financing Administration, *1999 HCFA Statistics: Providers/Suppliers*, 1999. All numbers are rounded to the nearest 100. Available at www.hcfa.gov/stats.

38. Statement of William Scanlon, *Twenty-first Century Challenges Prompt Fresh Thinking about Program's Administrative Structure* (Washington, D.C.: GAO, May 4, 2000), 4.

39. MedPAC, *Reducing Medicare Complexity and Regulatory Burden* (Washington, D.C.: MedPAC, December 2001), ix, 7.

40. National Academy of Social Insurance (NASI), *Medicare Claims Handling: The Consumer Perspective* (Washington, D.C.: NASI, April 1993). The report is useful in that it presents case examples of insurance claims problems faced by beneficiaries.

41. Richard J. Margolis, *Risking Old Age in America* (Boulder, Colo.: Westview Press, 1990), 61.

42. Charles B. Inlander and Charles MacKay, *Medicare Made Easy* (Allentown, Penn.: People's Medical Society, 1996).

43. Connacht Cash, *The Medicare Answer Book*, 3d ed. (Provincetown, Mass.: Race Point Press, 1999).

44. Centers for Medicare and Medicaid Services, *Medicare and You 2002* (Baltimore: CMS, September 2001). The complexity of this guide is discussed in MedPAC, *Reducing Medicare Complexity and Regulatory Burden*, 27.

45. Legislation to regulate physician incentive plans was first enacted in the Omnibus Budget Reconciliation Acts (OBRA) of 1986 and 1987. In 1990, these laws were superseded by a new OBRA. Further changes were enacted with the Medicare+Choice Program. See Medicare Regulations, part 422, of June 26, 1998, with the final rule in July 2000, including requirements for physician incentive program disclosure at sections 42 CFR 422.208/210.

46. Theda Skocpol, "Pundits, People, and Medicare Reform," in *Medicare: Preparing for the Challenges of the Twenty-first Century*, ed. Robert D. Reischauer, Stuart Butler, and Judith R. Lave (Washington, D.C.: National Academy of Social Insurance, dist. by the Brookings Institution, 1998), 21.

47. Jacob S. Hacker, *The Road to Nowhere* (Princeton, N.J.: Princeton University Press, 1997); Haynes Johnson and David S. Broder, *The System* (Boston: Little, Brown, 1996); and Theda Skocpol, *Boomerang* (New York: W. W. Norton, 1996).

48. Paul Starr, *The Social Transformation of American Medicine* (New York: Basic Books, 1982), 375.

49. For an insightful discussion of the divide between analyses of health politics and contemporary health policy, see Jacob Hacker's review essay, "A Tale of Editions: Marmor's *The Politics of Medicare* and the Study of Health Politics after 30 Years," *Journal of Health Politics, Policy, and Law* 26, no. 1 (February 2001): 120–38.

50. See Marilyn Moon, *Searching for Savings in Medicare* (Menlo Park, Calif.: Henry J. Kaiser Family Foundation, December 1995).

51. Concord Coalition, *A Primer on Medicare* (Washington, D.C.: June 2000), i.

52. David Cutler, "What Does Medicare Spending Buy Us?" in *Medicare Reform: Issues and Answers*, ed. Andrew Rettenmaier and Thomas R. Saving (Chicago: University of Chicago Press, 1999), 131–52.

53. The basic concept of a contract as a form of promise is developed in Charles Fried, *Contract As Promise* (Cambridge, Mass.: Harvard University Press, 1977); for an overview of old-age policy as an intergenerational contract, see Vern L. Bengtson and W. Andrew Achenbaum, eds., *The Changing Contract across Generations* (New York: Aldine de Gruyter, 1993).

54. The most recent systematic attempt to distill and articulate the nature of the social contract underlying Medicare was produced by a committee of the National Academy of Social Insurance (*Medicare and the American Social Contract: Final Report of the Study Panel on Medicare's Larger Social Role* [Washington, D.C.: NASI, February 1999]). The committee was asked to answer the question, "What social values is the nation trying to pursue through Medicare, recognizing that the government maintains other programs to help the aged and disabled?" The committee made a valuable contribution to the debate on long-term reform of Medicare, but by necessity it articulated very broad principles for understanding and discussing reform options—financial security, equity, efficiency, long-term affordability, political accountability, political sustainability, and maximizing individual liberty—principles which together raise a host of trade-offs and even internal contradictions. The strongest conceptual

notion of a social contract in the committee's report is a classic restatement and reaffirmation of the underpinning of social insurance for Medicare.

Chapter Two

1. Eric Patashnik and Julian Zelizer, "Paying for Medicare: Benefits, Budgets, and Wilbur Mill's Policy Legacy," *Journal of Health Politics, Policy and Law* 26, no. 1 (February 2001): 7–36.

2. Robert M. Ball, "What Medicare's Architects Had in Mind," *Health Affairs* 14, no. 4 (winter 1995): 62–63.

3. An extensive account of the influence of organized medicine, especially the AMA, on the politics and implementation of Medicare was contained in a *New Yorker* "Annals of Legislation" series: Richard Harris, "The Real Voice," parts 1–3, *New Yorker* 40 (March 14, 1965): 48–50+; (March 21, 1965): 75–76+; (March 28, 1965), 46–48+. See also Harris, *A Sacred Trust* (New York: New American Library, 1966).

4. W. J. Cohen, "Reflections on the Enactment of Medicare and Medicaid," *Health Care Financing Review*, annual supplement (1985): 8.

5. Stuart Altman, quoted in Emily Friedman, "The Compromise and the Afterthought: Medicare and Medicaid after 30 Years," *JAMA* 274, no. 3 (July 19, 1995): 280. For an extended discussion of the accommodations to the hospital industry in Medicare, see Judith Feder, *The Politics of Federal Health Insurance* (Lexington, Mass.: Lexington Books, 1977).

6. Starr, *The Social Transformation of American Medicine*, 375.

7. Ball, "What Medicare's Architects Had in Mind," 65.

8. Patashnik and Zelizer, "Paying for Medicare."

9. This administrative evolution is traced in Lawrence D. Brown, "Technocratic Corporatism and Administrative Reform in Medicare," *Journal of Health Policy, Politics, and Law* 10, no. 3 (fall 1985): 579–99.

10. For an extensive and highly personalized account of the activities and philosophy of this group, the apparatus, see Edward D. Berkowitz, *Mr. Social Security: The Life of Wilbur J. Cohen* (Lawrence: University of Kansas Press, 1995).

11. National Academy of Social Insurance, *Medicare and the American Social Contract*, 51–52.

12. John Oberlander, "Medicare and the American State: The Politics of Federal Health Insurance, 1965–1995" (Ph.D. diss., Yale University, 1995); and Robert Hudson, "The Evolution of the Welfare State: Shifting Rights and Responsibilities for the Old," in *Critical Gerontology: Perspectives from Political and Moral Economy*, ed. Meredith Minkler and Carroll Estes (New York: Baywood, 1997), 329–43.

13. Public Law 89-97, *Health Insurance for the Aged and Medical Assistance*, 89th Cong., HR 6675, July 30, 1965.

14. National Academy of Social Insurance, *Medicare and the American Social Contract*, 29.

15. David G. Smith, *Paying for Medicare: The Politics of Reform* (New York: Aldine de Gruyter, 1992).

16. Theodore Marmor, "Coping with a Creeping Crisis: Medicare at Twenty," in Theodore Marmor and Jerry Mashaw, eds., *Social Security: Beyond the Rhetoric of Crisis* (Princeton, N. J.: Princeton University Press, 1988), 182.

17. Carroll Estes, *The Aging Enterprise* (San Francisco: Josey Bass, 1979).

18. Richard Himelfarb, *Catastrophic Politics: The Rise and Fall of the Medicare Catastrophic Coverage Act of 1988* (University Park: Pennsylvania State University Press, 1995), 33–42, 95–103.

19. The history here is obviously rich and complicated. The Pharmaceutical Manufacturing Association lobbied heavily because of potential downstream limitations on prescription drug payments. Senior citizens' groups such as the National Committee for the Preservation of Social Security and Medicare as well as groups mobilized just for this purpose objected to the financing provisions. Members of the Congress shifted their positions as revised cost and budgetary estimates became available. Excellent accounts of this story are contained in Marilyn Moon, *Medicare Now and in the Future;* and the Kennedy School of Government, *Catastrophic Health Insurance for the Elderly* (Cambridge, Mass.: Kennedy School of Government Case Program, 1995).

20. For a vivid account of the backlash to the Medicare Catastrophic Coverage Act and Rostenkowski's encounter, see Annetta Miller, "The Elderly Duke It Out," *Newsweek,* September 1, 1989, 42–43.

21. Christine L. Day, "Older Americans' Attitudes toward the Medicare Catastrophic Coverage Act of 1988," *Journal of Politics* 55, no. 1 (February 1993): 167–77.

22. Nancy McCall, Treva Rice, and Judith A. Sangl, "A Consumer Knowledge of Medicare and Supplemental Health Insurance Benefits," *Health Services Research* 1 (February 1986): 633.

23. Thomas Rice, Katherine Desmond, and Jon Gabel, "The Medicare Catastrophic Coverage Act: A Post-Mortem," *Health Affairs* 9, no. 3 (fall 1990): 75–87.

24. Ibid.

25. Robin Toner and Robert Pear. "In Budget Talks, No Hint of Pact on Health Issues," *New York Times,* December 4, 1995, sec. A, 1.

26. Marmor, *The Politics of Medicare,* 124.

27. Marmor, "Coping with a Creeping Crisis," 182.

28. Health Care Financing Administration, *Distribution of Medicare+Choice Provider Payments under the Medicare, Medicaid, and SCHIP Benefit Improvement and Protection Act 2000* (Baltimore: HCFA, n.d.).

29. For an introduction to the institutionalists' perspective on health reform, see Mark Peterson, "Institutional Change and the Politics of the 1990s," *American Behavioral Scientist* 36 (1993): 782–801; and Sven Steinmo and Jon Watts, "It's the Institutions, Stupid! Why Comprehensive National Health Insurance Always Fails in America," *Journal of Health Politics, Policy, and Law* 20, no. 2 (summer 1995): 329–72.

30. Jack Hoadley, quoted in Thomas Oliver, "Analysis, Advice, and Congressional Leadership: The Physician Payment Commission and the Politics of Medicare," *Journal of Health Politics, Policy, and Law* 18, no. 1 (spring 1993): 141–42.

31. This account is drawn from unpublished commission documents, as well as Beth Fuchs and Lisa Poetz, "The Breaux-Thomas Proposal," in *Competition with Constraints,* ed. Marilyn Moon (Washington, D.C.: Urban Institute, 2000), 155–85.

32. Stuart Butler et al., "Crisis Facing HCFA and Millions of Americans," *Health Affairs* 18, no. 1 (January/February 1999): 8–10.

33. For a detailed presentation on this implementation, see National Academy on Social Insurance, *Reflections on Implementing Medicare* (Washington, D.C.: NASI, January 2001).

34. Discussed in Joseph A. Califano, *Governing America: An Insider's Report from the White House and the Cabinet* (New York: Simon & Schuster, 1981), 43–45.

35. Brown, "Technocratic Corporatism and Administrative Reform in Medicare."

36. Ibid., 584.

37. Congressional Research Service.

38. Scanlon, *Twenty-first Century Challenges Prompt Fresh Thinking,* 4.

39. GAO, *Medicare Transactions System: Success Depends upon Correcting Critical Managerial and Technical Weaknesses* (Washington, D.C.: GAO, May 16, 1997).

40. Scanlon, *Twenty-first-Century Challenges Prompt Fresh Thinking,* 6–7.

41. Lynn Etheredge, "Medicare's Structure and Governance: A Proposal," *Health Affairs* 19, no. 5 (September/October 2000): 60–71.

42. Barbara Cooper and Bruce Vladeck, "Bringing Competitive Pricing to Medicare: Theory Meets Reality, and Reality Wins," *Health Affairs* 19, no. 5 (September/October 2000): 49–54.

43. MedPAC, *Reducing Medicare Complexity and Regulatory Burden,* 9.

44. Johnson and Broder, *The System;* and Skocpol, *Boomerang.*

45. For an example of this critique, see Bill Thomas, "1965–1995: Medicare at a Crossroads," *JAMA* 274, no. 3 (July 19, 1995): 276–78.

46. Robert H. Binstock, "Older People and Voting Participation: Past and Future," *Gerontologist* 40, no. 1 (2000): 18–31; and Robert B. Hudson, "The History and Place of Age-Based Public Policy," in *The Future of Age-Based Public Policy,* ed. Robert B. Hudson (Baltimore: Johns Hopkins University Press, 1997).

47. The Kaiser-Harvard Program on the Public and Health/Social Policy, in *Survey on Medicare* (Menlo Park, Calif.: Kaiser Family Foundation, June 1995).

48. For an extensive review of the public opinion data on Medicare, see National Academy of Social Insurance, *Medicare and the American Social Contract,* 63–83.

49. Physician Payment Review Commission, *Monitoring Access for Medicare Beneficiaries* (Washington, D.C.: PPRC, May 1995).

50. See Edward Lawlor, "Hard Choices, Unfair Choices, and Tragic Choices," in *Paying for Health Care,* ed. Lawrence Joseph (Chicago: Chicago Assembly and the University of Illinois Press, 1990).

51. Robert Pear, "New Money for H.M.O.'s Isn't Going As Congress Intended," *New York Times,* January 26, 2001.

52. This importance of connecting policy analysis to politics in this way is described in Jacob Hacker's essay "A Tale of Two Editions." The classic formulation of path dependence is found in Paul Pierson, "When Effect Becomes Cause: Policy Feedback and Politics," *World Politics* 45 (1993): 595–628; and Pierson, "Increasing Returns, Path Dependence, and the Study of Politics," *American Political Science Review* 94, no. 2 (June 2000): 251–67.

53. Brown, "Technocratic Corporatism and Administrative Reform in Medicare," 579–80.

Chapter Three

1. Mark Pauly, *Medical Care at Public Expense* (New York: Praeger, 1977).

2. Charles Fried, *Contract As Promise.*

3. The economic theory of agency is generally traced back to Stephen A. Ross's "An Economic Theory of Agency: The Principal's Problem," *American Economic Review* 62, no. 2 (May 1973): 134–39; Michael Jensen and William Meckling, "Theory of the Firm: Managerial Behavior, Agency Costs, and Ownership Structure," *Journal of Financial Economics* 3, no. 4 (October 1976): 305–60. The legal literature on agency arises out of the law of agency, which specifies rights and responsibilities of principals and agents, usually emanating from voluntary contractual relations.

4. An example from my street illustrates this point: a neighbor approached a real estate agent to sell his house and revealed his reservation price. The real estate agent offered to pay this price and bought the house herself. Besides the questionable professional ethics of the agent's behavior, there are significant questions about the efficacy of the contract itself; the principal's and agent's interests were clearly not aligned, and no steps were taken either to monitor the agent's behavior or assure that the best outcome in terms of price had been achieved.

5. Kenneth J. Arrow, "The Economics of Agency," in *Principals and Agents,* ed. John W. Pratt and Richard J. Zeckhauser (1985; reprint, with a new preface, Boston: Harvard Business School Press, 1991), 37–51.

6. See, for example, Joseph Stiglitz, "Risk Sharing and Incentives in Sharecropping," *Review of Economic Studies* 61 (1974): 219–55; and Mark Cohen, "Optimal Enforcement Strategy to Prevent Oil Spills: An Application of a Principal Agent Model with Moral Hazard," *Journal of Law and Economics* 30 (April 1987): 23–51; Stefan Reichelstein, "Constructing Incentive Schemes for Government Contracts: An Application of Agency Theory," *Accounting Review* 67, no. 4 (October 1982): 712–31; and Mark McCabe, "Principals, Agents, and the Learning Curve: The Case of Steam Electric Power Plant Design and Construction," *Journal of Industrial Economics* 44, no. 4 (December 1996): 357–75.

7. Arrow, "The Economics of Agency," 50.

8. For a review of this literature, see Candice Prendergast, "The Provision of Incentives in Firms," *Journal of Economic Literature* 37 (March 1998): 7–63; Robert Gibson, "Incentives in Organizations," *Journal of Economic Perspectives* 12, no. 4 (fall 1998): 115–32; and Bengt Holmstrom and John Roberts, "The Boundaries of the Firm Revisited," *Journal of Economic Perspectives* 12, no. 4 (fall 1998): 73–94.

9. It is important to note that, in the social sciences, there is considerable debate about whether agency theory exists at all, what its central premises are, and what, if any, utility it provides in understanding problems of organization, compensation, and control.

10. Harrison C. White, "Agency As Control," in *Principals and Agents: The Structure of Business,* ed. John W. Pratt and Richard J. Zeckhauser (1985; reprint, with a new preface, Boston: Harvard Business School Press, 1991), 188.

11. For an excellent translation of this theory to public bureaucracy, see Terry Moe, "The New Economics of Organization," *American Journal of Political Science* 28, no. 4 (November 1984): 739–77.

12. See, for example, Anthony Scott and Sandra Vick, "Patients, Doctors, and Contracts: An Application of Principal-Agent Theory to the Doctor-Patient Relationship," *Scottish Journal of Political Economy* 46, no. 2 (May 1999): 111–34.

13. Mark Satterthwaite, "Consumer Information, Equilibrium Industry Prices, and the Number of Sellers," *Bell Journal of Economics* 10 (fall 1979): 483–502.

14. David Dranove and William White, "Agency and the Organization of Health Care Delivery," *Inquiry* 24, no. 4 (winter 1987): 410–11.

15. Schlesinger, "Countervailing Agency," 48.

16. J. Gregory Dees, "Principals, Agents, and Ethics," in *Ethics and Agency Theory: An Introduction,* ed. Norman Bowie and R. Edward Freeman (New York: Oxford University Press, 1992), 35.

17. David Mechanic, "Changing Medical Organization and the Erosion of Trust," *Milbank Quarterly* 24, no. 2 (1996): 171–89.

18. Marc A. Rodwin, *Medicine, Money and Morals: Physicians' Conflicts of Interest* (New York: Oxford University Press, 1995).

19. An extensive discussion of the shortcomings of Medicare's cost-sharing arrange-

ments is contained in William Scanlon's testimony before the House Ways and Means Committee: *Cost-Sharing Policies Problematic for Beneficiaries and the Program* (Washington, D.C.: GAO, May 9, 2001).

20. Testimony of Leslie Aronovitz, Associate Director GAO, U.S. Senate Committee on Governmental Affairs, Permanent Subcommittee on Investigations, June 26, 1997.

21. Pauly, *Medical Care at Public Expense,* 21–35.

22. Brook et al., "Appropriateness of Acute Medical Care for the Elderly."

23. Stephen Jencks et al., "Quality of Care Delivered to Medicare Beneficiaries."

24. GAO, *Health Care Quality: Implications of Purchaser's Experiences for HCFA* (Washington, D.C.: GAO, June 1998).

25. Kathleen M. Eisenhardt, "Agency Theory: An Assessment and Review," *Academy of Management Review* 14, no. 1 (1989): 71.

26. This simple case assumes that the agent and the principal have different objectives and that the agent is more risk averse than the principal is. For example, the agent would have greater risk aversion if his or her employment options were limited and the principal's contracting options were virtually unlimited.

27. Steven Shavell, "Risk Sharing and Incentives in the Principal and Agent Relationship," *Bell Journal of Economics* 10 (spring 1979): 55–73.

28. Despite the seemingly overwhelming obstacles to outcome-based reimbursement as a way of structuring agency in health services, there has been continuing interest in specific applications. In long-term care, for example, there has been a strong movement, led primarily by Robert Kane, to reward nursing homes on the basis of the outcomes of their program of care. See chapter 5.

29. Overcautious practice is precisely the result that David Mechanic ("Changing Medical Organization and the Erosion of Trust") describes in his analysis of defensive medicine, and the exit from practice has been observed in obstetrics, where risks of malpractice actions have driven many physicians out of the specialty. Although both of these results are primarily influenced by the malpractice environment, the same sanctions could be reproduced by a public agent.

30. This account is drawn from Ann Wozencraft, "It's a Baby or It's Your Money Back: Fertility Clinics Test Consumer Rebates," *New York Times,* August 25, 1996, sec. 3, 1, 10–11.

31. For a depiction of medical practice in these terms see Harold Bursztajn et al., *Medical Choices, Medical Chances: How Patients, Families, and Physicians Can Cope with Uncertainty* (New York: Routledge, 1990).

32. See Kathleen M. Eisenhardt, "Control: Organizational and Economic Approaches," *Management Science* 31, no. 2 (February1985): 134–44; and Eisenhardt, "Agency- and Institutional-Theory: The Case of Retail Sales Compensation," *Academy of Management Journal* 31, no. 3 (September 1988): 488–511.

33. Clark C. Havighurst, *Health Care Choices* (Washington, D.C.: AEI Press, 1995), 228.

34. Katie Merrell, Edward Lawlor, Kathleen Cagney, Kenneth Langa, and Robert Willis. "Medicare Beneficiaries As Medicare+Choice Consumers: A Framework" (Chicago: Center for Health Administration Studies, 2000).

35. A. Dale Taussing and Martha A. Wojtowycz, "The Agency Role of Physicians in Ireland, Britain, and the U.S.A.," *Policy Sciences* 19 (1986): 275–96.

36. Mark Schlesinger has made the broader case that there is a societal interest in all health services, including employer-sponsored health in managed care plans. He traces through the issues in promoting effective agency in these arrangements, primarily through

regulatory approaches. See Schlesinger, "Countervailing Agency." In Medicare, the public interest is much more explicit. In the formal literature, multiple-principal problems have received significant attention. See, for example, Pablo Spiller, "Politicians, Interest Groups, and Regulators: A Multiple-Principals Agency Theory of Regulation (or 'Let Them be Bribed')," Stanford Center for Economic Policy Research Discussion Paper 131 (Stanford, Calif.: Stanford University, 1988).

37. These happen to be the public criteria employed in designing the list for coverage in the Oregon Medicaid Waiver program.

38. See the discussion of *Shalala v. Grijalva* in chapter 4.

39. Stuart Guterman, "Risk Adjustment in a Competitive Medicare System with Premium Support," in *Competition with Constraints,* ed. Marilyn Moon (Washington, D.C.: Urban Institute, 2000), 119–34.

40. Stuart Hagen, "Hospital Response to Medicare Reimbursement Incentives: Hospital-Based Skilled Nursing Facilities and Their Impact on Discharge Behavior" (Ph.D. diss., University of Chicago, 1998).

41. A worker in a state Medicaid program described to me the dissatisfaction that many recipients felt about their experiences with the Medicaid HMO program. They felt they were being shortchanged in the number of prescriptions they were being offered. Recipients who had been acclimated to Medicaid fee-for-service provision (and fee-for-prescription diagnosis) reported that they left the doctor with "shopping bags" of prescription drugs. Under a capitated plan, when they were sent home with few or no prescription drugs, the perception was that they were cheated by their physicians, that they had received inferior care under the HMO. If patients were predisposed to believe that medical care tended to iatrogenic outcomes, a very different pattern of behavior and demands would be expected.

42. A vivid exposition of this phenomenon is provided in Bruce Vladeck's *Unloving Care* (New York: Basic Books, 1977).

43. The tort system offers both insurance for at-risk patients and some check on the performance of negligent and incompetent providers. The degree to which the tort system influences risk taking, preventative behavior, and quality consciousness is a critical question for thinking about the design of the contract for medical care. Although there is little empirical evidence about the influence of the tort system on provider behavior, there is some evidence that this system does not operate optimally. Patricia Danzon has demonstrated that the simple functions of risk pooling and compensation can be more efficiently provided by health, disability, and life insurance policies. See Patricia Danzon, *Medical Malpractice: Theory, Evidence, and Public Policy* (Cambridge, Mass.: Harvard University Press, 1985).

44. Daniel P. Kessler and Mark McClellan, "Do Doctors Practice Defensive Medicine?" *Quarterly Journal of Economics* 111, no. 2 (May 1996): 353–90.

45. Carol A. Heimer, *Reactive Risk and Rational Action: Managing Moral Hazard in Insurance Contracts* (Berkeley: University of California Press, 1989), 11.

46. Ibid., 11.

47. Even if there were meaningful copayments and deductibles, it is not clear how functional they would be, because of the dominance of provider interests in most medical decision making. The experience with DRGs, for example, has demonstrated the limited applicability of copayments, because the incentives for providers to limit length of stay are by themselves so powerful that imposing cost sharing on the patient is an essentially moot strategy.

48. In theory, there is an optimal level of information gathering, however imperfect, which weighs the benefits of further monitoring against the expected changes in behavior, all in the context of some knowledge about the propensities for risk taking by the agent. This is

something like the problem that confronts the Internal Revenue Service, where the number and intensity of audits are weighed against the expected returns in revenues and the political fallout that would accompany a strategy that is either too aggressive or too lenient.

Even if it were possible to prescribe care and monitor effort perfectly, it is doubtful that society would want to structure a medical system as rigid and inelastic as a version of pure protocol medicine. To illustrate our reticence about enforcement in the health care arena, consider the problem of enforcing speed limits on the highways. Individuals drive cars fast in order to cut down the time spent in the car, to enjoy the aesthetic pleasure that speed and driving intrinsically provide, and perhaps even as an outlet for some competitive urges. Thus, the speeding enforcement problem is more subtle than merely limiting all traffic to a prescribed speed limit. As a society, we apparently do not want to eliminate speeding; if we did there are a number of straightforward technical and legal instruments available that would allow us to prevent anyone from going over the speed limit. We could mandate governors on automobiles, we could employ technical devices such as photographic radar enforcement, or we could impose catastrophic penalties for driving over the speed limit. However, we do not go to these lengths because we accept that there are benefits as well as risks that are associated with driving fast. Instead, we enforce selectively, we levy fines that graduate proportionally to both the number of infractions and the severity of the infraction, and we enforce catastrophic sanctions (loss of license) only in a small number of serious cases. In other words, we encourage a calculus that forces drivers to evaluate the potential harms against the benefits of speeding, all in a probabilistic environment. So, too, the problem of enforcing health provider behavior involves a complex (significantly more complex than the speeding example) trade-off between the "benefits" of idiosyncratic physician and provider behavior—including rogue provider behavior—and the interests of uniformity, standardization, and quality assurance in medical care.

49. GAO, *Medicare: Information Systems Modernization Needs Stronger Management and Support* (Washington, D.C.: GAO, September 2001).

50. GAO, *Medicare: Millions Could Be Saved by Screening Claims for Overused Services* (Washington, D.C.: GAO, January 1996).

51. See, for example, Maria Goddard, Russell Mannion, and Peter Smith, "Enhancing Performance in Health Care: A Theoretical Perspective on Agency and the Role of Information," *Health Economics* 9 (2000): 95–107.

52. Smith, *Paying for Medicare.*

53. For example, see Oliver E. Williamson, *Economic Organization: Firms, Markets, and Policy Control* (New York: New York University Press, 1986); and Williamson, *The Mechanisms of Governance* (New York: Oxford University Press, 1996).

54. *The Medicare Preservation and Improvement Act of 1999*, S.R. 1895, 106th Cong., 1st session.

55. Etheredge, "Medicare's Governance and Structure."

Chapter Four

1. James Robinson, "The End of Managed Care," *JAMA* 285, no. 20 (May 23–30, 2001), 2622–28.

2. Randall Brown and Rachel Thompson, *Medicare Beneficiaries and HMOs: A Case Study of the Los Angeles Market* (Menlo Park, Calif.: Kaiser Family Foundation, January 1998); Marsha Gold and Anna Aizer, *Medicare Beneficiaries and HMOs: A Case Study of the New York City Market* (Menlo Park, Calif.: Kaiser Family Foundation, January 1998).

3. For an overview, see John Oberlander, "Managed Care and Medicare Reform," in *Healthy Markets? The New Competition in Medical Care,* ed. Mark Peterson (Durham, N.C.: Duke University Press, 1998), 255–83.

4. Louise B. Russell, *Is Prevention Better Than Cure?* Studies in Social Economics (Washington, D.C.: Brookings Institution, 1986).

5. D. G. Safran, A. R. Tarlov, and W. H. Rogers, "Primary Care Performance in Fee-for-Service and Prepaid Health Care Systems: Results from the Medical Outcomes Study," *JAMA* 271, no. 20 (May 25, 1994): 1579–86.

6. Dranove and White, "Agency and the Organization of Health Care Delivery."

7. Dranove and White point out that an extension of this informational function may be the emergence of brand marketing and loyalty among the national HMO chains.

8. Michael Millenson, *Demanding Medical Excellence: Doctors and Accountability in the Information Age* (Chicago: University of Chicago Press, 1997).

9. Louis F. Rossiter, *Understanding Medicare Managed Care* (Chicago: Health Administration Press, 2001), 135–79; and James C. Robinson, "Physician-Hospital Organization and the Theory of the Firm," *Medical Care Research and Review* 54 (1997): 3–24.

10. William T. Gormley Jr., and David L. Weimer, *Organizational Report Cards* (Cambridge, Mass.: Harvard University Press, 1999).

11. Obviously, these cost contracts provided few incentives to limit care or the use of resources.

12. Robert Berenson, "Medicare + Choice: Doubling or Disappearing?" *Health Affairs, Web Exclusives* supplement (November 28, 2001): W65–W82.

13. W. Pete Welch, "Growth in HMO Market Share of the Medicare Market, 1989–1994," *Health Affairs* 15, no. 1 (fall 1996): 201–14.

14. GAO, *Medicare + Choice: Recent Payment Increases Had Little Effect on Benefits or Plan Availability in 2001* (Washington, D.C.: GAO, November 2001).

15. Berenson, "Medicare + Choice"; GAO, *Medicare + Choice: Payments Exceed Costs of Benefits in Fee-for-Service, Adding Billions to Spending* (Washington, D.C.: GAO, August 2000).

16. Geraldine Dallek, *Medicare Managed Care: Securing Beneficiary Protections* (Washington, D.C.: Families USA Foundation, April 1997).

17. Gerald Riley, Eric Feuer, and James Lubitz, "Disenrollment of Medicare Cancer Patients from Health Maintenance Organizations," *Medical Care* 38, no. 4 (August 1996): 826–36.

18. Mathematica/PPRC, *Access to Care in Medicare Managed Care: Results from a 1996 Survey of Enrollees and Disenrollees,* External Research Series no. 7 (Washington, D.C.: Physician Payment Review Commission, November 1996), 66–124.

19. Robert H. Miller and Harold S. Luft, "Managed Care Performance since 1980: A Literature Analysis," *JAMA* 271, no. 19 (May 18, 1994); Miller and Luft, "Does Managed Care Lead to Better or Worse Quality of Care?" *Health Affairs* 16, no. 5 (September/October 1997): 7–25; and Miller and Luft, "HMO Plan Performance Update: An Analysis of the Literature, 1997–2001," *Health Affairs* 21, no. 4 (July/August 2002): 63–86.

20. For a review of recent trends in Medicare managed care, see Marsha Gold and Lori Achman, *Trends in Premiums, Cost-Sharing, and Benefits in Medicare + Choice Health Plans, 1999–2001* (New York: Commonwealth Fund, April 2001).

21. Thomas Kornfield and Marsha Gold, *Is There More or Less Choice?* Monitoring Medicare + Choice: Fast Facts (Washington, D.C.: Mathematica Policy Research, December 1999).

22. Marsha Gold and Natalie Justh, *Forced Exit: Beneficiaries in Plans Terminating in 2000,* Monitoring Medicare + Choice: Fast Facts (Washington, D.C.: Mathematica Policy Research, September 2000).

23. Michelle Casey, Astrid Knott, and Ira Moscovice, "Medicare Minus Choice: The Impact of HMO Withdrawals on Rural Medicare Beneficiaries," *Health Affairs* 21, no. 3 (May/June 2002): 192–99.

24. Amanda Cassidy and Marsha Gold, *Medicare+Choice in 2000: Will Enrollees Spend More and Receive Less?* (New York: Commonwealth Fund, July 2000).

25. Robert Pear, "Medicare Shift towards H.M.O.'s Is Planned, *New York Times,* June 5, 2001, sec. A, 19.

26. Marsha Gold, "Medicare+Choice: An Interim Report Card," *Health Affairs* 20, no. 4 (July/August 2001): 132.

27. Medicare Payment Advisory Commission, *Report to Congress: Medicare Payment Policy* (Washington, D.C.: MedPAC, March 2002), 124–26.

28. Dranove and White, "Agency and the Organization of Health Care Delivery," 412–13.

29. *Shalala v. Grijalva,* 526 U.S. 1096 (May 3, 1999).

30. *Cantazano v. Dowling,* 60 F.3d 113 (2d Cir. 1995); and *J. K. v. Dillenberg,* 836 F. Supp. 694 (D. Ariz. 1993); discussed in *Shalala v. Grijalva.*

31. *Shalala v. Grijalva.*

32. Spencer Rich, "Rules to Bolster Appeal Rights in Medicare HMOs," *Washington Post,* November 5, 1996, sec. A, 4.

33. The court has found elsewhere, however, that carriers and intermediaries can be the alter ego for day-to-day administration of the Medicare program. See *Himmler v. Califano,* 611 F.2d 137, 140 (6th Cir. 1979); and *Vorster v. Bowen,* 709 F. Supp. 934, 946–47 (C.D. Cal. 1989).

34. *Jass v. Prudential Health Care Plan, Inc.,* 88 F.3d 1482 (July 8, 1996).

35. *Pegram v. Herdrich,* 530 U.S. 211 (January 12, 2000); *Pappas v. Asbel,* 564 Pa. 407 (April 3, 2001); *Przybowski v. U.S. Healthcare, Inc.,* 64 F. Supp. 2d 361 (September 7, 1999).

36. The content and the implications of the *Pegram* decision are discussed in detail in M. Gregg Bloche and Peter D. Jacobson, "The Supreme Court and Bedside Rationing, "*JAMA* 284, no. 21 (December 6, 2000): 2776–79.

37. *McCall v. PacifiCare of California, Inc.,* 25 Cal. 4th 412 (May 3, 2001).

38. Harriet Chiang, "Medicare Patients Allowed to Sue HMOs: Top State Court Rules in Denial-of-Care Case," *San Francisco Chronicle,* May 4, 2001, sec. A, 1.

39. Sara Rosenbaum, *An Overview of Managed Care Liability: Implications for Patient Rights and Federal and State Reform* (Washington, D.C.: AARP Public Policy Institute, March 2001).

40. For a more extensive discussion of the legal challenge surrounding managed care reform, see W. L. Sage, "Regulation through Information: Disclosure Laws and American Health Care," *Columbia Law Review* 99, no. 7 (1999): 1701–829; Clark Havighurst, "Vicarious Liability: Relocating Responsibility for the Quality of Care," *American Journal of Law and Medicine* 26, no. 1 (2000): 7–29; and Havighurst, "Consumers versus Managed Care: The New Class Actions," *Health Affairs* (July/August 2001): 8–27.

41. The *Contract with Eligible Medicare+Choice Organizations Pursuant to Sections 1851 to 1859 of the Social Security Act for the Operation of a Medicare+Choice Coordinated Care Plan(s)* is available at www.hcfa.gov.

42. Scott Geron, "Managed Care and Care Management for Older Adults," in *Managed Care Services: Policy, Programs, and Research,* ed. Nancy Veeder and Wilma Peebles-Wilkins (New York: Oxford University Press, 2001), 150–62.

43. Christopher P. Tompkins et al., "Applying Disease Management Strategies to Medicare," *Milbank Quarterly* 77, no. 4 (December 1999): 461–84.

44. For an extended discussion of the model and its early implementation, see Walter N. Leutz et al., *Changing Health Care for an Aging Society: Planning for the Social Health Maintenance Organization* (Lexington, Mass.: Lexington Books, 1985); Robert L. Kane et al., "S/HMOs, the Second Generation: Building on the Experience of the First Social Health Maintenance Organization Demonstrations," *Journal of the American Geriatrics Society* 45, no. 1 (January 1997): 101–7.

45. Robert Newcomer et al., "Case Mix Controlled Service Use and Expenditures in the Social Health Maintenance Organization Demonstration," *Journal of Gerontology: Medical Sciences* 50A, 1 (1995): 111–19.

46. Robert Newcomer, Charlene Harrington, and Rosalie Kane, "Implementing the Second-Generation Social Health Maintenance Organization," *Journal of the American Geriatric Society* 48, no. 7 (July 2000): 829–34.

47. Judith Wooldridge, *Social Health Maintenance Organizations: Transition into Medicare+Choice* (Princeton, N.J.: Mathematica Policy Research, January 5, 2001).

48. Alan J. White et al., *Evaluation of the Program of All-Inclusive Care for the Elderly Demonstration: A Comparison of the PACE Capitation Rates to the Projected Costs of the Program in the First Year of Enrollment* (Cambridge, Mass.: Abt Associates, October 27, 2000).

49. For a discussion of the criticisms of this study and the authors' response, see Randall Brown, *Does Managed Care Work for Medicare? An Evaluation of the Risk Contract Program for HMOs* (Princeton, N.J.: Mathematica Policy Research, July 24, 1995).

50. For a review, see Richard Kronick and Joy de Beyer, "The Problem of Risk Selection in Medicare Risk-Based HMOs," in *Medicare HMOs: Making Them Work for the Chronically Ill,* ed. Richard Kronick and Joy de Beyer (Chicago: Health Administration Press, 1999), 9–26.

51. For summaries of this work, see *A Comparison of Alternative Approaches to Risk Measurement,* Selected External Research Series no. 1 ([Washington, D.C.]: Physician Payment Review Commission, December 1994); Randall Ellis et al., "Diagnosis-Based Risk Adjustment for Medicare Capitation Payment," *Health Care Financing Review* 17, no. 3 (spring 1996): 101–28.

52. It is important to note that it is statistically impossible to capture all of the sources of variation in use for a population with a simple set of risk adjusters, because some of the variation arises from individual (within person) random elements. See Joseph Newhouse et al., "Adjusting Capitation Rates Using Objective Health Measures and Prior Utilization," *Health Care Financing Review* 10, no. 3 (1989): 41–54. Analysts at Physician Payment Review Commission (PPRC) have estimated that basic demographic factors explain about 21 percent of maximum R^2, whereas a set of best available adjusters explains almost 60 percent of the maximum expected variance between individuals.

53. For an example and discussion of this problem in the context of high-risk chronically ill children, see Elizabeth Fowler and Gerald Anderson, "Capitation Adjustment for Pediatric Populations," *Pediatrics* 98, no. 1 (July 1996): 10–17.

54. Louis F. Rossiter, Henrng-Chia Chiu, and Sheau-Hwa Chen, "Strengths and Weaknesses of the AAPCC: When Does Risk Adjustment Become Cost Reimbursement?" in *HMOs and the Elderly,* ed. Harold S. Luft (Ann Arbor, Mich.: Health Administration Press, 1994), 251–69.

55. Kronick and de Beyer, "The Problem of Risk Selection in Medicare Risk-Based HMOs."

56. Kaiser Family Foundation (Focus Group), "Medicare Beneficiaries Consider Abil-

ity to Keep Their Physician As Most Important Factor in Deciding to Keep an HMO" (Menlo Park, Calif.: Kaiser Family Foundation, May 2, 1995).

57. Author's analysis of HCFA data.

58. Judith Hibbard, Paul Slovic, and Jacquelyn Jewett, "Informing Consumer Decisions in Health Care: Implications from Decision-Making Research," *Milbank Quarterly* 75, no. 3 (1997): 408.

59. Ibid.

60. Carol Cronin, "Reaching and Educating Medicare Beneficiaries about Choice," in *Improving the Medicare Market: Adding Choice and Protections,* ed. Stanley B. Jones and Marion Ein Lewin (Washington, D.C.: National Academy of Sciences, 1996), 236–69.

61. Robert L. Kane and Rosalie A. Kane, "What Older People Want from Long-Term Care, and How They Can Get It," *Health Affairs* 20, no. 8 (November/December 2001): 119.

62. Kronick and de Beyer, "The Problem of Risk Selection in Medicare Risk-Based HMOs."

Chapter Five

1. See, for example, Victor Fuchs, *The Future of Health Policy* (Cambridge, Mass.: Harvard University Press, 1993).

2. Joseph Newhouse, "Medical Care Costs: How Much Welfare Loss?" *Journal of Economic Perspectives* 6, no. 3 (1992): 3–21.

3. Richard A. Rettig, "Medical Innovation Duels Cost Containment," *Health Affairs* 13, no. 3 (summer 1994): 15.

4. Richard A. Rettig, "End-Stage Renal Disease and the Cost of Medical Technology," in *Medical Technology: The Culprit behind Health Care Costs?* ed. Stuart H. Altman and Robert Blendon (Washington, D.C.: U.S. Dept. of Health, Education, and Welfare, 1979), 88–115.

5. Mark Pauly, "Taxation and Health Insurance," *Journal of Economic Literature* 24, no. 2 (1986): 629–75.

6. Kenneth Arrow, "Economic Welfare and the Allocation of Resources for Invention," in *The Rate and Direction of Inventive Activity,* ed. Richard Nelson (Princeton, N.J.: Princeton University Press, 1962), 609–25.

7. For an extended discussion of the concept and issues of using QALYs for policy and clinical decision making, see John La Puma and Edward F. Lawlor, "Quality-Adjusted Life-Years: Ethical Implications for Physicians and Policymakers," *JAMA* 263, no. 21 (June 6, 1990): 2917–21; and George Tolley, Donald Kenkel, and Robert Fabian, eds., *Valuing Health for Policy: An Economic Approach* (Chicago: University of Chicago Press, 1994).

8. This is independent of the methodology used. Jerry Avorn has demonstrated how human-capital approaches to valuing benefits in an older population compound this problem because there are few years of earnings in addition to few years of life expectancy. See Jerry Avorn, "Benefit and Cost in Geriatric Care: Turning Age Discrimination into Policy," *New England Journal of Medicine* 310, no. 20 (May 17, 1984): 1294–1301.

9. David Meltzer, "Accounting for Future Costs in Medical Cost-Effectiveness Analysis," *Journal of Health Economics* 16, no. 1 (February 1997): 33–64.

10. Peter Neumann and Magnus Johannesson, "From Principle to Public Policy: Using Cost Effectiveness Analysis," *Health Affairs* 13, no. 3 (summer 1994): 206–14.

11. Susan Bartlett Foote, "Coexistence, Conflict, and Cooperation: Public Policy towards Medical Devices," *Journal of Health Politics, Policy, and Law* 11, no. 3 (fall 1986): 501–23.

12. A history of federal efforts to institutionalize technology assessment is contained

in Richard A. Rettig, "Technology Assessment: An Update," *Investigational Radiology* 26 (1991): 165–73.

13. The history is recounted in Richard Merrill, "Regulation of Drugs and Devices: An Evolution," *Health Affairs* 13, no. 3 (summer 1994): 48–69.

14. Seymour Perry and Mae Thamer, "Medical Innovation and the Critical Role of Health Technology Assessment," *JAMA* 282, no. 19 (November 17, 1999): 1869–72.

15. Susan B. Foote, "Why Medicare Cannot Promulgate a National Coverage Rule: A Case of Regula Mortis," *Journal of Health Politics, Policy, and Law* 27, no. 5 (October 2002): 707–30.

16. This adjustment is more fully described in Prospective Payment Assessment Commission, *Report and Recommendation to Congress,* March 1, 1997, 85–90. ProPAC also makes recommendations about changes in payment for productivity growth and associated changes in service mix. Much of the gain in hospital productivity can be attributed to changes in technology, particularly information systems. Interestingly, ProPAC recommended changes of between –1 and –3 percent for changes in productivity.

17. David Lee, "Estimating the Effect of New Technology on Medicare Part B Expenditure and Volume Growth," *Advances in Health Economics and Health Services Research* 13 (1992): 43–64.

18. For an extended discussion of Medicare treatment of technology in inpatient and outpatient payment systems, see MedPAC, *Report to Congress: Medicare Payment Policy* (Washington, D.C.: MedPAC, March 2001), 34–45.

19. For the criteria and policies for these pass-through payments, see ibid., 37–38.

20. Ibid., 41–44.

21. *Federal Register,* 54: 4304–9.

22. Kathleen Buto, "Can Medicare Keep Pace with Cutting Edge Technology?" *Health Affairs* 13, no. 3 (summer 1994): 137–40.

23. For a review of this early experience and the potential of evidence-based technology assessment, see Alan Garber, "Evidence-Based Coverage Policy," *Health Affairs* 20, no. 5 (September/October 2001): 62–82; and Sean Tunis and Jeffrey Kang, "Improvements in Medicare Coverage of New Technology," *Health Affairs* 20, no. 5 (September/October 2001): 83–85.

24. Daniel Goldstein, Mahmet Oz, and Eric Rose, "Implantable Left Ventricular Assist Devices," *New England Journal of Medicine* 339, no. 21 (November 13, 1999): 1522–33.

25. "Senators Doctors Kennedy and Hatch," editorial, *New York Times,* July 15, 1988, A-30.

26. Institute of Medicine, *The Total Artificial Heart: Prototypes, Policies, and Patients* (Washington, D.C.: National Academy of Sciences: 1991).

27. Elliot Marshal, "Artificial Heart: The Beat Goes On," *Science* 253 (August 2, 1991): 500–502.

28. Jack G. Copeland et al., "Bridge to Transplantation with the CardioWest Total Artificial Heart: The International Experience 1993–1995," *Journal of Heart and Lung Transplantation* 15, no. 1 (January 1996): 94–99.

29. Associated Press, "Kentucky Patient Receives Mechanical Heart Replacement," July 3, 2001.

30. Lynne Cohen, "Banking on the Artificial Heart," *Canadian Medical Association Journal* 157, no. 2 (July 15, 1997): 128.

31. Ronald Ozminkowski, Bernard Friedman, and Zachary Taylor, "Access to Heart and Liver Transplantation in the Late 1980s," *Medical Care* 31, no. 11 (1993): 1027–42.

32. Institute of Medicine, *Total Artificial Heart*, 65–84.

33. National Heart, Lung, and Blood Institute, *Expert Panel Review of the NHLBI Total Artificial Heart Program*, June 1998–November 1999.

34. Associated Press, "Doctors to Implant First Self-Contained Total Artificial Heart," April 19, 2001.

35. Institute of Medicine, *Total Artificial Heart*, 270–71. These results are quite sensitive to the actual quality adjustment used.

36. Gregory de Lissovoy, "Medicare and Heart Transplants: Will Lightening Strike Twice?" *Health Affairs* 7, no. 4 (fall 1988): 61–72.

37. Daniel Callahan, "The Artificial Heart: Bleeding Us Dry," *New York Times*, September 17, 1988, 20.

38. Institute of Medicine, *Total Artificial Heart*, 85–102.

39. Jon Van, "Artificial Hearts May Return As Transplant Alternative for Elderly," *Chicago Tribune*, November 19, 1995.

40. For a discussion of this phenomenon, see Thomas C. Schelling, "The Life You Save May Be Your Own," in *Choice or Consequence* (Cambridge, Mass.: Harvard University Press, 1986), 113–46.

41. In the regular course of technology diffusion, some inventions will have high initial cost-benefit ratios but eventually will look much more attractive as costs come down and, at the same time, the intervention becomes more reliable and effective.

42. Richard A. Rettig, "Medical Innovation Duels Cost Containment," in *Medical Technology: The Culprit behind Health Care Costs?* ed. Stuart H. Altman and Robert Blendon (Washington, D.C.: U.S. Dept. of Health, Education, and Welfare, 1979), 16–19.

43. Pascale Lehoux and Stuart Blume, "Technology Assessment and the Sociopolitics of Health Technologies," *Journal of Health Politics, Policy, and Law* 25, no. 6 (December 2000): 1083–120.

44. Ibid., 1108.

45. Charles Phelps and Steven Parente, "Priority Setting in Medical Technology and Medical Practice Assessment," *Medical Care* 28 (1990): 703–23.

46. Richard A. Rettig, *Health Care in Transition: Technology Assessment in the Private Sector* (Santa Monica, Calif.: RAND, 1997).

47. Burton Weisbrod, "The Health Care Quadrilemma: An Essay on Technological Change, Insurance, Quality of Care, and Cost Containment," *Journal of Economic Literature* 29 (June 1991): 523–52.

48. Rettig, *Health Care in Transition*.

49. John Eisenberg, "Ten Lessons for Evidence-Based Technology Assessment," *JAMA* 282, no. 19 (November 17, 1999): 1865–69.

50. This example is taken from Nancy M. Kane and Paul D. Manoukian, "The Effect of the Medicare Prospective Payment System on the Adoption of New Technology: The Case of Cochlear Implants," *New England Journal of Medicine* 321, no. 20 (November 16, 1989): 1378–83.

51. Eisenberg, "Ten Lessons," 1868.

52. Vallee Willman, "Workshop Conclusions and Recommendations," in *Report of the Workshop on the Artificial Heart: Planning for Evolving Technologies*, by National Heart, Lung, and Blood Institute (Bethesda, Md.: NHLBI, 1994): 127–29.

53. Institute of Medicine, *Total Artificial Heart*, 160.

Chapter Six

1. I am indebted to Nicholas Christakis for helping me frame this concept of a "good death." Other notions of a good death include the living of a "natural life span," the completion of a "biographical narrative," or the maintenance of a reasonable quality of life or functional status. Some would argue that a good death requires ample advance notice (others would argue the opposite). The Institute of Medicine committee defined a good death as "one that is free from avoidable distress and suffering for patients, families, and caregivers; in general accord with patients' and families' wishes; and reasonably consistent with clinical, cultural, and ethical standards" (Marilyn J. Field and Christine Cassel, eds., *Approaching Death: Improving Care at the End of Life*, report by the Institute of Medicine, Committee on Care at the End of Life [Washington, D.C.: National Academy Press, 1997], 4). A comprehensive framework for a good death is presented in Ezekiel J. Emanuel and Linda L. Emanuel, "The Promise of a Good Death," *Lancet* 351, no. 9114 (May 16, 1998): SII21-9.

2. David Eddy, "Conversation with my Mother," *JAMA* 272, no. 3 (July 20, 1994): 180.

3. Mortality Follow-Back Study results reported in Last Acts Financing Task Force, *The Challenge of End-of-Life Care: Moving toward Metanoia?* (Washington, D.C.: Last Acts, October 1998).

4. Literature reviewed in Nicholas Christakis, *Death Foretold: Prophecy and Prognosis in Medical Care* (Chicago: University of Chicago Press, 2000), 24.

5. See Christopher Hogan et al., "Medicare Beneficiaries Cost in the Last Year of Life," *Health Affairs* 20, no. 4 (July/August 2001): 188–95; and Hogan et al., *Medicare Beneficiaries Cost and Use of Care in the Last Year of Life*, Contractors Research Series Report no. 00-1 (Washington, D.C.: MedPAC, May 2000).

6. Harold R. Lentzner et al., "The Quality of Life in the Year before Death," *American Journal of Public Health* 82 (August 1992): 1093–98.

7. For an extensive review of the implications of Medicare reimbursement features, see Nicole Makowsky, Fowler Lynn, and Joanne Lynn, *Potential Medicare Reimbursements for Services to Patients with Chronic Fatal Illnesses* (Washington, D.C.: George Washington University Center to Improve Care of the Dying, July 6, 1999).

8. J. Lubitz and R. Prihoda, "The Use and Costs of Medicare Services in the Last Two Years of Life," *Health Care Financing Review* (spring 1984): 117–31.

9. J. D. Lubitz and G. F. Riley, "Trends in Medicare Payments in the Last Year of Life," *New England Journal of Medicine* 328, no. 15 (April 15, 1993): 1092–96.

10. M. Gornick, A. McMillan, and J. Lubitz, "A Longitudinal Perspective on Patterns of Medicare Payments," *Health Affairs* (summer 1993): 140–50; Bernard Lo, "End-of-Life after Termination of Support," *Hastings Center Report Special Supplement* (November/December 1995): S6–S8.

11. Anne A. Scitovsky, "The High Cost of Dying Revisited," *Milbank Quarterly* 72, no. 4 (1994): 561–91

12. For an overall review of this literature, see Ezekiel Emanuel, "Cost Savings at the End of Life: What Do the Data Show?" *JAMA* 275, no. 24 (June 26, 1996): 1907–14. Emanuel discusses the major methodological shortcomings of this literature: selection, problems of timing and censorship of the data, accounting for costs, and generalizing beyond cancer patients.

13. Christopher Chambers et al., "Relationship of Advance Directives to Hospital Charges in a Medicare Population," *Archives of Internal Medicine* 154 (1994): 541–47.

14. Vincent Mor and David Kidder, "Cost Savings in Hospice: Final Results from the National Hospice Study," *Health Services Research* 20 (1985): 407–22.

15. William A. Knaus et al., "A Controlled Trial to Improve Care for Seriously Ill Hospitalized Patients," *JAMA* 274, no. 20 (November 22/29, 1995): 1591–98; Robert Kane et al., "A Randomized Controlled Trial of Hospice Care," *Lancet*, no. 8382 (April 7, 1984): 890–94.

16. David Kidder, "The Effect of Hospice Coverage on Medicare Expenditures," *Health Services Research* 27 (June 1992): 213.

17. Ezekiel J. Emanuel and Linda L. Emanuel, "The Economics of Dying: The Illusion of Cost Savings at the End of Life," *New England Journal of Medicine* 330, no. 8 (February 24, 1994): 540–44.

18. A. L. Jones, Division of Health Care Statistics, National Center for Health Statistics, "Hospices and Home Health Agencies: Data from the 1991 National Health Provider Inventory," *Advance Data* 257 (November 3, 1994): 1–8.

19. Vincent Mor, David S. Greer, and Robert Kastenbaum, *The Hospice Experiment* (Baltimore: Johns Hopkins University Press, 1988).

20. Kidder, "Effect of Hospice Coverage."

21. Maria K. Goddard, "The Importance of Assessing the Effectiveness of Care: The Case of Hospices," *Journal of Social Policy* 22 (1993): 1–17.

22. Nicholas Christakis and Jose Escarce, "Survival of Medicare Patients after Enrollment in Hospice Programs," *New England Journal of Medicine* 335, no. 3 (July 18, 1996): 172–78.

23. See Jeremy Sugarman, Neil Powe, Dorothy Brillantes, and Melanie Smith, "The Costs of Ethics Legislation: A Look at the Patient Self-Determination Act," *Kennedy Institute of Ethics Journal* 3, no. 4 (1993): 387–99.

24. John La Puma, David Orentlicher, and Robert Moss, "Advance Directives on Admission: Clinical Implications and Analysis of the Patient Self-Determination Act of 1990," *JAMA* 266, no. 3 (July 17, 1991): 402–5.

25. Charles Sabatino, "Surely the Wizard Will Help Us, Toto? Implementing the Patient Self-Determination Act." *Hastings Center Report* 23, no. 1 (January/February 1993): 12–16.

26. Mathy Mezey and Beth Latimer, "The Patient Self-Determination Act: An Early Look at Implementation," *Hastings Center Report* 23, no. 1 (January/February 1993): 16–20.

27. Gavin Hougham, "Advance Directives, Self, and Social Role Preservation: Health Policy Innovations As Institutionalized Legitimation Mechanisms" (Ph.D. diss. proposal, University of Chicago, 1996).

28. Scitovsky, "High Cost of Dying Revisited."

29. For a complete account of the SUPPORT findings, see Knaus et al., "Controlled Trial to Improve Care for Seriously Ill Hospitalized Patients."

30. Ellen H. Moskowitz and James Lindemann Nelson, "The Best Laid Plans," *Hastings Center Report Special Supplement* (November/December 1995): S3–S5.

31. Bernard Lo, "End-of-Life Care after Termination of SUPPORT."

32. Patricia A. Marshall, "The Support Study: Whose Talking," *Hastings Center Report Special Supplement* (November/December 1995): S9–S11.

33. George Annas, "How We Lie," *Hastings Center Report Special Supplement* (November/December 1995): S13.

34. Franklin Miller and Joseph Fins, "A Proposal to Restructure Hospital Care for Dying Patients," *New England Journal of Medicine* 334, no. 26 (June 27, 1996): 1740–42.

35. Charles F. von Gunten et al., "Recommendations to Improve End-of-Life Care through Regulatory Change in U.S. Health Care Financing," *Journal of Palliative Medicine* 5, no. 1 (February 2002): 35–41.

36. Franklin G. Miller et al., "Regulating Physician-Assisted Death," *New England Journal of Medicine* 331, no. 2 (July 14, 1994): 119.

37. An informative analysis of this risk in the Netherlands is contained in Carlos Gomez, *Regulating Death: Euthanasia and the Case of the Netherlands* (New York: Free Press, 1991).

38. Robert J. Blendon, Ulrike S. Szalay, and Richard A. Knox, "Should Physicians Assist Their Patients in Dying? The Public Perspective," *JAMA* 267, no. 19 (May 20, 1992): 2658–62.

39. Jonathan Cohen, Stephan Fihn, Edward Boyko, Albert Jonsen, and Robert Wook, "Attitudes toward Physician-Assisted Suicide and Euthanasia in Washington State," *New England Journal of Medicine* 331, no. 2 (July 14, 1994): 89–94.

40. The Institute of Medicine, Committee on Care at the End of Life report (Field and Cassel, *Approaching Death*) recommended the following:

- People with advanced, potentially fatal illnesses and those close to them should be able to expect and receive reliable, skillful, and supportive care.
- Providers must commit themselves to improving care for dying patients and to using existing knowledge effectively to prevent and relieve pain and other symptoms.
- Revise financing mechanisms to encourage good end-of-life care, and reform burdensome drug prescription laws and regulations that impede good care.
- Initiate changes in education programs for providers to ensure that practitioners have relevant attitudes, knowledge, and skills to care well for dying patients.
- Ensure that palliative care becomes a defined area of expertise, education, and research.
- Define and implement priorities for strengthening the knowledge base in end-of-life care.
- Encourage public discussion about the experience of dying, the options available to patients and families, and the obligations of communities to those approaching death.

41. Linda Emanuel et al., "Advance Directives for Medical Care: A Case for Greater Use," *New England Journal of Medicine* 324, no. 13 (March 28, 1991): 889–95; Joel Tsevat et al., "Health Values of the Seriously Ill," *Annals of Internal Medicine* 122 (1995): 514–20.

42. Susan W. Tolle, Diane L. Elliot, and David H. Hickam, "Physician Attitudes and Practices at the Time of Death," *Archives of Internal Medicine* 144 (1984): 2389–91; Susan W. Tolle and Donald E. Girard, "Physicians' Role in the Events Surrounding Patient Death," *Archives of Internal Medicine* 143 (1983): 1447–49.

43. F. Southwick, "Who Was Caring for Mary?" *Annals of Internal Medicine* 118 (1993): 146–48.

44. Lawrence J. Markson et al., "Implementing Advance Directives in the Primary Care Setting," *Archives of Internal Medicine* 154 (October 24, 1994): 2321–27.

45. Daniel Callahan, *The Troubled Dream of Life* (New York: Simon & Schuster, 1993), 44.

46. Christakis, *Death Foretold*.

47. Michael Rabow et al., "End-of-Life Care Content in 50 Textbooks from Multiple Specialties," *JAMA* 283, no. 6 (February 9, 2000): 771–78.

48. Sherwin B. Nuland, *How We Die: Reflections on Life's Final Chapter* (New York: Knopf, 1994), 84.

49. Field and Cassel, *Approaching Death*, 7.

50. As a matter of policy in Social Security, we force savings for retirement in part because younger workers are myopic. However, we only encourage, but do not enforce, planning and foresight to prepare for care and decision making at the time of death, in spite of the probability of reaching this state.

51. This "option demand" for a good contract at the end of life suggests that there is actually a public-good character to the existence of these arrangements. The idea of an option demand imagines that individuals benefit from the knowledge that the option is going to be there if and when they need it, whether or not they actually use the service.

52. Jonathan Stewart, "Diagnosing and Treating Depression in the Hospitalized Elderly," *Geriatrics* 46 (January 1991): 64–72.

53. For a discussion of these requirements see Linda Emanuel, "Advance Directives: What Have We Learned So Far?" *Journal of Clinical Ethics* 4 (spring 1993): 8–16, and Joanne Lynn and Joan M. Teno, "After the Patient Self-Determination Act: The Need for Empirical Research on Formal Advance Directives," *Hastings Center Report* (January/February 1993): 20–24.

54. Maria J. Silveira et al., "Patients' Knowledge of Options at the End of Life," *JAMA* 284, no. 19 (November 15, 2000): 2483–94.

55. Donald J. Murphy et al., "Outcomes of Cardiopulmonary Resuscitation in the Elderly," *Annals of Internal Medicine* 111 (1989): 199–205.

56. See, for example, George Annas, "The Health Care Proxy and Living Will," *New England Journal of Medicine* 324 (1991): 1210–13; and A. Seckler et al., "Substituted Judgment: How Accurate Are Proxy Predictions?" *Annals of Internal Medicine* 115 (1991): 92–98; and J. Ely et al., "The Physician's Decision to Use Tube Feedings: The Role of the Family, the Living Will, and the Cruzan Decision," *Journal of the American Geriatrics Society* 40 (1992): 471–75; A. V. Luddington, "The Death Control Dilemma: Who Is to Make End-of-Life Decisions: You and Your Patient, or 'the System'?" *Geriatrics* 48 (1993): 72–77; J. Slomaka, "The Negotiation of Death: Clinical Decision Making at the End of Life," *Social Science and Medicine* 35 (1992): 251–59.

57. For an example of such a process, see Joanne Lynn, "Serving Patients Who May Die Soon and Their Families," *JAMA* 285, no. 7 (February 21, 2001): 925–32.

58. Linda L. Emanuel et al., "Advance Care Planning As a Process: Structuring the Discussion in Practice," *Journal of the American Geriatrics Society* 43 (1995): 440–46.

59. As a policy matter, it is worth questioning whether physicians are appropriate agents for end-of-life decisions. One could imagine alternative models using social workers, spiritual counselors, clinical teams, or even lay volunteers, as occurs in some hospice approaches. However, physicians are positioned to make the key clinical decisions and are both legally and ethically mandated to serve the interests of the patient. Even the designation of when a patient is terminal, and the resulting order for hospice care, depend on a physician's determination.

60. M. F. Morrison, "Obstacles to Doctor-Patient Communication at the End-of-Life," in *End-of-Life Decisions: A Psychosocial Perspective,* ed. M. D. Steinberg and S. J. Youngner (Washington, D.C.: American Psychiatric Press, 1998), 109–36.

61. Mildred Solomon et al., "Decisions Near the End of Life: Professional Views on Life-Sustaining Treatments," *American Journal of Public Health* 83 (January 1993): 14–23.

62. Nicholas Christakis, "Prognostication and Death in Medical Thought and Practice" (Ph.D. diss., University of Pennsylvania, 1995).

63. Nicholas Christakis and David Asch, "Biases in How Physicians Choose to Withdraw Life Support," *Lancet* 342 (September 11, 1993): 642–46.

64. Joanne Lynn, "Caring at the End of Our Lives," *New England Journal of Medicine* 335, no. 3 (July 18, 1996): 202.

65. Steven Miles, Eileen Weber, and Robert Koepp, "End-of-Life Treatment in Managed Care," *Western Journal of Medicine* 163, no. 3 (September 1995): 302–5.

66. Peter Fox, *End-of-Life Care in Managed Care Organizations* (Washington, D.C.: AARP Public Policy Institute, July 1999).

67. Daniel Cher and Leslie Lenert, "Method of Medicare Reimbursement and the Rate of Potentially Ineffective Care of Critically Ill Patients," *JAMA* 278, no. 12 (September 24, 1997): 1001–7.

68. For a review of these plans and practices, see Fox, *End-of-Life Care in Managed Care Organizations*, 9–10, 13–15.

69. Field and Cassel, *Approaching Death;* and Foundation for Accountability, *Quality of Care at the End of Life: Proposed Measurement Set,* available at www.facct.org/

70. National Hospice Organization, *Medical Guidelines for Determining Prognosis in Selected Non-Cancer Diagnoses* (Alexandria, Va.: NHO, 1966).

71. Lynn, "Serving Patients."

72. L. Emanuel et al., "Advance Care Planning As a Process."

73. Ronald Cranford traces the evolution of medical futility and other standards of care (e.g., brain death, artificial nutrition) from narrow clinical standards to broader socially and legally accepted concepts. See Ronald Cranford, "Medical Futility: Transforming a Clinical Concept into Legal and Social Policies," *Journal of the American Geriatrics Society* 42 (August 1994): 894–98.

74. Robert Veatch and Carol Mason Spicer, "Medically Futile Care: The Role of the Physician in Settings Limits," *American Journal of Law and Medicine* 18 (1992): 15–36.

75. See Linda Johnson White, "Clinical Uncertainty, Medical Futility, and Practice Guidelines," *Journal of the American Geriatrics Society* 42 (1994): 899–901; and Donald Murphy, "Can We Set Futile Care Policies? Institutional and Systemic Challenges," *Journal of the American Geriatrics Society* 42 (1994): 890–93.

76. The "Santa Monica Hospital Medical Center Guidelines for Futile Care":

1.0 The attending physician should take the time to carefully explain the nature of the ailment, the options, and the prognosis to the aware patient and to the family. The doctor should explain that abandoning treatment does not mean abandoning the patient in terms of comfort, dignity, and psychological support.

2.0 The attending physician should provide the names of appropriate consultants to provide an independent opinion.

3.0 The assistance of the nurses, chaplain, patient care representative, and social services should be offered to the patient's family. A joint conference with the doctor is desirable.

4.0 At the attending physician's request, the bioethics committee may be called in to consider the matter and offer advice and counsel to the physician or family.

5.0 Adequate time should be given so that the patient and family can consider this information.

6.0 If all of these steps are taken and the family remains unconvinced, neither the doctor nor the hospital is required to provide care that is not medically indicated, and the family may be offered a substitute physician (if one can be found) and another hospital (if one is available).

7.0 If it is determined that the patient can no longer benefit from an acute hospital stay and the patient insists on staying, or the family insists that the patient remain, the mechanism for personal payment can be invoked.

These guidelines were published in *Hospitals and Health Networks* (Chicago: American Hospital Publishing, February 20, 1994), 28.

77. See Lawlor and Raube, "Social Interventions and Outcomes in Medical Effectiveness Research."

78. Neil MacDonald, "Oncology and Palliative Care: The Case for Co-ordination," *Cancer Treatment Reviews* 19 (1993): 29–41; and Ada Jacox , Daniel B. Carr, and Richard Payne, "New Clinical-Practice Guidelines for the Management of Pain in Patients with Cancer," *New England Journal of Medicine* 330, no. 9 (March 3, 1994): 651–55.

79. Callahan, *Troubled Dream of Life.*

80. Dale Larson and Daniel Tobin, "End-of-Life Conversations: Evolving Practice and Theory," *JAMA* 284, no. 12 (September 27, 2000): 1573–78.

81. E. Emanuel, "Cost Savings at the End of Life."

82. Linda Emanuel, "Structured Advance Planning: Is It Finally Time for Physician Action and Reimbursement?" *JAMA* 274, no. 6 (August 9, 1995): 503.

83. Susan Tolle, personal communication.

84. Beth Virnig et al., "Geographic Variation in Hospice Use Prior to Death," *Journal of the American Geriatrics Society* 48 (September 2000): 1117–25.

85. R. S. Prichard et al., "Influence of Patient Preferences and Local Health System Characteristics in the Place of Death," *Journal of the American Geriatrics Society* 46 (October 1998): 1320–21.

Chapter Seven

1. John E. Chubb and Terry M. Moe, *Politics, Markets, and America's Schools* (Washington, D.C.: Brookings Institution, 1990), 18.

2. See, for example, GAO, *Medicare: Private Payer Strategies Suggest Options to Reduce Rapid Spending Growth* (Washington, D.C., GAO, 1996).

3. For a review of these initiatives, see Jack Meyer, Sean Sullivan, and Sharon Silow-Carroll, *Private Sector Initiatives: Controlling Health Care Costs* (Washington, D.C.: Health Care Leadership Council, March 1991).

4. For case studies of employer coalitions and their practices, see Jack Meyer, Sharon Silow-Carroll, Ingrid Tillman, and Lise Rybowski, *Employer Coalition Initiatives in Health Care Purchasing,* 2 vols. (Washington, D.C.: Economic and Social Research Institute, February 1996).

5. These observations are taken from case studies of the Midwest Business Group on Health, *Public-Private Healthcare Purchasing Partnerships* (Chicago: MBGH, October 1996).

6. David B. Kendall, *A New Deal for Medicare and Medicaid: Building a Buyer's Market for Health Care* (Washington, D.C.: Progressive Policy Institute, September 22, 1995).

7. Elliot K. Wicks and Mark A. Hall, "Purchasing Cooperatives for Small Employers: Performance and Prospects," *Milbank Quarterly* 78, no. 4 (2000): 511–46.

8. Institute for Health Policy Solutions, *Resource Manual: Implementing Healthplan Purchasing Cooperatives* (Washington, D.C.: IHPS, 1994).

9. However, James Morone, in considering the complexities of the regional risk adjustment function for alliances, argued that these "nonpolitical" outcomes were neither feasible nor necessarily desirable: "In the real world of health politics, there is no Archimedean

point from which these choices can be made in a rational and dispassionate manner. On the contrary, such choices are fundamentally political. Groups will lobby. So will payers with an economic stake in the outcomes. Just picture the scene when the risk raters take up the question of people who have tested HIV-positive. And what will they say to the Blue Cross contention that telephone workers (whom it happens to insure) cost more to cover and should be reimbursed at a higher rate? Will elected officials sit still for the process?" ("Hidden Complications: Why Health Care Competition Needs Regulation," *American Prospect* 3, no. 10 [summer 1992]: 46). Morone is correct, but it is not necessarily undesirable for political forces to be unleashed in these kinds of regional political/administrative forays. Indeed, the question is not whether politics will occur or not, but rather what are the expected properties of these politics at higher or lower levels of the intergovernmental hierarchy. This is a complex question that has been debated in this country since the Federalist Papers, but it is at least reasonable to imagine a net improvement in the representation of beneficiary interests in administration (as opposed to resources and policy) as the sponsorship devolves from Washington and Baltimore to closer and smaller regional jurisdictions.

10. Calculated from information in Timothy Jost, "Governing Medicare," *Administrative Law Review* 51, no. 1 (1999): 70. For a comprehensive analysis of the dimensions and implications of divided government for Medicare policy making and administration, see Jost, "Governing Medicare," 70–81.

11. For an extensive review of committee structure and its implications for health, see John W. Hardin, "An In-Depth Look at Congressional Committee Jurisdictions Surrounding Health Issues," *Journal of Health Politics, Policy, and Law* 23 (1998): 517–50.

12. Oliver, "Analysis, Advice, and Congressional Leadership," 143–44. He quotes James MacGregor Burns, *The Deadlock of Democracy* (Englewood Cliffs, N.J.: Prentice Hall, 1963); and Smith, *Paying for Medicare*, 129.

13. Interestingly, Guzmano and Schlesinger argue for expanding some of Medicare's collateral responsibilities in the name of more comprehensively and proactively controlling a health agenda. See Michael Guzmano and Mark Schlesinger, "The Social Roles of Medicare: Assessing Medicare's Collateral Benefits," *Journal of Health Politics, Policy, and Law* 26, no. 1 (February 2001): 36–79.

14. Public Law 89-97, *Health Insurance for the Aged and Medical Assistance,* 89th Cong., HR 6675, July 30, 1965.

15. The GAO has been persistent and visible in analyzing the administrative performance of HCFA and CMS. See, for example, William J. Scanlon, *Medicare Management: Current and Future Challenges,* Testimony before the Senate Finance Committee (Washington, D.C.: GAO, June 19, 2001); GAO, *Medicare Management: CMS Faces Challenges to Sustain Progress and Address Weaknesses* (Washington, D.C.: GAO, July 2001); and Scanlon, *Medicare: Successful Reform Requires Meeting Key Management Challenges,* Testimony before the House Committee on the Budget (Washington, D.C.: GAO, July 25, 2001).

16. Jost, "Governing Medicare," 43.

17. Thomas H. Hammond and Jack H. Knott, "Who Controls the Bureaucracy? Presidential Power, Congressional Dominance, Legal Constraints, and Bureaucratic Autonomy in a Model of Multi-institutional Policy-Making," *Journal of Law, Economics, and Organization* 12, no. 1 (April 1996): 119–66.

18. The intellectually exciting challenge here is to build an administrative reform project on the foundation of an empirical understanding of the properties of effective public management. For an overview of the state of the art and possibilities for administrative reform, see Laurence E. Lynn Jr., Carolyn J. Heinrich, and Carolyn J. Hill, *Improving Governance: A New Logic for Empirical Research* (Washington, D.C.: Georgetown University Press, 2001).

19. Scanlon, *Medicare: Successful Reform,* 8.

20. Scanlon, *Medicare Management,* 3.

21. CMS regional apparatus does not currently have the expertise and infrastructure to support such a regional orientation. See, for example, Health and Human Services, Office of the Inspector General, *Medicare's Oversight of Managed Care: Implications for Regional Staffing* (Washington, D.C.: Office of the Inspector General, April 1998).

22. In the history of managed competition, various terms have been applied to these organizational entities: *sponsors, purchasing cooperatives,* and *alliances.* This framework builds on Enthoven's original concept of the public sponsor, though it contains some of the more active purchasing philosophy of health insurance purchasing cooperatives and regulatory elements of alliances. See Alain Enthoven and Richard Kronick, "A Consumer-Choice Health Plan for the 1990s," parts 1 and 2, *New England Journal of Medicine* 320, no. 1 (January 5, 1989): 29–37, 320; no. 2 (January 12, 1989): 94–101; and Enthoven, "The History and Principles of Managed Competition," *Health Affairs,* 12 (1993 supplement): 4–48.

23. Jonathan Skinner, Elliot Fisher, and John Wennberg, *The Efficiency of Medicare,* NBER Working Paper 8395 (Cambridge, Mass.: NBER, July 2001).

24. Oliver Williamson, "Franchise Bidding for Natural Monopolies—in General and with Respect to CATV," in *Economic Organization: Firms, Markets, and Policy Control* (New York: New York University Press, 1986), 258–97.

25. Pamela Brown Drumheller, "Medicare and Innovative Insurance Plans," in *Renewing the Promise: Medicare and Its Reform,* ed. David Blumenthal, Mark Schlesinger, and Pamela Brown Drumheller (New York: Oxford University Press, 1988), 138; and David Blumenthal et al., "The Future of Medicare," *New England Journal of Medicine* 314, no. 11, special report (March 13, 1986): 722–28. In addition to regional budgeting, the Harvard plan called for major reductions in deductibles and coinsurance for beneficiaries. The hospital deductible would have been cut in half, the physician deductible would be eliminated, and several of the coinsurance provisions would be eliminated or reduced. Unlike acute care, long-term care benefits would have required cost sharing, although if designed in a progressive way that is unlikely to affect utilization. An overall ceiling on liabilities would have been set at $1,000. The authors reason that the current mechanisms for controlling utilization were more than enough and that the cost-sharing provisions of Medicare place an onerous burden on beneficiaries. Premiums would increase to cover the lost revenues from these reduced cost-sharing provisions and would vary according to ability to pay.

26. Rashi Fein, *Medical Care, Medical Costs* (Cambridge, Mass.: Harvard University Press, 1986), 200.

27. Ibid., 201.

28. See, for example, Mark Alan Hughes, *The Administrative Geography of Devolving Social Welfare Programs* (Washington, D.C.: Brookings Institution, 1997).

29. Ibid., 5.

30. Havighurst, *Health Care Choices,* 228.

31. William Cass McCaughrin, "Antecedents of Optimal Decision Making for Client Care in Health Services Delivery Organizations," *Medical Care Review* 48, no. 3 (fall 1991): 331–62; Michael Klinkman, "The Process of Choice of Health Care Plan and Provider: Development of an Integrated Analytic Framework," *Medical Care Review* 48, no. 3 (fall 1991): 295–330; Hibbard, Slovic, and Jewett, "Informing Consumer Decisions in Health Care"; Susan Edgman-Levitan and Paul D. Cleary, "What Information Do Consumers Want and Need?" *Health Affairs* 15, no. 4 (winter 1996): 42–56; Catherine McLaughlin," Health Care Consumers: Choices and Constraints," *Medical Care Research and Review* 56, supplement 1 (1999): 24–59; and James S. Lubalin and Lauren D. Harris Kojetin, "What Do Consumers Want and

Need to Know in Making Health Care Choices," *Medical Care Research and Review* 56, supplement 1 (1999): 67–102.

32. Shoshanna Sofaer and Margo-Lea Hurwicz, "When Medical Group and HMO Part Company: Disenrollment Decisions in Medicare HMOs," *Medical Care* 31, no. 9 (1993): 801–21.

33. Susan C. Reinhard and Marisa Scala, *Navigating the Long-Term Care Maze: New Approaches to Information and Assistance in Three States* (Washington, D.C.: AARP Public Policy Institute, 2001).

34. Perry and Thamer, "Medical Innovation and the Critical Role of Health Technology Assessment," 1870.

BIBLIOGRAPHY

Altman, Stuart H., and Robert Blendon. *Medical Technology: The Culprit behind Health Care Costs?* Washington, D.C.: U.S. Dept. of Health, Education, and Welfare, 1979.

Annas, George J. "The Health Care Proxy and Living Will." *New England Journal of Medicine* 324 (1991): 1210–13.

———. "How We Lie." *Hastings Center Report Special Supplement.* November/ December 1995: S12–S14.

Aronovitz, Leslie, Associate Director, General Accounting Office (GAO). Testimony to U.S. Senate Committee on Governmental Affairs, Permanent Subcommittee on Investigations, June 26, 1997.

Arrow, Kenneth. "The Economics of Agency." In *Principals and Agents: The Structure of Business,* edited by John W. Pratt and Richard J. Zeckhauser, 37–51. 1985. Reprint, with a new preface, Boston: Harvard Business School Press, 1991.

———. "Economic Welfare and the Allocation of Resources for Invention." In *The Rate and Direction of Inventive Activity,* edited by Richard Nelson, 609–25. Princeton, N.J.: Princeton University Press, 1962.

Asch, Steven M., E. M. Sloss, C. Hogan, R. H. Brook, and R. L. Kravitz. "Measuring Underuse of Necessary Care among Elderly Medicare Beneficiaries Using Inpatient and Outpatient Claims." *JAMA* 284, no. 18 (November 8, 2000): 2325–33.

Associated Press. "Doctors to Implant First Self-Contained Total Artificial Heart," April 19, 2001.

———. "Kentucky Patient Receives Mechanical Heart Replacement," July 3, 2001.

Avorn, Jerry. "Benefit and Cost in Geriatric Care: Turning Age Discrimination into Policy." *New England Journal of Medicine* 310, no. 20 (May 17, 1984): 1294–301.

Ball, Robert M. "What Medicare's Architects Had in Mind." *Health Affairs* 14, no. 4 (winter 1995): 62–72.

Bengtson, Vern L., and W. Andrew Achenbaum, eds. *The Changing Contract across Generations.* New York: Aldine de Gruyter, 1993.

Berenson, Robert. "Medicare+Choice: Doubling or Disappearing?" *Health Affairs, Web Exclusives* supplement (November 28, 2001): W65–W82.

Berkowitz, Edward D. *Mr. Social Security: The Life of Wilbur J. Cohen.* Lawrence: University of Kansas Press, 1995.

Binstock, Robert H. "Older People and Voting Participation: Past and Future." *Gerontologist* 40, no. 1 (2000): 18–31.

Blakeslee, Sandra. "Therapies Push Injured Brains and Spinal Cords into New Paths." *New York Times,* August 5, 2001, sec. D, 6.

Blendon, Robert J., Ulrike S. Szalay, and Richard A. Knox. "Should Physicians Assist Their Patients in Dying? The Public Perspective." *JAMA* 267, no. 19 (May 20, 1992): 2658–62.

Bloche, M. Gregg, and Peter D. Jacobson. "The Supreme Court and Bedside Rationing." *JAMA* 284, no. 21 (December 6, 2000): 2776–79.

Blumenthal, David, Mark Schlesinger, and Pamela Brown Drumheller, eds. *Renewing the Promise: Medicare and Its Reform.* New York: Oxford University Press, 1988.

Blumenthal, David, Mark Schlesinger, Pamela Brown Drumheller, and the Harvard Medicare Project. "The Future of Medicare." *New England Journal of Medicine* 314, no. 11, special report (March 13, 1986): 722–28.

Bowie, Norman, and R. Edward Freeman, eds. *Ethics and Agency Theory.* New York: Oxford University Press, 1992.

Brook, Robert H., Caren J. Kamberg, Allison Mayer-Oakes, Mark H. Beers, Kristiana Raube, and Andrea Steiner. "Appropriateness of Acute Medical Care for the Elderly: An Analysis of the Literature." *Health Policy* 14, no. 3 (May 1990): 225–42.

———. "Predicting the Appropriate Use of Carotid Endarterectomy, Upper Gastrointestinal Endoscopy, and Coronary Angiography." *New England Journal of Medicine* 323, no. 17 (October 25, 1990): 1173–77.

Brown, Lawrence D. "Technocratic Corporatism and Administrative Reform in Medicare." *Journal of Health Politics, Policy, and Law* 10, no. 3 (fall 1985): 579–99.

Brown, Randall. *Does Managed Care Work for Medicare? An Evaluation of the Risk Contract Program for HMOs.* Princeton, N.J.: Mathematica Policy Research, July 24, 1995.

Brown, Randall, and Rachel Thompson. *Medicare Beneficiaries and HMOs: A Case Study of the Los Angeles Market.* Menlo Park, Calif.: Kaiser Family Foundation, January 1998.

Burns, James MacGregor. *The Deadlock of Democracy.* Englewood Cliffs, N.J.: Prentice Hall, 1963.

Bursztajn, Harold, Richard I. Feinbloom, Robert M. Hamm, and Archie Brodsky. *Medical Choices, Medical Chances: How Patients, Families, and Physicians Can Cope with Uncertainty.* New York: Routledge, 1990.

Butler, Stuart, Patricia M. Danzon, Bill Gradison, et al. "Crisis Facing HCFA and Millions of Americans." Open Letter to Congress and the Executive. *Health Affairs* 18, no. 1 (January/February 1999): 8–10.

Buto, Kathleen. "Can Medicare Keep Pace with Cutting Edge Technology?" *Health Affairs* 13, no. 3 (summer 1994): 137–40.

Califano, Joseph A. *Governing America: An Insider's Report from the White House and the Cabinet.* New York: Simon & Schuster, 1982.

Callahan, Daniel. "The Artificial Heart: Bleeding Us Dry." *New York Times,* September 17, 1988, 20.

———. *The Troubled Dream of Life.* New York: Simon & Schuster, 1993.

Calvert, Randall L., Matthew D. McCubbins, and Barry R. Weingast. "A Theory of Political

Control and Agency Discretion." *American Journal of Political Science* 33, no. 3 (August 1989): 588–611.

Cantazano v. Dowling. 60 F.3d 113 (2d Cir. 1995).

Casey, Michelle, Astrid Knott, and Ira Moscovice. "Medicare Minus Choice: The Impact of HMO Withdrawals on Rural Medicare Beneficiaries." *Health Affairs* 21, no. 3 (May/June 2002): 192–99.

Cash, Connacht. *The Medicare Answer Book,* 3d ed. Provincetown, Mass.: Race Point Press, 1999.

Cassidy, Amanda, and Marsha Gold. *Medicare+Choice in 2000: Will Enrollees Spend More and Receive Less?* New York: Commonwealth Fund, July 2000.

Centers for Medicare and Medicaid Services (CMS). *Medicare and You, 2002.* Baltimore: CMS, September 2001.

Chambers, Christopher, James J. Diamond, Robert L. Perkel, and Lori A Lasch. "Relationship of Advance Directives to Hospital Charges in a Medicare Population." *Archives of Internal Medicine* 154 (1994): 541–47.

Cher, Daniel, and Leslie Lenert. "Method of Medicare Reimbursement and the Rate of Potentially Ineffective Care of Critically Ill Patients." *JAMA* 278, no. 12 (September 24, 1997): 1001–7.

Chiang, Harriet. "Medicare Patients Allowed to Sue HMOs: Top State Court Rules in Denial-of-Care Case." *San Francisco Chronicle,* May 4, 2001, sec. A, 1.

Christakis, Nicholas A. *Death Foretold: Prophecy and Prognosis in Medical Care.* Chicago: University of Chicago Press, 2000.

———. "Prognostication and Death in Medical Thought and Practice." Ph.D. diss., University of Pennsylvania, 1995.

Christakis, Nicholas A., and David Asch. "Biases in How Physicians Choose to Withdraw Life Support." *Lancet* 342 (September 11, 1993): 642–46.

Christakis, Nicholas A., and Jose Escarce. "Survival of Medicare Patients after Enrollment in Hospice Programs." *New England Journal of Medicine* 335, no. 3 (July 18, 1996): 172–78.

Chubb, John E., and Terry M. Moe. *Politics, Markets, and America's Schools.* Washington, D.C.: Brookings Institution, 1990.

Cohen, Jonathan, Stephan Fihn, Edward Boyko, Albert Jonsen, and Robert Wook. "Attitudes toward Physician-Assisted Suicide and Euthanasia in Washington State." *New England Journal of Medicine* 331, no. 2 (July 14, 1994): 89–94.

Cohen, Lynne. "Banking on the Artificial Heart." News and Analysis. *Canadian Medical Association Journal* 157, no. 2 (July 15, 1997): 128.

Cohen, Mark. "Optimal Enforcement Strategy to Prevent Oil Spills: An Application of a Principal Agent Model with Moral Hazard." *Journal of Law and Economics* 30 (April 1987): 23–51.

Cohen, W. J. "Reflections on the Enactment of Medicare and Medicaid." *Health Care Financing Review,* annual supplement (1985): 3–11.

A Comparison of Alternative Approaches to Risk Measurement. Selected External Research Series no 1. [Washington, D.C.]: Physician Payment Review Commission, December 1994.

Concord Coalition. *A Primer on Medicare.* Washington, D.C.: June 2000.

Contract with Eligible Medicare+Choice Organizations Pursuant to Sections 1851 to 1859 of the Social Security Act for the Operation of a Medicare+Choice Coordinated Care Plan(s). Available at cms.hhs.gov.

Cooper, Barbara, and Bruce Vladeck. "Bringing Competitive Pricing to Medicare: Theory Meets Reality, and Reality Wins." *Health Affairs* 19, no. 5 (September/October 2000): 49–54.

Cooper, Gregory S., Zhong Yuan, Amitabh Chak, and Alfred A. Rimm. "Geographic and Patient Variation among Medicare Beneficiaries in the Use of Follow-Up Testing after
Surgery for Nonmetastatic Colorectal Carcinoma." *Cancer* 85, no. 10 (May 15, 1999):
2124–31.

Copeland, Jack G., A. Pavie, D. Duveau, W. J. Keon, R. Masters, R. Pifarre, R. G. Smith, and
F. A. Arabia. "Bridge to Transplantation with the CardioWest Total Artificial Heart: The
International Experience 1993–1995." *Journal of Heart and Lung Transplantation* 15,
no. 1 (January 1996): 94–99.

Cowper, Patricia A., Elizabeth R. DeLong, Eric D. Peterson, Joseph Lipscomb, Lawrence H.
Muhlbaier, James G. Jollis, David B. Pryor, and Daniel B. Mark for the IAD Port Inves-
tigators. "Geographic Variation in Resource Use for Coronary Artery Bypass Surgery."
Medical Care 35, no. 4 (April 1997): 320–33.

Cranford, Ronald. "Medical Futility: Transforming a Clinical Concept into Legal and Social
Policies." *Journal of the American Geriatrics Society* 42 (August 1994): 894–98.

Cronin, Carol. "Reaching and Educating Medicare Beneficiaries about Choice." In *Improving
the Medicare Market: Adding Choice and Protections,* edited by Stanley B. Jones and Marion Ein Lewin, 236–69. Washington, D.C.: National Academy of Sciences, 1996.

Cutler, David. "What Does Medicare Spending Buy Us?" In *Medicare Reform: Issues and Answers,* edited by Andrew Rettenmaier and Thomas R. Saving, 131–52. Chicago: University of Chicago Press, 1999.

Cutler, David, Kenneth G. Manton, and James W. Vaupel. "Survival after the Age of 80 in the
United States, Sweden, France, England, and Japan." *New England Journal of Medicine*
333, no. 18 (November 2, 1995): 1232–35.

Dallek, Geraldine. *Consumer Protections in Medicare+Choice.* Menlo Park, Calif.: Kaiser Family
Foundation, December 1998.

———. *Medicare Managed Care: Securing Beneficiary Protections.* Washington, D.C.: Families
USA Foundation, April 1997.

Danzon, Patricia. *Medical Malpractice: Theory, Evidence, and Public Policy.* Cambridge, Mass.:
Harvard University Press, 1985.

Dartmouth Medical School, Center for the Evaluative Clinical Sciences. *Dartmouth Atlas of
Health Care.* Chicago: American Hospital Publishing, 1998.

Davis, Karen, and Diane Rowland. *Medicare Policy: New Directions for Health and Long-Term
Care.* Baltimore: Johns Hopkins University Press, 1986.

Day, Christine L. "Older Americans' Attitudes toward the Medicare Catastrophic Coverage Act
of 1988." *Journal of Politics* 55, no. 1 (February 1993): 167–77.

Dees, J. Gregory. "Principals, Agents, and Ethics." In *Ethics and Agency Theory: An Introduction,* edited by Norman Bowie and R. Edward Freeman. New York: Oxford University
Press, 1992.

de Lissovoy, G. "Medicare and Heart Transplants: Will Lightning Strike Twice?" *Health Affairs*
7, no. 4 (fall 1988): 61–72.

Dowd, Bryan, Robert Coulam, and Roger Feldman. "A Tale of Four Cities: Medicare Reform
and Competitive Pricing." *Health Affairs* 19, no. 5 (September/October 2000): 9–29

Dowd, Bryan, Roger Feldman, and Jon Christianson. *Competitive Pricing for Medicare.* Washington, D.C.: AEI Press, 1996.

Dranove, David, and William White. "Agency and the Organization of Health Care Delivery."
Inquiry 24, no. 4 (winter 1987): 405–15.

Drumheller, Pamela Brown. "Medicare and Innovative Insurance Plans." In *Renewing the*

Promise: Medicare and Its Reform, edited by David Blumenthal, Mark Schlesinger, and Pamela Brown Drumheller. New York: Oxford University Press, 1988.

Eddy, David. "A Conversation with My Mother." *JAMA* 272, no. 3 (July 20, 1994): 179–81.

Edgman-Levitan, Susan, and Paul D. Cleary. "What Information Do Consumers Want and Need?" *Health Affairs* 15, no. 4 (winter 1996): 42–56.

Eisenberg, John. "Ten Lessons for Evidence-Based Technology Assessment." *JAMA* 282, no. 19 (November 17, 1999): 1865–69.

Eisenhardt, Kathleen M. "Agency- and Institutional-Theory: The Case of Retail Sales." *Academy of Management Journal* 31, no. 3 (September 1988): 488–511.

———. "Agency Theory: An Assessment and Review." *Academy of Management Review* 14, no. 1 (1989): 57–74.

———. "Control: Organizational and Economic Approaches." *Management Science* 31, no. 2 (February1985): 134–44.

Ellis, Randall P., G. C. Pope, L. I. Iezzoni, J. Z. Ayanian, D. W. Bates, H. Burstin, and A. S. Ash, "Diagnosis-Based Risk Adjustment for Medicare Capitation Payment." *Health Care Financing Review* 17, no. 3 (spring 1996): 101–28.

Ely, John W., Philip G. Peters Jr., Steven Zweig, Nancy Elder, and F. David Scheider. "The Physician's Decision to Use Tube Feedings: The Role of the Family, the Living Will, and the Cruzan Decision." *Journal of the American Geriatrics Society* 40 (1992): 471–75.

Emanuel, Ezekiel J. "Cost Savings at the End of Life: What Do the Data Show?" *JAMA* 275, no. 24 (June 26, 1996): 1907–14.

Emanuel, Ezekiel J., and Linda L. Emanuel. "The Economics of Dying: The Illusion of Cost Savings at the End of Life." *New England Journal of Medicine* 330, no. 8 (February 24, 1994): 540–44.

———. "The Promise of a Good Death." *Lancet* 351, no. 9114, supplement 2 (May 16, 1998): 21–29.

Emanuel, Linda L. "Advance Directives: What Have We Learned So Far?" *Journal of Clinical Ethics* 4 (spring 1993): 8–16.

———. "Structured Advance Planning: Is It Finally Time for Physician Action and Reimbursement?" *JAMA* 274, no. 6 (August 9, 1995): 501–3.

Emanuel, Linda L., Marion Danis, Robert A. Pearlman, and Peter A. Singer. "Advance Care Planning As a Process: Structuring the Discussion in Practice." *Journal of the American Geriatrics Society* 43 (1995): 40–46.

Emanuel, Linda L., Michael J. Barry, John D. Stoeckle, Lucy M. Ettelson, and Ezekiel J. Emanuel. "Advance Directives for Medical Care: A Case for Greater Use." *New England Journal of Medicine* 324, no. 13 (March 28, 1991): 889–95.

Enthoven, Alain. "The History and Principles of Managed Competition." *Health Affairs* 12 (1993 supplement): 4–48.

Enthoven, Alain, and Richard Kronick. "A Consumer-Choice Health Plan for the 1990s." Parts 1 and 2. *New England Journal of Medicine* 320, no. 1 (January 5, 1989): 29–37; no. 2 (January 12, 1989): 94–101.

Epstein, David, and Sharyn O'Halloran. "Administrative Procedures, Information, and Agency Discretion." *American Journal of Political Science* 38, no. 3 (August 1994): 697–722.

Estes, Carroll. *The Aging Enterprise.* San Francisco: Josey Bass, 1979.

Etheredge, Lynn. "Medicare's Structure and Governance: A Proposal." *Health Affairs* 19, no. 5 (September/October 2000): 60–71.

Feder, Judith. *The Politics of Federal Health Insurance.* Lexington, Mass.: Lexington Books, 1977. *Federal Register,* 54: 4304–9.

Fein, Rashi. *Medical Care, Medical Costs.* Cambridge, Mass.: Harvard University Press, 1986.

Field, Marilyn J., and Christine Cassel, eds. *Approaching Death: Improving Care at the End of Life.* Report by the Institute of Medicine, Committee on Care at the End of Life. Washington, D.C.: National Academy Press, 1997.

Fisher, Elliot S., David E. Wennberg, Thérèse A. Stukel, Daniel J. Gottlieb, F. L. Lucas, and Étoile L. Pinder. "The Implications of Regional Variations in Medicare Spending. Part 1: The Content, Quality, and Accessibility of Care." *Annals of Internal Medicine* 138, no. 4 (February 18, 2003): 273–87.

———. "The Implications of Regional Variations in Medicare Spending. Part 2: Health Outcomes and Satisfaction with Care." *Annals of Internal Medicine* 138, no. 4 (February 18, 2003): 288–98.

Fisher, Elliot S., John E. Wennberg, Thérèse A. Stukel, Jonathan S. Skinner, Sandra M. Sharp, Jean L. Freeman, and Alan M. Gittelsohn. "Associations among Hospital Capacity, Utilization, and Mortality of U.S. Medicare Beneficiaries, Controlling for Sociodemographic Factors." *Health Services Research* 34, no. 6 (February 2000): 1351–62.

Foote, Susan Bartlett. "Coexistence, Conflict, and Cooperation: Public Policy towards Medical Devices." *Journal of Health Politics, Policy, and Law* 11, no. 3 (fall 1986): 501–23.

———. "Why Medicare Cannot Promulgate a National Coverage Rule: A Case of Regula Mortis." *Journal of Health Politics, Policy, and Law* 27, no. 5 (October 2002): 707–30.

Foundation for Accountability. *Quality of Care at the End of Life: Proposed Measurement Set.* Available at www.facct.org.

Fowler, Elizabeth, and Gerald Anderson. "Capitation Adjustment for Pediatric Populations." *Pediatrics* 98, no. 1 (July 1996): 10–17.

Fox, Peter. *End-of-Life Care in Managed Care Organizations.* Washington, D.C.: AARP Public Policy Institute, July 1999.

Fried, Charles. *Contract As Promise.* Cambridge, Mass: Harvard University Press, 1986.

Friedman, Emily. "The Compromise and the Afterthought: Medicare and Medicaid after 30 Years." *JAMA* 274, no. 3 (July 19, 1995): 278–81.

Fuchs, Beth, and Lisa Poetz. "The Breaux-Thomas Proposal." In *Competition with Constraints,* edited by Marilyn Moon, 155–85. Washington, D.C.: Urban Institute, 2000.

Fuchs, Victor. *The Future of Health Policy.* Cambridge, Mass.: Harvard University Press, 1993.

Gage, Barbara, Marilyn Moon, and Sang Chi. "State-Level Variation in Medicare Spending." *Health Care Financing Review* 21, no. 2 (winter 1999): 85–98.

Garber, Alan. "Evidence-Based Coverage Policy." *Health Affairs* 20, no. 5 (September/October 2001): 62–82.

General Accounting Office (GAO). *Health Care Quality: Implications of Purchaser's Experiences for HCFA.* Washington, D.C.: GAO, June 1998.

———. *Medicare: Home Health Care Utilization Expands While Controls Deteriorate.* Washington, D.C.: GAO, March 1996.

———. *Medicare: Information Systems Modernization Needs Stronger Management and Support.* Washington, D.C.: GAO, September 2001.

———. *Medicare: Millions Could Be Saved by Screening Claims for Overused Services.* Washington, D.C.: GAO, January 1996.

———. *Medicare: Private Payer Strategies Suggest Options to Reduce Rapid Spending Growth.* Washington, D.C., GAO, 1996.

———. *Medicare+Choice: Payments Exceed Costs of Benefits in Fee-for-Service, Adding Billions to Spending.* Washington, D.C.: GAO, August 2000.

———. *Medicare+Choice: Recent Payment Increases Had Little Effect on Benefits or Plan Availability in 2001.* Washington, D.C.: GAO, November 2001.

———. *Medicare Home Health Agencies: Closures Continue, but Little Evidence Beneficiary Access Is Impaired.* Washington, D.C.: GAO, May 1999.

———. *Medicare Home Health Care: Prospective Payment System Could Reverse Recent Declines in Spending.* Washington, D.C.: GAO, September 2000.

———. *Medicare Management: CMS Faces Challenges to Sustain Progress and Address Weaknesses.* Washington, D.C.: GAO, July 2001.

———. *Medicare Transactions System: Success Depends upon Correcting Critical Managerial and Technical Weaknesses.* Washington, D.C.: GAO, May 16, 1997.

Geron, Scott. "Managed Care and Care Management for Older Adults." In *Managed Care Services: Policy, Programs, and Research,* edited by Nancy Veeder and Wilma Peebles-Wilkins, 150–62. New York: Oxford University Press, 2001.

Gibson, Robert. "Incentives in Organizations." *Journal of Economic Perspectives* 12, no. 4 (fall 1998): 115–32.

Goddard, Maria K. "The Importance of Assessing the Effectiveness of Care: The Case of Hospices." *Journal of Social Policy* 22 (1993): 1–17.

Goddard, Maria, Russell Mannion, and Peter Smith. "Enhancing Performance in Health Care: A Theoretical Perspective on Agency and the Role of Information." *Health Economics* 9 (2000): 95–107.

Gold, Marsha. "Medicare+Choice: An Interim Report Card." *Health Affairs* 20, no. 4 (July/August 2001): 120–38.

Gold, Marsha, and Anna Aizer. *Medicare Beneficiaries and HMOs: A Case Study of the New York City Market.* Menlo Park, Calif.: Kaiser Family Foundation, January 1998.

Gold, Marsha, and Lori Achman. *Trends in Premiums, Cost-Sharing, and Benefits in Medicare+Choice Health Plans, 1999–2001.* New York: Commonwealth Fund, April 2001.

Gold, Marsha, and Natalie Justh. *Forced Exit: Beneficiaries in Plans Terminating in 2000.* Monitoring Medicare+Choice: Fast Facts. Washington, D.C.: Mathematica Policy Research, September 2000.

Goldstein, Daniel, Mahmet Oz, and Eric Rose. "Implantable Left Ventricular Assist Devices." *New England Journal of Medicine* 339, no. 21 (November 13, 1999): 1522–33.

Gomez, Carlos. *Regulating Death: Euthanasia and the Case of the Netherlands.* New York: Free Press, 1991.

Gormley, William T., Jr., and David L. Weimer. *Organizational Report Cards.* Cambridge, Mass.: Harvard University Press, 1999.

Gornick, M., A. McMillan, and J. Lubitz. "A Longitudinal Perspective on Patterns of Medicare Payments." *Health Affairs* (summer 1993): 140–50.

Green, Lisa. *Medicare State Profiles: State and Regional Data on Medicare and the Population It Serves.* Menlo Park, Calif.: Henry J. Kaiser Family Foundation, September 1999.

Gunten, Charles F. von, Frank D. Ferris, Robert D'Antuono, and Linda L. Emanuel. "Recommendations to Improve End-of-Life Care through Regulatory Change in U.S. Health Care Financing." *Journal of Palliative Medicine* 5, no. 1 (February 2002): 35–41.

Guterman, Stuart. "Risk Adjustment in a Competitive Medicare System with Premium Support." In *Competition with Constraints,* edited by Marilyn Moon, 119–34. Washington, D.C.: Urban Institute, 2000.

Guzmano, Michael, and Mark Schlesinger. "The Social Roles of Medicare: Assessing Medicare's Collateral Benefits." *Journal of Health Politics, Policy, and Law* 26, no. 1 (February 2001): 36–79.

Hacker, Jacob S. *The Road to Nowhere.* Princeton, N.J.: Princeton University Press, 1997.

———. "A Tale of Editions: Marmor's *The Politics of Medicare* and the Study of Health Politics after 30 Years." *Journal of Health Politics, Policy, and Law* 26, no. 1 (February 2001): 120–38.

Hadley, Jack, Jean M. Mitchell, and Jeanne Mandelblatt. "Medicare Fees and Small Area Variations in Breast-Conserving Surgery among Elderly Women." *Medical Care Research and Review* 58, no. 3 (September 2001): 334–60.

Hagen, Stuart. "Hospital Response to Medicare Reimbursement Incentives: Hospital-Based Skilled Nursing Facilities and Their Impact on Discharge Behavior." Ph.D. diss., University of Chicago, 1998.

Hammond, Thomas H., and Jack H. Knott. "Who Controls the Bureaucracy? Presidential Power, Congressional Dominance, Legal Constraints, and Bureaucratic Autonomy in a Model of Multi-institutional Policy-Making." *Journal of Law, Economics, and Organization* 12, no. 1 (April 1996): 119–66.

Hardin, John W. "An In-Depth Look at Congressional Committee Jurisdictions Surrounding Health Issues." *Journal of Health Politics, Policy, and Law* 23 (1998): 517–50.

Harris, Richard. "Annals of Legislation: The Real Voice." Parts 1–3. *New Yorker* 40, March 14, 1965, 48–50+; March 21, 1965, 75–76+; March 28, 1965, 46–48+.

———. *A Sacred Trust.* New York: New American Library, 1966.

Havighurst, Clark C. "Consumers versus Managed Care: The New Class Actions." *Health Affairs* (July/August 2001): 8–27.

———. *Health Care Choices.* Washington, D.C.: AEI Press, 1995.

———. "Vicarious Liability: Relocating Responsibility for the Quality of Care." *American Journal of Law and Medicine* 26, no. 1 (2000): 7–29.

Health and Human Services, Office of the Inspector General. *Medicare's Oversight of Managed Care: Implications for Regional Staffing.* Washington, D.C.: Office of the Inspector General, April 1998.

"Health Care Consumers: Choices and Constraints." *Medical Care Research and Review* 56, supplement 1 (1999): 24–59.

Health Care Financing Administration (HCFA). *1999 HCFA Statistics: Providers/Suppliers.* Available at cms.hhs.gov/researchers/statsdata.asp.

———. *Distribution of Medicare+Choice Provider Payments under the Medicare, Medicaid, and SCHIP Benefit Improvement and Protection Act 2000.* Baltimore: HCFA, n.d.

———, Office of Strategic Planning. *Medicare Current Beneficiary Survey.* Available from CMS in digital format.

Heimer, Carol A. *Reactive Risk and Rational Action: Managing Moral Hazard in Insurance Contracts.* Berkeley: University of California Press, 1989.

Hibbard, Judith, Paul Slovic, and Jacquelyn J. Jewett. "Informing Consumer Decisions in Health Care: Implications from Decision-Making Research." *Milbank Quarterly* 75, no. 3 (1977): 395–417.

Himelfarb, Richard. *Catastrophic Politics: The Rise and Fall of the Medicare Catastrophic Coverage Act of 1988.* University Park: Pennsylvania State University Press, 1995.

Himmler v. Califano. 611 F.2d 137, 140 (6th Cir. 1979).

Hogan, Christopher, Joanne Lynn, Jon Gabel, June Lunney, Ann O'Mara, and Ann Wilkinson.

Medicare Beneficiaries' Cost and Use of Care in the Last Year of Life. Contractors Research Series Report no. 00-1. Washington, D.C.: MedPAC, May 2000.

Hogan, Christopher, June Lunney, Jon Gabel, and Joanne Lynn. "Medicare Beneficiaries' Cost in the Last Year of Life." *Health Affairs* 20, no. 4 (July/August 2001): 188–95.

Holmstrom, Bengt, and John Roberts. "The Boundaries of the Firm Revisited." *Journal of Economic Perspectives* 12, no. 4 (fall 1998): 73–94.

Hospitals and Health Networks. Chicago: American Hospital Publishing, February 20, 1994.

Hougham, Gavin. "Advance Directives, Self, and Social Role Preservation: Health Policy Innovations As Institutionalized Legitimation Mechanisms." Ph.D. diss. proposal, University of Chicago, 1996.

Hudson, Robert B. "The Evolution of the Welfare State: Shifting Rights and Responsibilities for the Old." In *Critical Gerontology: Perspectives from Political and Moral Economy,* edited by Meredith Minkler and Carroll Estes, 329–43. New York: Baywood, 1997.

———. "The History and Place of Age-Based Public Policy." In *The Future of Age-Based Public Policy,* edited by Robert B. Hudson, 1–22. Baltimore: Johns Hopkins University Press, 1997.

Hughes, Mark Alan. *The Administrative Geography of Devolving Social Welfare Programs.* Washington, D.C.: Brookings Institution, 1997.

Inlander, Charles B., and Charles MacKay. *Medicare Made Easy.* Allentown, Penn.: People's Medical Society, 1996.

Institute for Health Policy Solutions. *Resource Manual: Implementing Healthplan Purchasing Cooperatives.* Washington, D.C.: IHPS, 1994.

Institute of Medicine. *The Total Artificial Heart: Prototypes, Policies, and Patients.* Washington, D.C.: National Academy of Sciences, 1991.

J. K. v. Dillenberg. 836 F. Supp. 694 (D. Ariz. 1993).

Jacox, Ada, Daniel B. Carr, and Richard Payne. "New Clinical-Practice Guidelines for the Management of Pain in Patients with Cancer." *New England Journal of Medicine* 330, no. 9 (March 3, 1994): 651–55.

Jass v. Prudential Health Care Plan, Inc. 88 F.3d 1482 (July 8, 1996).

Jencks, Stephen F., Timothy Cuerdon, Dale R. Burman, Barbara Fleming, Peter M. Houck, Annette E. Kussmaul, David S. Nilasera, Diana L. Ordin, and David R. Arday. "Quality of Medical Care Delivered to Medicare Beneficiaries: A Profile at State and National Levels." *JAMA* 284, no. 13 (October 4, 2000): 1670–76.

Jensen, Michael, and William Meckling. "Theory of the Firm: Managerial Behavior, Agency Costs, and Ownership Structure." *Journal of Financial Economics* 3, no. 4 (October 1976): 305–60.

Johnson, Haynes, and David S. Broder. *The System.* Boston: Little, Brown, 1996.

Joint Economic Committee. *1999 Greenbook .*Washington, D.C.: U.S. Congress JEC, 2000.

Jones, Stanley B., and Marion Ein Lewin, eds. *Improving the Medicare Market: Adding Choice and Protections.* Washington, D.C.: National Academy of Sciences, 1996.

Jost, Timothy. "Governing Medicare." *Administrative Law Review* 51, no. 1 (1999): 39–116.

Kaiser Family Foundation (Focus Group). "Medicare Beneficiaries Consider Ability to Keep Their Physician As Most Important Factor in Deciding to Keep an HMO." Menlo Park, Calif.: Kaiser Family Foundation, May 2, 1995.

The Kaiser-Harvard Program on the Public and Health/Social Policy. *Survey on Medicare.* Menlo Park, Calif.: Kaiser Family Foundation, June 1995.

Kane, Nancy M., and Paul D. Manoukian. "The Effect of the Medicare Prospective Payment

System on the Adoption of New Technology: The Case of Cochlear Implants." *New England Journal of Medicine* 321, no. 20 (November 16, 1989): 1378–83.

Kane, Robert L., and Rosalie A. Kane. "What Older People Want from Long-Term Care, and How They Can Get It." *Health Affairs* 20, no. 6 (November/December 2001): 114–27.

Kane, Robert L., Jeffrey Wales, Leslie Bernstein, Arleen Liebowitz, and Stevan Kaplan. "A Randomized Controlled Trial of Hospice Care." *Lancet*, no. 8382 (April 7, 1984): 890–94.

Kane, Robert L., Rosalie A. Kane, Michael Finch, Charlene Harrington, Robert Newcomer, Nancy Miller, and Melissa Hulbert. "S/HMOs, the Second Generation: Building on the Experience of the First Social Health Maintenance Organization Demonstrations." *Journal of the American Geriatrics Society* 45, no. 1 (January 1997): 101–7.

Katz, Barry P., Deborah A. Freund, David A. Heck, Robert S. Dittus, John E. Paul, James Wright, Peter Coyte, Eleanor Holleman, and Gillian Hawker. "Demographic Variation in the Rate of Knee Replacement: A Multi-Year Analysis." *Health Services Research* 31, no. 2 (June 1996): 125–40.

Kendall, David B. *A New Deal for Medicare and Medicaid: Building a Buyer's Market for Health Care.* Washington, D.C.: Progressive Policy Institute, September 22, 1995.

Kennedy School of Government. *Catastrophic Health Insurance for the Elderly.* Cambridge, Mass.: Kennedy School of Government Case Program, 1995.

Kessler, Daniel P., and Mark McClellan. "Do Doctors Practice Defensive Medicine?" *Quarterly Journal of Economics* 111, no. 2 (May 1996): 353–90.

Kidder, David. "The Effect of Hospice Coverage on Medicare Expenditures." *Health Services Research* 27 (June 1992): 195–217.

Klinkman, Michael. "The Process of Choice of Health Care Plan and Provider: Development of an Integrated Analytic Framework." *Medical Care Review* 48, no. 3 (fall 1991): 295–330.

Knaus, William A., Alfred F. Connors, Neal V. Dawson, Norman A. Derbiens, William J. Fulkerson, Lee Goldman, Joanne Lynn, and Robert K Oye. "A Controlled Trial to Improve Care for Seriously Ill Hospitalized Patients." *JAMA* 274, no. 20 (November 22/29, 1995): 1591–98.

Kornfield, Thomas, and Marsha Gold. *Is There More or Less Choice?* Monitoring Medicare+Choice: Fast Facts. Washington, D.C.: Mathematica Policy Research, December 1999.

Krakauer, Henry, R. Clifton Bailey, Harold Cooper, Wai-Kouk Yu, Kimberley J. Skellan, and George Kattakkuzhy. "The Systematic Assessment of Medical Practice Variations and Their Outcomes." *Public Health Reports* 110, no. 1 (January/February 1995): 2–12.

Kronick, Richard, and Joy de Beyer. "The Problem of Risk Selection in Medicare Risk-Based HMOs." In *Medicare HMOs: Making Them Work for the Chronically Ill,* edited by Richard Kronick and Joy de Beyer, 9–26. Chicago: Health Administration Press, 1999.

———, eds. *Medicare HMOs: Making Them Work for the Chronically Ill.* Chicago: Health Administration Press, 1999.

La Puma, John, and Edward F. Lawlor. "Quality-Adjusted Life-Years: Ethical Implications for Physicians and Policymakers." *JAMA* 263, no. 21 (June 6, 1990): 2917–21.

La Puma, John, David Orentlicher, and Robert Moss. "Advance Directives on Admission: Clinical Implications and Analysis of the Patient Self-Determination Act of 1990." *JAMA* 266, no. 3 (July 17, 1991): 402–5.

Larson, Dale, and Daniel Tobin. "End-of-Life Conversations: Evolving Practice and Theory." *JAMA* 284, no. 12 (September 27, 2000): 1573–78.

Last Acts Financing Task Force. *The Challenge of End-of-Life Care: Moving toward Metanoia?* Washington, D.C.: Last Acts, October 1998.

Lawlor, Edward. "Hard Choices, Unfair Choices, and Tragic Choices." In *Paying for Health Care,* edited by Lawrence Joseph. Chicago: Chicago Assembly and the University of Illinois Press, 1990.

Lawlor, Edward F., and Kristiana Raube. "Social Interventions and Outcomes in Medical Effectiveness Research." *Social Service Review* 69, no. 3 (September 1995): 383–404.

Lee, David. "Estimating the Effect of New Technology on Medicare Part B Expenditure and Volume Growth." *Advances in Health Economics and Health Services Research* 13 (1992): 43–64.

Lehoux, Pascale, and Stuart Blume. "Technology Assessment and the Sociopolitics of Health Technologies." *Journal of Health Politics, Policy, and Law* 25, no. 6 (December 2000): 1083–120.

Lentzner, Harold R., Elsie R. Pamok, Elaine Rhodenheiser, Richard Rothenberg, and Eve Powell-Griner. "The Quality of Life in the Year before Death." *American Journal of Public Health* 82 (August 1992): 1093–98.

Leutz, Walter N., et al. *Changing Health Care for an Aging Society: Planning for the Social Health Maintenance Organization.* Lexington, Mass.: Lexington Books, 1985.

Lo, Bernard. "End-of-Life after Termination of Support." *Hastings Center Report Special Supplement* 25, no. 6 (November/December 1995): S6–S8.

Lubalin, James S., and Lauren D. Harris Kojetin. "What Do Consumers Want and Need to Know in Making Health Care Choices?" *Medical Care Research and Review* 56, supplement 1 (1999): 67–102.

Lubitz, J., and R. Prihoda. "The Use and Costs of Medicare Services in the Last Two Years of Life." *Health Care Financing Review* (spring 1984): 117–31.

Lubitz, J. D., and G. F. Riley. "Trends in Medicare Payments in the Last Year of Life." *New England Journal of Medicine* 328, no. 15 (April 15, 1993): 1092–96.

Lucas, F. L., D. E. Wennberg, and D. J. Malenka. "Variation in the Use of Echocardiography." *Effective Clinical Practice* 2, no. 2 (March/April 1999): 71–75.

Luddington, A. V. "The Death Control Dilemma: Who Is to Make End-of-Life Decisions: You and Your Patient, or 'the System'?" *Geriatrics* 48 (1993): 72–77.

Luft, Harold S., ed. *HMOs and the Elderly.* Ann Arbor, Mich.: Health Administration Press, 1994.

Lynn, Joanne. "Caring at the End of Our Lives." Editorial. *New England Journal of Medicine* 335, no. 3 (July 18, 1996): 201–2.

———. "Serving Patients Who May Die Soon and Their Families." *JAMA* 285, no. 7 (February 21, 2001): 925–32.

Lynn, Joanne, and Joan M. Teno. "After the Patient Self-Determination Act: The Need for Empirical Research on Formal Advance Directives." *Hastings Center Report* (January/February 1993): 20–24.

Lynn, Laurence E., Jr., Carolyn J. Heinrich, and Carolyn J. Hill. *Improving Governance: A New Logic for Empirical Research.* Washington, D.C.: Georgetown University Press, 2001.

MacDonald, Neil. "Oncology and Palliative Care: The Case for Co-ordination." *Cancer Treatment Reviews* 19 (1993): 29–41.

Makowsky, Nicole, Fowler Lynn, and Joanne Lynn. *Potential Medicare Reimbursements for Services to Patients with Chronic Fatal Illnesses.* Washington, D.C.: George Washington University Center to Improve Care of the Dying, July 6, 1999.

Markson, Lawrence J., James Fanale, Knight Steel, David Kern, and George Annas. "Implementing Advance Directives in the Primary Care Setting." *Archives of Internal Medicine* 154 (October 24, 1994): 2321–27.

Margolis, Richard J. *Risking Old Age in America*. Boulder, Colo.: Westview Press, 1990.

Marmor, Theodore R.. "Coping with a Creeping Crisis: Medicare at Twenty." In *Social Security: Beyond the Rhetoric of Crisis*, edited by Theodore Marmor and Jerry Mashaw. Princeton, N.J.: Princeton University Press, 1988.

———. *The Politics of Medicare*. 2d ed. New York: Aldine de Gruyter, 2000.

Marmor, Theodore, and Jerry Mashaw, eds. *Social Security: Beyond the Rhetoric of Crisis*. Princeton, N.J.: Princeton University Press, 1988.

Marshal, Elliot. "Artificial Heart: The Beat Goes On." News & Comments. *Science* 253 (August 2, 1991): 500–502.

Marshall, Patricia A. "The Support Study: Who's Talking." *Hastings Center Report Special Supplement* 25, no. 4 (November/December 1995): S9–S11.

Mathematica/PPRC. *Access to Care in Medicare Managed Care: Results from a 1996 Survey of Enrollees and Disenrollees*. External Research Series no. 7. Washington, D.C.: Physician Payment Review Commission, November 1996.

McCabe, Mark. "Principals, Agents, and the Learning Curve: The Case of Steam Electric Power Plant Design and Construction." *Journal of Industrial Economics* 44, no. 4 (December 1996): 357–75.

McCall, Nancy, Treva Rice, and Judith A. Sangl. "A Consumer Knowledge of Medicare and Supplemental Health Insurance Benefits." *Health Services Research* 20, no. 6, pt. 1 (February 1986): 633–57.

McCall v. PacifiCare of California, Inc. 25 Cal. 4th 412 (May 3, 2001).

McCaughrin, William Cass. "Antecedents of Optimal Decision Making for Client Care in Health Services Delivery Organizations." *Medical Care Review* 48, no. 3 (fall 1991): 331–62.

McCormack, Lauren, et al. "Health Insurance Knowledge among Medicare Beneficiaries." October 20, 1999. Draft.

McLaughlin, Catherine. "Health Care Consumers: Choices and Constraints." *Medical Care Research and Review* 56, supplement 1 (1999): 24–59.

Mechanic, David. "Changing Medical Organization and the Erosion of Trust." *Milbank Quarterly* 24, no. 2 (1996): 171–89.

Medicare Payment Advisory Commission (MedPAC). *Reducing Medicare Complexity and Regulatory Burden*. Washington, D.C.: MedPAC, December 2001.

———. *Report to Congress: Medicare in Rural America* (Washington, D.C.: MedPAC, June 2001).

———. *Report to Congress: Medicare Payment Policy*. Washington, D.C.: MedPAC, March 2001.

———. *Report to Congress: Medicare Payment Policy*. Washington, D.C.: MedPAC, March 2002.

Medicare Preservation and Improvement Act of 1999, S.R. 1895. 106th Cong., 1st sess.

Medicare Regulations. Part 422, of June 26, 1998; final rule in July 2000.

Meltzer, David. "Accounting for Future Costs in Medical Cost-Effectiveness Analysis." *Journal of Health Economics* 16, no. 1 (February 1997): 33–64.

Merrell, Katie, Edward Lawlor, Kathleen Cagney, Kenneth Langa, and Robert Willis. "Medicare Beneficiaries As Medicare+Choice Consumers: A Framework." Chicago: Center for Health Administration Studies, 2000.

Merrill, Richard. "Regulation of Drugs and Devices: An Evolution." *Health Affairs* 13, no. 3 (summer 1994): 48–69.

Meyer, Jack, Sean Sullivan, and Sharon Silow-Carroll. *Private Sector Initiatives: Controlling Health Care Costs.* Washington, D.C.: Health Care Leadership Council, March 1991.

Meyer, Jack, Sharon Silow-Carroll, Ingrid Tillman, and Lise Rybowski. *Employer Coalition Initiatives in Health Care Purchasing.* 2 vols. Washington, D.C.: Economic and Social Research Institute, February 1996.

Mezey, Mathy, and Beth Latimer. "The Patient Self-Determination Act: An Early Look at Implementation." *Hastings Center Report* 23, no. 1 (January/February 1993): 16–20.

Midwest Business Group on Health. *Public-Private Healthcare Purchasing Partnerships.* Chicago: MBGH, October 1996.

Miles, Steven, Eileen Weber, and Robert Koepp. "End-of-Life Treatment in Managed Care." *Western Journal of Medicine* 163, no. 3 (September 1995): 302–5.

Millenson, Michael. *Demanding Medical Excellence: Doctors and Accountability in the Information Age.* Chicago: University of Chicago Press, 1997.

Miller, Annetta. "The Elderly Duke It Out." *Newsweek,* September 1, 1989, 42–43.

Miller, Franklin, and Joseph Fins. "A Proposal to Restructure Hospital Care for Dying Patients." *New England Journal of Medicine* 334, no. 26 (June 27, 1996): 1740–42.

Miller, Franklin G., Timothy E. Quill, Howard Brody, John C. Fletcher, Lawrence O. Gostin, and Diane E. Meier. "Regulating Physician-Assisted Death." *New England Journal of Medicine* 331, no. 2 (July 14, 1994): 119–23.

Miller, Robert H., and Harold S. Luft. "Does Managed Care Lead to Better or Worse Quality of Care?" *Health Affairs* 16, no. 5 (September/October 1997): 7–25.

———. "HMO Plan Performance Update: An Analysis of the Literature, 1997–2001." *Health Affairs* 21, no. 4 (July/August 2002): 63–86.

———. "Managed Care Performance since 1980: A Literature Analysis." *JAMA* 271, no. 19 (May 18, 1994): 1512–19.

Minkler, Meredith, and Carroll Estes. *Critical Gerontology: Perspectives from Political and Moral Economy.* New York: Baywood, 1997.

Moe, Terry. "The New Economics of Organization." *American Journal of Political Science* 28, no. 4 (November 1984): 739–77.

Moon, Marilyn. *Medicare Now and in the Future.* 2d ed.. Washington, D.C.: Urban Institute, 1996.

———. *Searching for Savings in Medicare.* Menlo Park, Calif.: Henry J. Kaiser Family Foundation, December 1995.

———, ed. *Competition with Constraints.* Washington, D.C.: Urban Institute, 2000.

Mor, Vincent, and David Kidder. "Cost Savings in Hospice: Final Results from the National Hospice Study." *Health Services Research* 20 (1985): 407–22.

Mor, Vincent, David S. Greer, and Robert Kastenbaum. *The Hospice Experiment.* Baltimore: Johns Hopkins University Press, 1988.

Morone, James. "Hidden Complications: Why Health Care Competition Needs Regulation." *American Prospect* 3, no. 10 (summer 1992): 40–48.

Morrison, M. F. "Obstacles to Doctor-Patient Communication at the End-of-Life." In *End-of-Life Decisions: A Psychosocial Perspective,* edited by M. D. Steinberg and S. J. Youngner, 109–36. Washington, D.C.: American Psychiatric Press, 1998.

Moskowitz, Ellen H., and James Lindemann Nelson. "The Best Laid Plans." *Hastings Center Report Special Supplement* 25, no. 4 (November/December 1995): S3–S6.

Murphy, Donald. "Can We Set Futile Care Policies? Institutional and Systemic Challenges." *Journal of the American Geriatrics Society* 42 (1994): 890–93.

Murphy, Donald J., Anne M. Murray, Bruce E. Robinson, and Edward W. Campion. "Outcomes of Cardiopulmonary Resuscitation in the Elderly." *Annals of Internal Medicine* 111 (1989): 199–205.

National Academy of Social Insurance (NASI). *Medicare and the American Social Contract: Final Report of the Study Panel on Medicare's Larger Social Role.* Washington, D.C.: NASI, February 1999.

———. *Medicare Claims Handling: The Consumer Perspective.* Washington, D.C.: NASI, April 1993.

———. *Reflections on Implementing Medicare.* Washington, D.C.: NASI, January 2001.

Jones, A. L., Division of Health Care Statistics, National Center for Health Statistics. "Hospices and Home Health Agencies: Data from the 1991 National Health Provider Inventory." *Advance Data* 257 (November 3, 1994): 1–8.

National Heart, Lung, and Blood Institute. *Expert Panel Review of the NHLBI Total Artificial Heart Program.* National Heart, Lung, and Blood Institute, June 1998–November 1999.

National Hospice Organization. *Medical Guidelines for Determining Prognosis in Selected Non-Cancer Diagnoses.* Alexandria, Va.: NHO, 1966.

Neuman, Patricia, Diane Rowland, and Elaine Puleo. "Understanding the Diverse Needs of the Medicare Population: Implications for Medicare Reform." *Journal of Aging and Social Policy* 10, no. 4 (1999): 25–50.

Neumann, Peter, and Magnus Johannesson. "From Principle to Public Policy: Using Cost Effectiveness Analysis." *Health Affairs* 13, no. 3 (summer 1994): 206–14.

Newcomer, Robert, Charlene Harrington, and Rosalie Kane. "Implementing the Second-Generation Social Health Maintenance Organization." *Journal of the American Geriatric Society* 48, no. 7 (July 2000): 829–34.

Newcomer, Robert, Kenne H. Manton, Charlene Harrington, Carrleen Yordi, and James Ventrees. "Case Mix Controlled Service Use and Expenditures in the Social Health Maintenance Organization Demonstration." *Journal of Gerontology: Medical Sciences* 50A, no. 1 (1995): 111–19.

Newhouse, Joseph. "Medical Care Costs: How Much Welfare Loss?" *Journal of Economic Perspectives* 6, no. 3 (1992): 3–21.

Newhouse, Joseph, W. G. Manning, E. B. Keeler, and E. M. Sloss. "Adjusting Capitation Rates Using Objective Health Measures and Prior Utilization." *Health Care Financing Review* 10, no. 3 (1989): 41–54.

Nuland, Sherwin B. *How We Die: Reflections on Life's Final Chapter.* New York: Knopf, 1994.

Oberlander, John. "Managed Care and Medicare Reform." In *Healthy Markets? The New Competition in Medical Care,* edited by Mark Peterson, 255–83. Durham, N.C.: Duke University Press, 1998.

———. "Medicare and the American State: The Politics of Federal Health Insurance, 1965–1995." Ph.D. diss., Yale University, 1995.

Oliver, Thomas. "Analysis, Advice, and Congressional Leadership: The Physician Payment Commission and the Politics of Medicare." *Journal of Health Politics, Policy, and Law* 18, no. 1 (spring 1993): 141–44.

Ozminkowski, Ronald, Bernard Friedman, and Zachary Taylor. "Access to Heart and Liver Transplantation in the Late 1980s." *Medical Care* 31, no. 11 (1993): 1027–42.

Pappas v. Asbel. 564 Pa. 407 (April 3, 2001).

Patashnik, Eric, and Julian Zelizer. "Paying for Medicare: Benefits, Budgets, and Wilbur Mill's Policy Legacy." *Journal of Health Politics, Policy, and Law* 26, no. 1 (February 2001): 7–36.

Pauly, Mark. *Medical Care at Public Expense.* New York: Praeger, 1977.

———. "Taxation and Health Insurance." *Journal of Economic Literature* 24, no. 2 (1986): 629–75.

Pauly, Mark, and William Kissick, eds. *Lessons from the First Twenty Years of Medicare.* Philadelphia: University of Pennsylvania Press, 1988.

Pear, Robert. "Medicare Shift towards H.M.O.'s Is Planned." *New York Times,* June 5, 2001, sec. A, 19.

———. "Medicare Spending for Care at Home Plunges by 45 Percent." *New York Times,* April 21, 2000, 1.

———. "New Money for H.M.O.'s Isn't Going As Congress Intended." *New York Times,* January 26, 2001.

Pegram v. Herdrich. 530 U.S. 211 (January 12, 2000).

Perry, Seymour, and Mae Thamer. "Medical Innovation and the Critical Role of Health Technology Assessment." *JAMA* 282, no. 19 (November 17, 1999): 1869–72.

Peterson, Mark. "Institutional Change and the Politics of the 1990s." *American Behavioral Scientist* 36 (1993): 782–801.

———, ed. *Healthy Markets? The New Competition in Medical Care.* Durham, N.C.: Duke University Press, 1998.

Phelps, Charles, and Steven Parente. "Priority Setting in Medical Technology and Medical Practice Assessment." *Medical Care* 28 (1990): 703–23.

Physician Payment Review Commission. *Monitoring Access for Medicare Beneficiaries.* Washington, D.C.: PPRC, May 1995.

Pierson, Paul. "Increasing Returns, Path Dependence, and the Study of Politics." *American Political Science Review* 94, no. 2 (June 2000): 251–67.

———. "When Effect Becomes Cause: Policy Feedback and Politics." *World Politics* 45 (1993): 595–628.

Pratt, John W., and Richard J. Zeckhauser. *Principals and Agents: The Structure of Business.* 1985. Reprint, with a new preface, Boston: Harvard Business School Press, 1991.

Prendergast, Candice. "The Provision of Incentives in Firms." *Journal of Economic Literature* 37 (March 1998): 7–63.

Prichard, Robert S., Elliott S. Fisher, Joan M. Teno, Sandra M. Sharp, Douglas J. Reding, William A. Knaus, John E. Wennberg, and Joanne Lynn for the SUPPORT Investigation. "Influence of Patient Preferences and Local Health System Characteristics in the Place of Death." *Journal of the American Geriatrics Society* 46 (October 1998): 1242–50.

Prospective Payment Assessment Commission. *Report and Recommendation to Congress,* March 1, 1997.

Przybowski v. U.S. Healthcare, Inc. 64 F. Supp. 2d 361 (September 7, 1999).

Public Law 89-97. *Health Insurance for the Aged and Medical Assistance.* 89th Cong., HR 6675, July 30, 1965.

Rabow, Michael, Grace E. Hardie, Joan M. Fair, and Stephen J. McPhee. "End-of-Life Care Content in 50 Textbooks from Multiple Specialties." *JAMA* 283, no. 6 (February 9, 2000): 771–78.

Reichelstein, Stefan. "Constructing Incentive Schemes for Government Contracts: An Application of Agency Theory." *Accounting Review* 67, no. 4 (October 1982): 712–31.

Reinhard, Susan C., and Marisa Scala. *Navigating the Long-Term Care Maze: New Approaches to Information and Assistance in Three States.* Washington, D.C.: AARP Public Policy Institute, 2001.

Reischauer, Robert D., Stuart Butler, and Judith R. Lave, eds. *Medicare: Preparing for the Challenges of the Twenty-first Century.* Washington, D.C.: National Academy of Social Insurance, 1998.

Rettenmaier, Andrew, and Thomas R. Saving, eds. *Medicare Reform: Issues and Answers.* Chicago: University of Chicago Press, 1999.

Rettig, Richard A. "End-Stage Renal Disease and the Cost of Medical Technology." In *Medical Technology: The Culprit behind Health Care Costs?* edited by Stuart H. Altman and Robert Blendon, 88–115. Washington, D.C.: U.S. Dept. of Health, Education, and Welfare, 1979.

———. *Health Care in Transition: Technology Assessment in the Private Sector.* Santa Monica, Calif.: RAND, 1997.

———. "Medical Innovation Duels Cost Containment." *Health Affairs* 13, no. 3 (summer 1994): 7–27.

———. "Medical Innovation Duels Cost Containment." In *Medical Technology: The Culprit behind Health Care Costs?* edited by Stuart H. Altman and Robert Blendon, 16–19. Washington, D.C.: U.S. Dept. of Health, Education, and Welfare, 1979.

———. "Technology Assessment: An Update." *Investigational Radiology* 26 (1991): 165–73.

Rice, Thomas, Katherine Desmond, and Jon Gabel. "The Medicare Catastrophic Coverage Act: A Post-Mortem." *Health Affairs* 9, no. 3 (fall 1990): 75–87.

Rich, Spencer. "Rules to Bolster Appeal Rights in Medicare HMOs." *Washington Post,* November 5, 1996, sec. A, 4.

Riley, Gerald, Eric Feuer, and James Lubitz. "Disenrollment of Medicare Cancer Patients from Health Maintenance Organizations." *Medical Care* 38, no. 4 (August 1996): 826–36.

Robinson, James. "The End of Managed Care." *JAMA* 285, no. 20 (May 23–30, 2001), 2622–28.

Robinson, James C. "Physician-Hospital Organization and the Theory of the Firm." *Medical Care Research and Review* 54 (1997): 3–24.

Rodwin, Marc A. *Medicine, Money, and Morals: Physicians' Conflicts of Interest.* New York: Oxford University Press, 1995.

Rosenbaum, Sara. *An Overview of Managed Care Liability: Implications for Patient Rights and Federal and State Reform.* Washington, D.C.: AARP Public Policy Institute, March 2001.

Ross, Stephen A. "An Economic Theory of Agency: The Principal's Problem." *American Economic Review* 62, no. 2 (May 1973): 134–39.

Rossiter, Louis F. *Understanding Medicare Managed Care.* Chicago: Health Administration Press, 2001.

Rossiter, Louis F., Henrng-Chia Chiu, and Sheau-Hwa Chen. "Strengths and Weaknesses of the AAPCC: When Does Risk Adjustment Become Cost Reimbursement?" In *HMOs and the Elderly,* edited by Harold S. Luft. Ann Arbor, Mich.: Health Administration Press, 1994.

Russell, Louise B. *Is Prevention Better Than Cure?* Studies in Social Economics. Washington, D.C.: Brookings Institution, 1986.

Rybowski, Lise. *Employer Coalition Initiatives in Health Care Purchasing.* 2 vols. Washington, D.C.: Economic and Social Research Institute, February 1996.

Sabatino, Charles. "Surely the Wizard Will Help Us, Toto? Implementing the Patient Self-Determination Act." *Hastings Center Report* 23, no. 1 (January/February 1993): 12–16.

Safran, D. G., A. R. Tarlov, and W. H. Rogers. "Primary Care Performance in Fee-for-Service and Prepaid Health Care Systems: Results from the Medical Outcomes Study." *JAMA* 271, no. 20 (May 25, 1994): 1579–86.

Sage, William M. "Regulating through Information: Disclosure Laws and American Health Care." *Columbia Law Review* 99, no. 7 (1999): 1701–829.

Santa Monica Hospital Medical Center. "Guidelines for Futile Care." In *Hospitals and Health Networks*. Chicago: American Hospital Publishing, February 20, 1994.

Satterthwaite, Mark. "Consumer Information, Equilibrium Industry Prices, and the Number of Sellers." *Bell Journal of Economics* 10 (fall 1979): 483–502.

Scanlon, William J. *Cost-Sharing Policies Problematic for Beneficiaries and the Program.* Testimony before the House Ways and Means Committee. Washington, D.C.: GAO, May 9, 2001.

———. *Medicare: Successful Reform Requires Meeting Key Management Challenges.* Testimony before the House Committee on the Budget. Washington, D.C.: GAO, July 25, 2001.

———. *Medicare Management: Current and Future Challenges.* Testimony before the Senate Finance Committee. Washington, D.C.: GAO, June 19, 2001.

———. *Twenty-first Century Challenges Prompt Fresh Thinking about Program's Administrative Structure.* Washington, D.C.: GAO, May 4, 2000.

Schelling, Thomas C. "The Life You Save May Be Your Own." In *Choice or Consequence.* Cambridge, Mass.: Harvard University Press, 1986.

Schlesinger, Mark. "Countervailing Agency: A Strategy of Principaled Regulation under Managed Competition." *Milbank Quarterly* 7, no. 1 (1997): 35–87.

Schoen, Cathy. *Medicare Beneficiaries: A Population at Risk.* Menlo Park, Calif.: Henry J. Kaiser Family Foundation, December 1998.

Scitovsky, Anne A. "The High Cost of Dying Revisited." *Milbank Quarterly* 72, no. 4 (1994): 561–91.

Scott, Anthony, and Sandra Vick. "Patients, Doctors, and Contracts: An Application of Principal-Agent Theory to the Doctor-Patient Relationship." *Scottish Journal of Political Economy* 46, no. 2 (May 1999): 111–34.

Seckler, Allison B., Diane E. Meier, Michael Mulvihill, and Barbara E. Paris. "Substituted Judgment: How Accurate Are Proxy Predictions?" *Annals of Internal Medicine* 115 (1991): 92–98.

"Senators Doctors Kennedy and Hatch." Editorial. *New York Times,* July 15, 1988, A-30.

Shalala v. Grijalva. 526 U.S. 1096 (May 3, 1999).

Shavell, Steven. "Risk Sharing and Incentives in the Principal and Agent Relationship." *Bell Journal of Economics* 10 (spring 1979): 55–73.

Silveira, Maria J., Albert Di Piero, Martha S Gerrity, and Chris Feudtner. "Patients' Knowledge of Options at the End of Life." *JAMA* 284, no. 19 (November 15, 2000): 2483–94.

Simon, Herbert. *Models of Bounded Rationality.* Vol. 2. Cambridge, Mass.: MIT Press, 1982.

Skinner, Jonathan, and John E. Wennberg. *How Much Is Enough? Efficiency and Medicare Spending in the Last Six Months of Life.* National Bureau of Economic Research (NBER) Working Paper 6513. Cambridge, Mass.: NBER, April 1998.

Skinner, Jonathan, Elliot Fisher, and John Wennberg. *The Efficiency of Medicare.* NBER Working Paper 8395. Cambridge, Mass.: NBER, July 2001.

Skocpol, Theda. *Boomerang.* New York: W. W. Norton, 1996.

———. "Pundits, People, and Medicare Reform." In *Medicare: Preparing for the Challenges of the Twenty-first Century,* edited by Robert D. Reischauer, Stuart Butler, and Judith R. Lave. Washington, D.C.: National Academy of Social Insurance, distributed by Brookings Institution,1998.

Slomaka, J. "The Negotiation of Death: Clinical Decision Making at the End of Life." *Social Science and Medicine* 35 (1992): 251–59.

Smith, David G. *Paying for Medicare: The Politics of Reform*. New York: Aldine de Gruyter, 1992.

Sofaer, Shoshanna, and Margo-Lea Hurwicz. "When Medical Group and HMO Part Company: Disenrollment Decisions in Medicare HMOs." *Medical Care* 31, no. 9 (1993): 801–21.

Solomon, Mildred Z., Lydia O'Donnell, Bruce Jennings, Vivian Guilfoy, Susan M. Wolf, Kathleen Nolan, Rebecca Jackson, Dieter Koch-Weser, and Strachan Donnelley. "Decisions near the End of Life: Professional Views on Life-Sustaining Treatments." *American Journal of Public Health* 83 (January 1993): 14–23.

Southwick, F. "Who Was Caring for Mary?" *Annals of Internal Medicine* 118 (1993): 146–48.

Spiller, Pablo. "Politicians, Interest Groups, and Regulators: A Multiple-Principals Agency Theory of Regulation (or 'Let Them be Bribed')." Stanford Center for Economic Policy Research Discussion Paper 131. Stanford, Calif.: Stanford University, 1988.

Starr, Paul. *The Social Transformation of American Medicine*. New York: Basic Books, 1982.

Steinberg, M. D., and S. J. Youngner, eds. *End-of-Life Decisions: A Psychosocial Perspective*. Washington, D.C.: American Psychiatric Press, 1998.

Steinmo, Sven, and Jon Watts. "It's the Institutions, Stupid! Why Comprehensive National Health Insurance Always Fails in America." *Journal of Health Politics, Policy, and Law* 20, no. 2 (summer 1995): 329–72.

Stewart, Jonathan. "Diagnosing and Treating Depression in the Hospitalized Elderly." *Geriatrics* 46 (January 1991): 64–72.

Stiglitz, Joseph. "Risk Sharing and Incentives in Sharecropping." *Review of Economic Studies* 61 (1974): 219–55.

Sugarman, Jeremy, Neil Powe, Dorothy Brillantes, and Melanie Smith. "The Costs of Ethics Legislation: A Look at the Patient Self-Determination Act." *Kennedy Institute of Ethics Journal* 3, no. 4 (1993): 387–99.

Taussing, A. Dale, and Martha A. Wojtowycz. "The Agency Role of Physicians in Ireland, Britain, and the U.S.A.." *Policy Sciences* 19 (1986): 275–96.

Thomas, Bill. "1965–1995: Medicare at a Crossroads." *JAMA* 274, no. 3 (July 19, 1995): 276–78.

Tolle, Susan W., and Donald E. Girard. "Physicians' Role in the Events Surrounding Patient Death." *Archives of Internal Medicine* 143 (1983): 1447–49.

Tolle, Susan W., Diane L. Elliot, and David H. Hickam. "Physician Attitudes and Practices at the Time of Death." *Archives of Internal Medicine* 144 (1984): 2389–91.

Tolley, George, Donald Kenkel, and Robert Fabian, eds. *Valuing Health for Policy: An Economic Approach*. Chicago: University of Chicago Press, 1994.

Tompkins, Christopher P., Sarita Bhalotra, Michael Trisolini, Stanley S. Wallack, Scott Rasgon, and Hock Yeoh. "Applying Disease Management Strategies to Medicare." *Milbank Quarterly* 77, no. 4 (December 1999): 461–84.

Toner, Robin, and Robert Pear. "In Budget Talks, No Hint of Pact on Health Issues." *New York Times*, December 4, 1995, sec. A, 1.

Tsevat, Joel, E. Francis Cook, Michael L. Green, et al. "Health Values of the Seriously Ill." *Annals of Internal Medicine* 122 (1995): 514–20.

Tunis, Sean, and Jeffrey Kang. "Improvements in Medicare Coverage of New Technology." *Health Affairs* 20, no. 5 (September/October 2001): 83–85.

Van, Jon. "Artificial Hearts May Return As Transplant Alternative for Elderly." *Chicago Tribune*, November 19, 1995.

Veatch, Robert, and Carol Mason Spicer. "Medically Futile Care: The Role of the Physician in Settings Limits." *American Journal of Law and Medicine* 18 (1992): 15–36.

Veeder, Nancy, and Wilma Peebles-Wilkins, eds. *Managed Care Services: Policy, Programs, and Research*. New York: Oxford University Press, 2001.

Virnig, Beth A., Sara Kind, Marshall McBean, and Elliott Fisher. "Geographic Variation in Hospice Use Prior to Death." *Journal of the American Geriatrics Society* 48 (September 2000): 1117–25.

Vladeck, Bruce. *Unloving Care*. New York: Basic Books, 1977.

Vladeck, Bruce, and Barbara Cooper. *Making Medicare Work Better*. New York: Mt. Sinai Institute for Medicare Practice, March 2001.

Vogel, Ronald J. *Medicare: Issues in Political Economy*. Ann Arbor: University of Michigan Press, 1999.

Vorster v. Bowen. 709 F. Supp. 934, 946–47 (C.D. Cal. 1989).

Weisbrod, Burton. "The Health Care Quadrilemma: An Essay on Technological Change, Insurance, Quality of Care, and Cost Containment." *Journal of Economic Literature* 29 (June 1991): 523–52.

Welch, H. Gilbert, David Wennberg, and W. Pete Welch. "The Use of Medicare Home Health Services." *New England Journal of Medicine* 335, no. 5 (August 1, 1996): 324–29.

Welch, W. Pete. "Growth in HMO Market Share of the Medicare Market, 1989–1994." *Health Affairs* 15, no. 1 (fall 1996): 201–14.

Wennberg, John. "Understanding Geographic Variation in Health Care Delivery." *New England Journal of Medicine* 340, no. 1 (January 7, 1999): 32–39.

White, Alan J., et al. *Evaluation of the Program of All-Inclusive Care for the Elderly Demonstration: A Comparison of the PACE Capitation Rates to the Projected Costs of the Program in the First Year of Enrollment*. Cambridge, Mass.: Abt Associates, October 27, 2000.

White, Harrison C. "Agency As Control." In *Principals and Agents: The Structure of Business*, edited by John W. Pratt and Richard J. Zeckhauser. Reprint with new preface. Boston: Harvard Business School Press, 1991.

White, Joseph. *False Alarm*. Baltimore: Johns Hopkins University Press, 2001.

White, Linda Johnson. "Clinical Uncertainty, Medical Futility, and Practice Guidelines." *Journal of the American Geriatrics Society* 42 (1994): 899–901.

Wicks, Elliot K., and Mark A. Hall. "Purchasing Cooperatives for Small Employers: Performance and Prospects." *Milbank Quarterly* 78, no. 4 (2000): 511–46.

Williamson, Oliver E. *Economic Organization: Firms, Markets, and Policy Control*. New York: New York University Press, 1986.

———. "Franchise Bidding for Natural Monopolies—in General and with Respect to CATV." In *Economic Organization: Firms, Markets, and Policy Control*, 258–97. New York: New York University Press, 1986.

———. *The Mechanisms of Governance*. New York: Oxford University Press, 1996.

Willman, Vallee. "Workshop Conclusions and Recommendations." In *Report of the Workshop on the Artificial Heart: Planning for Evolving Technologies*, by National Heart, Lung, and Blood Institute. Bethesda, Md.: NHLBI, 1994

Wooldridge, Judith. *Social Health Maintenance Organizations: Transition into Medicare+ Choice*. Princeton, N.J.: Mathematica Policy Research, January 5, 2001.

Wozencraft, Ann. "It's a Baby or It's Your Money Back: Fertility Clinics Test Consumer Rebates." *New York Times*, August 25, 1996, sec. 3, 1, 10–11.